SCHEIN'S COMMON SENSE
Prevention and Management
of Surgical Complications

For surgeons, residents, lawyers, and even
those who *never have any complications*

Moshe Schein MD FACS
Paul N. Rogers MBChB MBA MD FRCS
Ari Leppäniemi MD

tfm Publishing Limited, Castle Hill Barns, Harley, Nr Shrewsbury, SY5 6LX, UK
Tel: +44 (0)1952 510061; Fax: +44 (0)1952 510192
E-mail: info@tfmpublishing.com;
Web site: www.tfmpublishing.com

Design & Typesetting: Nikki Bramhill BSc Hons Dip Law
First edition: © October 2013
Cartoons: © 2013 Evgeniy E. (Perya) Perelygin, MD
Front and back cover paintings: © 2013 Dan Schein (www.danschein.com)
"Before the operation" and "The mortality": oil on canvas

Paperback   ISBN: 978-1-903378-93-9

E-book editions: January 2014
ePub   ISBN: 978-1-903378-96-0
Mobi   ISBN: 978-1-903378-97-7
Web pdf   ISBN: 978-1-903378-98-4

Printed by Gutenberg Press Ltd., Gudja Road, Tarxien, PLA 19, Malta
Tel: +356 21897037; Fax: +356 21800069

Contents

Contributors   vii

Foreword   x

Editors' note   xi

Preface   xiii

Dedications   xvi

PART I — GENERAL CONSIDERATIONS   1

Chapter 1   3
What are complications?
Definitions, classification and ruminations
Moshe Schein, Paul N. Rogers, Ari Leppäniemi and Danny Rosin

Chapter 2   13
Preventing morbidity and mortality (M&M): general principles
Moshe Schein, Paul N. Rogers, Ari Leppäniemi and Danny Rosin

Chapter 3   39
Hemostasis and bleeding
Samir Johna and Moshe Schein

Chapter 4   57
Postoperative infections
Moshe Schein

Chapter 5   77
The wound, the wound...
Moshe Schein, Paul N. Rogers, Ari Leppäniemi and Danny Rosin

Chapter 6   91
Leaking gastrointestinal anastomoses

     Section 1.   **Basic considerations**   91
                         Moshe Schein
     Section 2.   **The esophagus**   106
                         John Hunter
     Section 3.   **Stomach and duodenum**   116
                         Wen-hao Tang
     Section 4.   **Small intestine**   128
                         Moshe Schein and Mark Cheetham
     Section 5.   **Large bowel and rectum**   134
                         Caitlin W. Hicks and Jonathan E. Efron

Chapter 7   145
Abdominal wall dehiscence
Moshe Schein, Paul N. Rogers, Ari Leppäniemi and Danny Rosin

Chapter 8   155
Ileus and early postoperative small bowel obstruction (EPSBO)
Moshe Schein

Chapter 9   169
Minimal access surgery
Danny Rosin

Chapter 10   183
Dealing with patients, families, lawyers and yourself
Avi Rubinstein and Moshe Schein

Chapter 11   203
The developing ('Third') World
B. Ramana

Chapter 12   217
Going to the country: the rural situation
Moshe Schein

Contents

PART II — SPECIFIC CONSIDERATIONS   229

Chapter 13   231
The Intensive Care Unit (ICU)
Ronald V. Maier

Chapter 14   257
Colon and rectum (and the humble anus)
Mark Cheetham

Chapter 15   291
Hernias
Danny Rosin

Chapter 16   315
The gallbladder and bile ducts
Danny Rosin, Paul N. Rogers and Moshe Schein

Chapter 17   345
The appendix
Moshe Schein

Chapter 18   361
The pancreas
Gregory Sergeant, Mickaël Lesurtel and Pierre-Alain Clavien

Chapter 19   377
The liver
Erik Schadde and Pierre-Alain Clavien

Chapter 20   393
The breast
Danny Rosin

Chapter 21   413
The thyroid, parathyroid and adrenal glands
Saba Balasubramanian

Chapter 22   431
Vascular surgery
Paul N. Rogers

Chapter 23   451
Bariatric surgery
Ahmad Assalia

Chapter 24   471
Trauma
Ari Leppäniemi

Chapter 25   497
Pediatric surgery
Graeme Pitcher

Chapter 26   519
Urology
Zohar A. Dotan

Epilogue   535
Lessons learned from surgical complications
David Dent

Index   539

Contributors

Ahmad Assalia MD Chief of Advanced and Bariatric Surgery, Rambam Health Care Campus, Haifa, Israel (⊙ Chapter 23)
assaliaa@gmail.com

Saba Balasubramanian MS FRCS PhD Consultant Endocrine Surgeon, Royal Hallamshire Hospital, Sheffield, UK (⊙ Chapter 21)
sababalasubramanian@gmail.com

Mark Cheetham BSc MD FRCS Consultant General and Colorectal Surgeon, Royal Shrewsbury Hospital, Shrewsbury, Shropshire, UK (⊙ Chapters 6 and 14)
markcheets@aol.com

Pierre-Alain Clavien MD PhD FACS FRCS (Ed.) Professor and Chairman of Surgery, Swiss HPB Center, Department of Surgery, University Hospital Zurich, Zurich, Switzerland (⊙ Chapters 18 and 19)
clavien@access.uzh.ch

David Dent ChM FRCS (Eng) FCS(SA) FRCP&S (Glas. Hon) Emeritus Professor of Surgery, University of Cape Town, South Africa (⊙ Epilogue)
dmdent2@mweb.co.za

Zohar A. Dotan MD PhD Head of Uro-oncology Service, Department of Urology, Sheba Medical Center, Tel Hashomer, Israel (⊙ Chapter 26)
zohar.dotan@sheba.health.gov.il

Jonathan E. Efron MD FACS FASCRS Associate Professor of Surgery, The Mark M. Ravitch MD Endowed Professorship in Surgery; Chief, Ravitch Division, Johns Hopkins University, Baltimore, Maryland, USA (⊙ Chapter 6, section 5)
jefron1@jhmi.edu

Caitlin W. Hicks MD MS Resident in Surgery, Johns Hopkins Hospital, Baltimore, Maryland, USA (⊙ Chapter 6, section 5)

John Hunter MDFACS Mackenzie Professor and Chairman of Surgery, Oregon Health & Science University, Portland, Oregon, USA (⟳ Chapter 6, section 2)
hunterj@ohsu.edu

Samir Johna MD FACS FICS Staff Surgeon, Southern California Permanente Medical Group; Clinical Professor of Surgery, Loma Linda University School of Medicine; Director, Arrowhead Regional — Kaiser Fontana General Surgery Residency Program, California, USA (⟳ Chapter 3)
samir.johna@gmail.com

Ari Leppäniemi MD Head of Trauma and Emergency Surgery, University of Helsinki, Finland (⟳ Chapters 1, 2, 5, 7 and 24)
ari.leppaniemi@hus.fi

Mickaël Lesurtel MD PhD SNF Förderungsprofessor, Swiss HPB Center, Department of Surgery, University Hospital Zurich, Zurich, Switzerland (⟳ Chapter 18)
mickael.lesurtel@usz.ch

Ronald V. Maier MD FACS Jane and Donald D. Trunkey Professor and Vice-Chair of Surgery, University of Washington; Surgeon-in-Chief, Harborview Medical Center, Seattle, USA (⟳ Chapter 13)
ronmaier@uw.edu

Graeme Pitcher MD FACS Pediatric Surgeon, Associate Professor of Surgery, University of Iowa, Iowa City, USA (⟳ Chapter 25)
graeme-pitcher@uiowa.edu

B. Ramana MS DNB FRCS Advanced Laparoscopic & Bariatric Surgeon, BMI (Bariatrics & Metabolism Initiative), Belle Vue Clinic, Kolkata, India (⟳ Chapter 11)
rambodoc@gmail.com

Paul N. Rogers MBChB MBA MD FRCS Consultant General and Vascular Surgeon, Western Infirmary, Glasgow, UK (⟳ Chapters 1, 2, 5, 7, 16 and 22)
pn.rogers@btinternet.com

Danny Rosin MD Attending General and Advanced Laparoscopic Surgeon, Sheba Medical Center, University of Tel Aviv, Israel (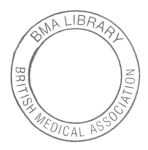 Chapters 1, 2, 5, 7, 9, 15, 16 and 20)
drosin@mac.com

Avi Rubinstein MD MSc Neurosurgeon, Advocate, Law Offices Rubinstein-Yakirevtch, Ramat Gan, Israel (Chapter 10)
avirubinstein88@gmail.com

Erik Schadde MD FACS Director HPB Fellowship, Swiss HPB Center, Department of Surgery, University Hospital Zurich, Zurich, Switzerland (Chapter 19)
erik.schadde@usz.ch

Moshe Schein MD FACS General Surgeon, Marshfield Clinic, Ladysmith, Wisconsin, USA (Chapters 1-8, 10, 12, 16 and 17)
mosheschein@gmail.com

Gregory Sergeant MD PhD HPB Fellow, Swiss HPB Center, Department of Surgery, University Hospital Zurich, Zurich, Switzerland (Chapter 18)
gregorysergeant@gmail.com

Wen-hao Tang MD PhD Professor & Chief Surgeon, Zhongda Hospital, Southeast University, Nanjing, P. R. China (Chapter 6, section 3)
tang_wh26@126.com

Foreword

All surgeons have complications. It is usually said that the more operations you do, the more complications you will get. This is only partly true. Age and experience bring an understanding of what can be achieved during a surgical procedure. A real understanding of surgery, however, comes only when you learn what you can get away with.

Surgeons learn about complications and how to avoid them from books, and during their apprenticeship, from watching their teachers. All surgeons love tips and tricks to make operations easier and more successful. These four Editors and their authors bring a wealth of knowledge and experience. They have assembled information in a way that is easily accessible to surgeons at all stages, and their style of delivery is unique, and about as far as it is possible to get away from the sober and evidential journals of surgery, with which most surgeons are familiar. Yet, surgery is theatre, and lessons learned from bold statements and cartoons live long and are hard to forget.

For authors to write about complications is a brave step; many find it preferable to write about triumphs, rather than tribulations. Yet teaching how to prevent complications has the potential to make a greater impact on patient care, since complications undermine all involved. The four horsemen of the apocalypse of complications have ridden again, and the Editors are to be congratulated on a stylish and valuable textbook.

Jonothan J. Earnshaw DM FRCS
Consultant Vascular Surgeon
Gloucestershire Royal Hospital
Gloucester, UK
Joint Chief Editor, *British Journal of Surgery*

Editors' note

The enthusiastic feedback received from readers of *Schein's Common Sense Emergency Abdominal Surgery* (now in its 3rd edition, translated to seven languages) inspired us to create a similar book dedicated to **surgical complications**: practical, non-formal, internationally relevant (to all types of practice and levels of hospitals), blunt, 'in your face' — with as little BS as possible — and a little humorous. For how can we preserve our sanity in the increasingly bureaucratic, restrictive, over-politically-correct medical environment without being able to smile and make a little fun of ourselves?

As in our previous book, we restrict the use of references to the absolute minimum and avoid citing figures and percentages as much as possible. You should consider the chapters in this book to be the opinion of experts — and indeed, we promise you that each of our contributors has a vast personal knowledge and clinical experience in the field he writes about.

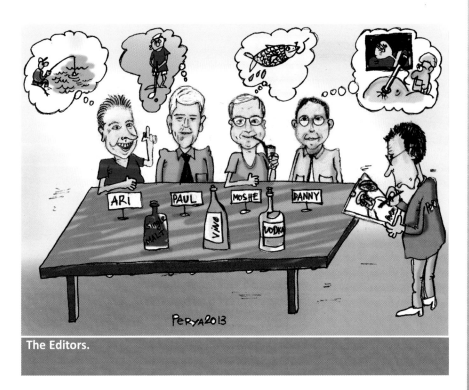

The Editors.

Please look again at the original painting (oil on canvas) depicted on the back cover. It is based on a photograph that one of us (MS) found some 30 years ago in a glossy magazine. What do you see? A dead patient, a distraught surgeon — death on the OR table is something we don't wish on even our worst enemy — blood dripping on the floor, an exhausted assistant; like a scene after a lost battle, from a war movie. How gloomy! But complications and deaths are woven into the fabric of our trade. We have to look death in the eye and avert it — this is our main task as surgeons. And this is what this book is all about.

We are grateful to our publisher, Nikki Bramhill (tfm publishing Ltd), for the meticulous production, to our illustrator, Dr. Evgeniy "Perya" Perelygin (Russia), for his apposite caricatures and to all the contributors who are also our friends. Thanks also to the members of SURGINET for their advice and support. And a special appreciation to Prof. Pierre-Alain Clavien and his team from Zurich for coming to our help at such short notice!

Moshe Schein MD FACS
Paul N. Rogers MBChB MBA MD FRCS
Ari Leppäniemi MD
Danny Rosin MD

Preface

The rule of "2": When you hear a surgeon telling his number of performed cases, <u>divide</u> it by two. When he tells you about his complication rate, <u>multiply</u> it by two.

Rick Paul

"Only those who don't operate don't experience complications." Surely you must be familiar with this ancient surgical aphorism, passed on with a fatalistic smirk by wrinkled surgeons to their disciples. And, in fact, complications are an integral component of our trade — whatever we do is associated with potential or actual complications. **Complications corrode the pleasure of our surgical life!**

Of course, other medical specialties produce as many complications as we do — if not more. But ours are much more visible. When a physician forgets to prescribe aspirin and the patient dies of stroke, everybody shrugs their shoulders: "Well, he was an old man, eh?" But when an old man dies of an anastomotic leak after a colectomy for cancer, his surgeon immediately comes under scrutiny, even if he is not directly blamed for the poor outcome. It is much easier, and consequently more tempting, for 'big brother' (whoever that is…) to 'red flag' and count our surgical complications, whether preventable or not, than those of our non-surgical colleagues. How effortless it is to tally the times we took a patient back to the operating room, as compared to the number of patients boxed in by errors in prescribing medications, or delays in diagnosis.

We start dreading complications as soon as we take our first steps in surgical life. In addition to hurting our surgical egos, complications, or the threat of them, exponentially increase the stress associated with our practice. Imagine operating on a ruptured aortic aneurysm without having to worry about the looming immediate and late dangers like bleeding, infection, thrombosis, renal failure, intestinal ischemia, abdominal compartment syndrome… oh, the list is so long… and death. How great would it be to practice surgery without having to explain/justify complications to the patient? Or if he or she is already dead, to the members of their family, who stare at you with accusing eyes, under the neon lights, at 5am. How serene would life be without having to be grilled by our Chief about the recent abdominal wound dehiscence? How tranquil would it be if none of our cases were ever to be presented at the morbidity and mortality conference? And only those who have been sued, frivolously or not, can bear true witness to the misery of the adversarial legal process and the agony of facing the plaintiff and jury in court.

It has been said: "**It is easier to stay out of trouble than to get out of it.**" **And: "Good surgeons operate well but *great* surgeons know how to manage their own complications**." And so, when discussing surgical complications the key words are PREVENTION and MANAGEMENT. Even if we cannot prevent all complications, we can at least truncate their damaging consequences by early recognition and proper treatment, thereby improving outcome… and saving our own butts. Let's be honest: when we lose a patient because of some terrible error, we do not feel sorry only for the stricken patient and his family; we feel sorry for ourselves and we worry about our reputation. Often, we look in the mirror, blame ourselves, and then try to forget the whole thing as quickly as possible.

This book deals with the **prevention** and **management** of surgical complications. It aims at distilling for you our *wisdom* (did you ever meet a modest surgeon? ☺) based on a combined experience of long years, practicing general, trauma, vascular and advanced laparoscopic surgery, in teaching hospitals, district hospitals and rural circumstances — in the UK, Australia, South Africa, Israel, the United States, Finland, Nigeria, Kenya, Sudan, Thailand, Pakistan and Tuvalu. But it is not a conventional book. A 'complete' book of surgical complications — which would cover the prevention and treatment of each and every possible complication, ranging from a leaking jejunoesophageal anastomosis after total gastrectomy to a recurrent ingrown toenail after nail ablation, from intraperitoneal bleeding after a Whipple procedure to a non-healing perineal wound after abdominoperineal resection of the rectum — would result in yet another giant textbook, and many such are available. Furthermore, these days if you wish to learn about a specific rare complication your best choice would be to do it through a Google search!

The aim of this little book, on the other hand, is to instill in you a knowledge of a range of basic core concepts — grounded in common sense and cemented by personal and collective experience — which should help make you a safer surgeon, one who constantly (subconsciously and consciously) strives to prevent misadventures and adverse outcomes. And if complications do develop (never say never in surgery!), the lessons embedded in these pages will help you rescue the patient and yourself.

This book will not nag you with the 'incidence' or 'prevalence' of (almost) anything; it will not exhaust you with elaborate 'flow-charts'; nor will it test your patience with the currently popular 'check lists' (we trust that you know to properly identify your patient and mark the correct limb to be amputated ☺). We are not going to encumber you with current politically-correct clichés — that "to err is human", and it is "human to be human" and that "patients come first" and that "all doctors are so compassionate". Instead, our narrative may seem a little harsh, rough, and 'in your face' — but don't you want to hear the truth? **It is targeted at your *juvenile* surgical soul, trying to strengthen it!** Why "juvenile"? Because this book is aimed largely at younger surgeons — those in their formative years. Older surgeons, the solid ones, should by now possess the wisdom, gained by trial and error. Those who lack such wisdom are probably more likely to continue reading the *Wall Street Journal* rather than seek self-improvement [1]. **Good surgical judgment comes from experience and experience comes from poor surgical judgment**. But while good surgeons learn from their own experience the really wise ones learn from the experience of others!

With due respect to *evidence-based medicine*, the practice of surgery is still an art and this requires to some degree *gut-based medicine*. So join us in the following chapters, which we believe you will be able to consume with some pleasure in a few days. And then please let us hear from you: are you already a little wiser and more mature? Are you sorry that you have not read this book before?

What is considered taboo by others is not taboo for us: here we'll discuss 'everything'!

> **"Nothing stands out so conspicuously, or remains so firmly fixed in our memory, as something in which we have blundered."**
>
> **Cicero**

---

[1] *After 33 years in surgery I observe a lot of very happy surgeons, most of them stopped reading medical journals after graduation, they have no complications, they know everything and they are informed only by company representatives or glossy brochures.* [Marian Littke].

Dedications

George Decker FRCS
1931-2013

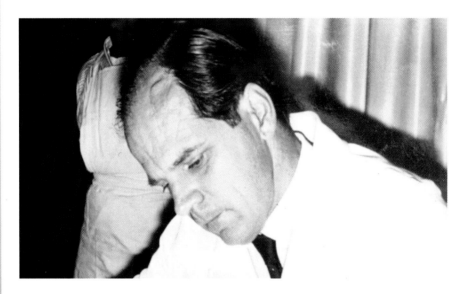

**I dedicate this book to Professor George Decker
of Johannesburg, South Africa.**
He taught me the ABC of surgery — obsessively and ruthlessly demanding
that we know and examine the "whole patient" and that each and every suture
is to be placed and tied correctly. I never saw any surgeon as dedicated to his
patients and as worried about their outcome. When I told him about the idea
of this book, he aptly commented: "this should be the perfect book for
surgeons who never have any complications!" He simply thought, said and did
what he believed to be right, irrespective of authorities, political correctness or
hierarchies. I will never forget his sweating forehead almost touching mine —
his sausage-like fingers guiding my hands to the neck of a juxtarenal abdominal
aortic aneurysm — hissing "be careful!" **He was my mentor.** Moshe Schein

**Surgery is my profession and vocation. Jackie, Lucy and Michael are my
life. This modest book is dedicated to them.** Paul Rogers

To my wife and fishing friend Eija. Ari Leppäniemi

To Gilly. Danny Rosin

PART I

General considerations

Chapter 1

What are complications?
Definitions, classification and ruminations

Moshe Schein, Paul N. Rogers, Ari Leppäniemi and Danny Rosin

We have our faults and our virtues; we meet with failures and achieve successes. Many of our faults are entirely unavoidable, and arise from the fact that medicine is not an exact science... some things are quite impossible, and our work is carried out upon a living, breathing, complexity called a man, and not upon a jar, a chemical mixture in a retort, or a wooden Indian from the front of a cigar store.

J. Chalmers Da Costa

What is a complication? It is anything happening with your patient that should not have happened — *any* adverse event. It includes any deviation from what we know, based on our collective experience, to be the *expected, uneventful* intra- and postoperative course. **Anything that 'goes wrong' is a complication!**

Take for example a case of **inguinal hernia repair with mesh** under local anesthesia and i.v. sedation. You expect the patient to return to his room fully awake, to stand up and pee; and a few hours later to *walk* to the car and be driven home. After 2-3 days you want him to require no analgesia, to defecate normally and to return to his normal activities except, of course, heavy lifting and/or vigorous sports. A week later, when you see him in your office, you expect his wound to be completely healed, his scrotum pink and not swollen and his testicles soft and non-tender. **Anything which deviates from the above, from normal, like wound *ecchymoses* or a 'scrotal eggplant' (*aubergine*) is a complication!** Even something as *minor* as a tiny bit of pestering subcuticular suture at the edge of the incision (i.e. an *aberration of healing* — ➲ Chapter 5) is a complication. "**A minor complication is one that happens to somebody else!**"

If we use such sensitive and all inclusive definitions of complications, and if we do search for them objectively and obsessively, and list them meticulously — almost all of our operations would be associated with complications: a strikingly high morbidity rate. Because when we cut, burn, tear, dissect, suture, staple or strangulate the human flesh, when we alter normal physiology — even for a short term — we and our patients are punished for it (■ Figure 1.1).

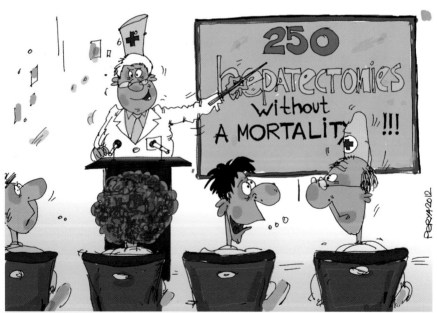

Figure 1.1. A young doc whispers to his neighbor: "Actually, we did 25 hepatectomies in our unit — the extra zero must be a mistake. We had a few mortalities, however, just a week or so, before and after the period of the study…"

For years surgical academicians have tried to introduce elaborate **classification systems of surgical complications**. The classification proposed by Professor Pierre Clavien of Zurich seems to have become the most popular, having been adapted to a wide range of procedures (■ Table 1.1). Other, perhaps more user-friendly systems have been suggested but none has any value in the practical management of the *individual* patient. They serve only as an academic or research tool: to increase uniformity in reporting outcomes, allowing comparison and analysis; they may be of value when used in departmental audits. But we, and you — not big researchers, nor technocrats — need something down to earth, more meaningful and practical.

Table 1.1. Clavien's classification of postoperative complications.
Modified from: Dindo D, Demartines N, Clavien PA. Classification of surgical complications: a new proposal with evaluation in a cohort of 6336 patients and results of a survey. Ann Surg 2004; 240: 205-13.

Grade	Subgrade	Definition
I		Any deviation from the normal postoperative course without the need for pharmacological treatment or surgical, endoscopic and radiological interventions. Allowed therapeutic regimens are drugs such as antiemetics, antipyretics, analgesics, diuretics, electrolytes and physiotherapy. This grade also includes wound infections opened at the bedside.
II		Requiring pharmacological treatment with drugs other than such allowed for grade I complications. Blood transfusions and total parenteral nutrition are also included.
III		Requiring surgical, endoscopic or radiological intervention:
	a.	- intervention not under general anesthesia
	b.	- intervention under general anesthesia
IV		Life-threatening complications (including CNS complications) requiring intensive care management:
	a.	- single organ dysfunction (including dialysis)
	b.	- multiorgan dysfunction
V		DEATH.

So, in practical terms, what questions should we ask when addressing any complication?

What is the cause? Was it a result of an error of judgment or a technical mishap?

Operating on a dying terminal cancer patient indicates that your *judgment* has been clouded. On the other hand, having to reoperate for bleeding after a laparoscopic cholecystectomy suggests that you did not achieve adequate hemostasis of the gallbladder bed at the first operation — a *technical* error. **Please note however that these two types of errors commonly occur in combination**: the patient with ischemic intestine died because his operation was delayed (poor judgment) and his colostomy has retracted, leaking back into the abdomen (poor technique). Often, however, it is impossible to decide exactly whether a *technical complication* (e.g. leaking anastomosis) has been caused by poor technique (technical error) or by patient-related factors, such as poor nutrition or long-term intake of steroids.

Was it an error of commission or omission?

If you operated too late, or not at all, on a patient with necrotic bowel, it is an error of **omission**; but if you operated too early, or unnecessarily, it becomes an error of **commission**. After the operation you either failed to reoperate for the abscess (**omission**) or operated unnecessarily when percutaneous drainage was possible (**commission**). It appears that the 'collective surgical psyche' tends to consider errors of omission more gravely than those of commission; the latter are looked upon with sympathy: "yes, in retrospect it may have been an unnecessary operation, but at least we know now what we are dealing with…"

Was the index operation (the one responsible for the complication) indicated at all?

It is always a trade-off: what happens if I don't operate? The graver the potential consequences of expectant management, the more acceptable it is to perform a high-risk operation, and conversely, the more minor the ailment, the higher the threshold should be for a risky operation.

"The lesser is the indication, the greater are the complications." We do enjoy this adage but are not sure how accurate it is. **What we know, however, is that a serious complication developing after an unnecessary, non-**

indicated, operation is a tragedy. Think about a common bile duct injury after a cholecystectomy for *asymptomatic* gallstones; imagine a death due to a missed bowel injury after repair of a minimally symptomatic incisional hernia in a morbidly obese patient. Some experts claim that up to a third of operative procedures performed across the world could be defined as *unnecessary*. The incidence of such procedures varies from country to country and place to place, depending on multiple factors — chief among the latter, we believe, are: **greed** (unnecessary surgery is more common where the 'fee for service' system exists and in locations with a higher density of surgeons) and **funktionslust** (in surgical terms: the pleasure of doing what one does best, or lives for — operating!). You will not find much about unnecessary surgery in textbooks. And rarely will you hear surgeons speaking about it openly. In some places, at morbidity and mortality meetings you will seldom observe anyone questioning the indication for the operation that led to the complication being discussed. So when a case of an infected aortic graft is presented, the discussion focuses on the etiology and management of this condition, but the notion that a 91-year-old patient suffering from a smallish, 5cm abdominal aortic aneurysm hadn't needed an operation at all would be, typically, ignored. **The truth is that, in many places, the subject of unwarranted, pointless, redundant surgery is still hushed — it is a *taboo* among surgeons and their 'managers'**. Why? Because the prevailing culture wants us to continue doing *more*, to earn money for the hospitals, group practices, and ourselves, to justify our existence and income. But beware — to the lawyers, advised by their surgical expert witnesses, this issue is not a taboo; and they will ask you: "Doc, why did you have to do that Nissen fundoplication? Did you try conservative treatment?" Your justification that the "patient wanted it", that "the family pressed you to proceed" and that "an informed consent was obtained", would not sound too convincing to the members of the jury... **So think about the indication all the time and avoid redundant surgery!** (⟳ Chapter 2).

Was the complication *reportable*?

An increasing number of hospitals, health organizations and credentialing bodies have come up with diverse lists of *reportable* complications: perioperative events which, by law, have to be 'flagged', 'tagged' and reported to 'big brother'. The rationale for such measures seems theoretically attractive: to measure the quality of hospitals and individual surgeons (weed out habitual wrongdoers) and take *corrective measures*, thus improving quality of care. But in daily practice such efforts do nothing more than pay lip service to popular demands. A few of the items listed as "serious reportable adverse events" do make sense (and sometimes TV headlines). For example: operating on (amputating!) the wrong limb or leaving behind a foreign body (e.g. instrument, sponge) within the patient's abdomen or chest. But other reportable complications make much less sense, if any at all. We see infection control nurses hunting for, and listing, reportable wound infections for individual surgeons; but how accurate is their definition and assessment of what exactly a wound infection is, especially given that nowadays most wound infections develop at home, days after the patient's discharge, and are diagnosed by the surgeon at his office on follow-up — thus easily hidden from scrutiny. Yet other reportable events are counterproductive — like an "unplanned return to the operating room". We have seen surgeons, afraid to be flagged, delaying a lifesaving emergency reoperation! While we must live with such administrative constraints we should recognize that in practice the measurement of such reportable complications has little value to us or our patients. **Avoiding complications is more important than using a lot of energy to record questionable 'near-misses'.**

Who was responsible for the complication?

Culpability is not the main issue. But we need to know on whom to focus *corrective actions* or educational efforts. Traditionally, the surgeon used to be the Captain of the ship, personally responsible for each and every aspect surrounding the care of his patients. But this has been changing over many years and today we have the SYSTEM. And some systems tend to fail and harm our patients [1] without us being able to do much about it.

According to Leo A. Gordon: "The only thing more complex than human pathology is the system we have designed to identify and to treat human pathology." And complex systems can be dysfunctional and prone to error and complications. **In many instances complications are caused by 'system failure',** which in practice means a malfunctioning chain of command, or other deficiencies in organization, supervision, education, morals and culture. For example: an old lady 'rots' for hours, partially attended, in the emergency room until somebody bothers to call you to assess her distended abdomen. You ask for a CT but the waiting list is long and her turn arrives only after a few hours. Meanwhile her i.v. infiltrates and she is not getting the fluids you have ordered. This, in combination with the intravenous contrast, damages her kidneys. You wish to discuss the CT results with the radiologist but he has left for lunch. When you finally, many hours later, take the patient to the operating room (you have to wait until all elective lists are done) you find out that the antibiotics you have asked for have not been given. And so on and so forth: the number of possible misfortunes is endless, and there is a limit to what an old lady with a surgical abdomen can tolerate.

---

[1] In fact, in the USA, hospitals earn an average $30,000 extra for a patient who suffers from surgical complications: the more complications the system generates, the more there is to do and earn!

The hospital is a dangerous place! — we see it every day. Of course there are constant efforts to make hospitals a safer place — "like the aviation industry". But hospitals are not Boeing 777s, and patients are more complex and much more unpredictable than an Airbus A380. We surgeons, who are often compared to pilots, must do whatever we can to fly our patients from the brink of death to recovery. But increasingly we have been reduced to a little cog within the great machine — the system, which is run and controlled by others, including politicians and consulting firms, who do not always share goals and priorities with us. **So who is responsible for the death of that old lady who eventually succumbs to multiple organ failure a week after the operation?** Can you blame the nurse who forgot something? Can you shift the responsibility to the resident who ignored the patient's dropping hemoglobin? Can you accuse the Head Nurse or the almighty CEO for running a cesspit? Of course not! At the end of the day you will have to take the blame: this will be recorded as *your* surgical mortality and so discussed by the hospital's quality assurance (QA) bodies and at the morbidity and mortality (M&M) conference. But hopefully not at any legal deposition nor in court.

While the 'system' is often the source of the problem, you have to master it and swim within it the best you can. Not only do you have to treat your patients but also you have to protect them from the vast army of people who surround them; in general they do not mean harm but are nevertheless potentially harmful. For example: do not assume that the nurse will inform you about the decreasing urine output of your patient but call her periodically to find out. Do not take for granted that the radiographer has noticed your request not to use i.v. contrast — speak to him directly. **Be proactive and vigilant in your endless struggle to tame the system**. As Vladimir Ilyich Lenin said: "Trust is good, control is better!"

Was the complication preventable?

This is an important and practical question. An experienced and knowledgeable surgeon should be able to come up with a definitive and learned answer of "yes", "no" or "maybe" after studying the case's details. Such evaluation is the chief task of the legal expert witnesses on both sides of the aisle; in a perfect world it would be included in the way QA or licensing bodies assess 'problem cases'. From an educational point of view this is also a key question to ask during M&M conferences. For instance:

A 90-year-old male patient dies of a massive myocardial infarction (MI) a day after an operation for a ruptured abdominal aortic aneurysm (AAA).

What do you think? Was his death preventable or not? Was it potentially preventable? Well, when you reach the end of this book (⮑ Chapter 22) you'll appreciate why any vascular surgeon asked about this case would immediately say: "this patient was doomed — **his death unpreventable**!"

And in the following instance:

> A 45-year-old lady sustains a major common bile duct (CBD) injury during laparoscopic cholecystectomy for biliary dyskinesia (i.e. acalculous biliary pain). In his operative report the surgeon wrote that the procedure was "uneventful".

Your verdict? Clearly this potentially devastating complication **could have been prevented** (⮑ Chapter 16).

Browsing through the following chapters you will appreciate that between these two extremes of 'clearly unpreventable' and 'obviously preventable' complications, there lies a wide gray area, which requires meticulous analysis by experts. With almost everything in surgery depending on a multitude of factors, and masked by a haze of uncertainty, the term 'potentially preventable' often becomes nebulous, controversial, open to diverse opinions and hard to decipher. Therefore, more often than not the 'system' will place your complication within this 'no man's land'. But this should not obviate your introspection: often, in self-analysis, you will come to a conclusion that what others shrugged off and defined as "it could have happened to anyone" was actually your own fault and preventable. **Wouldn't many complications of laparoscopic surgery be prevented by timely conversion to an open procedure?** (⮑ Chapter 9). One way to analyze complications is to **go through the case from one critical decision to the next** (pre- and intra-operative decisions that lead to actions), assess the information available to the surgeon at the time of decision, and evaluate if another decision could have been justified (based on the available information AT THE TIME). Such an analysis, of course, is often missing from legal deliberations where judgments can be clouded by the well-recognized phenomenon of hindsight bias, in which knowledge of the eventual outcome subliminally influences the opinion of the experts.

Was it a *real* complication or something which *simply happens*?

This question merges with the former. Many surgeons argue that what some would define as "complication" actually represents no more than recognized events, or potential mishaps, which are inherent and specific to any operative procedure. For example:

> After a 'difficult' laparoscopic cholecystectomy for acute cholecystitis the patient's hemoglobin dropped from 13.3 to 8.8g/dL. The patient did well and went home on postoperative day 3.

The gallbladder had been grossly inflamed and the dissection relatively 'bloody'. The surgeon did what he could — isn't some blood loss an integral part of some procedures? Surely you will say that this is not a complication. But what if the hemoglobin drops to say, 6.2g/dL, requiring a blood transfusion? What if the patient develops a major hemolytic reaction to the transfusion? And what if he suffers a heart attack? Aren't those direct consequences of the bleeding during laparoscopic cholecystectomy?

And in the following example:

> When separating dense adhesions during a laparotomy for adhesive small bowel obstruction you injure the small bowel. You recognize the enterotomy and repair it. The patient does well.

Surely this is not a real complication, one would say, not even a Clavien's grade I complication (■ Table 1.1). This could happen to anyone! But what if the enterotomy leaks, leading to severe postoperative peritonitis or enterocutaneous fistula, or even death? Of course now it is a horrendous complication, grade III or IV.

Now you see that what really matters is the OUTCOME. Mishaps occur all the time, even to the best of us, and are part of our life. How readily and competently we deal with it — how carefully did we repair that enterotomy — is crucial, determining whether this was just a non-significant and forgettable event or a real complication, and whether we will be sued or not.

As you see, definitions are not clear cut and a wide gray area exists. But let us conclude this chapter with a **unifying concept** — a practical one.

S**t happens/should not have happened [2]

Please forgive the coarse language but this is how weathered trench-dwelling surgeons tend to consider the recurring dilemma, how they look at and analyze complications, whether their own or produced by their colleagues. Any complication is either a known/potential consequence of the procedure and/or was unpreventable ("**s**t happens**") or the opposite is true: "**s**t should not have happened**." Each case should be analyzed individually and in some cases the answer remains unknown.

The rest of this book will help you to reduce the incidence of s**t happening and to deal with it when it does occur.

> "Use the knife and the cautery to cure the intumescence and moral necrosis which you will feel in the posterior parietal region... of self-esteem... after you have made a mistake in diagnosis."
>
> William Osler

---

[2] Dr. Barry Alexander of Australia commented (on SURGINET) on a negligent case (from another country) of thoracoscopy for spontaneous pneumothorax resulting in paralysis of the hemidiaphragm, Horner's syndrome and chylothorax: "Shit didn't happen, but it seems everything else did — phrenic n. injury, sympathetic n. injury and thoracic duct injury, each one could be shit but all three are definitely diarrhea."

Chapter 2

Preventing morbidity and mortality (M&M): general principles

Moshe Schein, Paul N. Rogers, Ari Leppäniemi and Danny Rosin

Surgery is the most dangerous activity of legal society.

P.O. Nyström

While surgeons tend to *exaggerate* their operative experience they commonly *understate* the number of their complications (■ Figure 2.1). This surely reflects a defense mechanism — denial. But even those who habitually deny having "any problems" understand that the undisputable key to a long and satisfying surgical career is avoiding/preventing M&M as much as possible.

Any reasonable surgeon with more than 20 years in practice is intimately familiar with all the principles to be discussed in this chapter. They know it reflectively and intuitively — it is in their bloodstream. We hope it will flow in your veins as well, not in 20 years from now but soon after reading this book. This chapter, because it deals with universal principles, applicable to surgery in general, is one of the longest chapters in this book. Please bear with us.

Determinants of M&M

We promise we won't be chatting about percentages, rates, uni- or multivariate analyses or p-values. We will focus only on common sense and

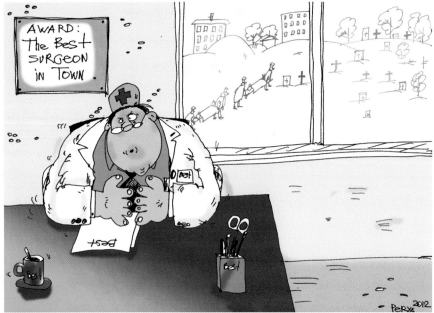

Figure 2.1. The 'best' surgeon in town: "Hell no! Those are not mine; they are Dr. Kumar's. I bury mine at night..."

established facts. **The following are the undeniable determinants of M&M** — associated with any operation:

- **The general health of your patient**: age, comorbidities, functional capacity and the status of his organs. "In general the patient's ability to survive a major operation is proportional to his productivity in society..." and: "There is nothing like a major operation to make someone show their real age."
- **The specific indication for operation**: what exactly is the pathology you are trying to cure or palliate? As Mark M. Ravitch said: "The lowest mortality and fewest complications result from the removal of normal tissue."
- **The magnitude of the operation: the more you do, the greater the dangers and potential complications!**
- **Your technical skills** in performing the operation — according to Max Thorek: "The two unforgivable sins of surgery: to operate unnecessarily and/or to undertake an operation for which the surgeon is not sufficiently skilled technically."
- **How adept you and your 'system' are in treating** any complications that develop. However: "An ounce of prevention is worth a pound of cure."

- **Luck!** Some believe that "It is better to be lucky than good, and the better you are — the luckier you become."

In general, the fate of your patient depends on how well you <u>think</u> and what you <u>do</u> — before, during and after the operation. Below, and in the following chapters, we'll try to follow this order of events.

Pre-operative considerations

Professor George Decker of Johannesburg (MS's mentor) always demanded an answer to each of the following three questions, before taking any patient to the operating room.

■ What is the indication? If any!

■ What is the correct operation — to fit the indication?

■ Is the patient fit for the planned operation? And if not what are the alternatives?

The correct answers to these three questions, which are always to be asked and answered — objectively and without bias — are the key to your success as a surgeon.

Without doubt, defining the *indication* for operation, and *tailoring* the most appropriate operation to the patient and his pathology are the chief intellectual tasks of the surgeon — at least as important, if not more important, than the surgeon's technical skills. Remember: first we learn how to operate, then we learn when to operate and finally we learn when not to operate. This is **judgment**: to be able to **select the right operation for the patient and the right patient for the operation**.

> *Poor judgment is responsible for much bad surgery, including the withholding of operations that are necessary or advisable, the performance of unnecessary and superfluous operations, and the performance of inefficient, imperfect, and wrongly chosen ones.*
>
> **Charles F.M. Saint**

Specific indications for the vast spectrum of maladies which could be helped by surgery are beyond the scope of this little book. But in general terms we should strive to avoid unwarranted, futile, excessive surgery — unnecessarily placing our patients at risk. **The punishment (the operation) should fit the crime (the disease) and the offender (the patient)**:

> *One should only advise surgery when there is a reasonable chance of success. To operate without having a chance means to prostitute the beautiful art and science of surgery.*
> **Theodor Billroth**

Clearly: **anything in surgery boils down to *risk* and *benefit!***

The general risk of morbidity and mortality (M&M) associated with any operation is represented in the following simplistic formula.

$$\text{M\&M} = \frac{\text{Complexity of operation* + patient's risk factors + acute/chronic health}}{\text{Surgeon's judgment, skills and quality of local health system}}$$

* Complexity: see below in the intra-operative section

How do we define the patient's risk?

Rather than boring you with elaborate protocols and figures (you probably have had enough of it) we'll stick to basics. To assess the risk **you have to know your patient**. Before operating on anyone you have to familiarize yourself with all aspects of his previous history and current status. No one has to know the patient better than his surgeon!

H & P (history and physical examination) are crucial

Even if the patient has just undergone H & P by an excellent internist you have to repeat it. Operating on someone with whose past and present medical details you are not familiar, or whom you did not examine thoroughly, is like embarking on a trip through the desert without a compass, map or GPS.

> *The undone, incomplete, unrepeated, physical assessment will get you, and the patient, into more trouble than any other problem.*

Review old records

Obtain and read old records. Study the operative report from 20 years ago. Otherwise how would you know that during the previous attempt to repair the ventral hernia the Mayo Clinic surgeon had placed the Marlex® mesh directly on the bowel, thus making your planned operation hazardous? The EMR (electronic medical record) allegedly improves our access to documentation but here, yet again, the human factor comes into play: **even electronic files have to be searched, opened and read by a human — yourself**. Again and again we see doctors oblivious to information which is just a click away. But even the best airplane is useless if the pilot is sloppy.

Age

Current teaching maintains that it is the **physiological** rather than the **chronological** age that matters. There is considerable truth in this line of thinking: some patients are already 'wrecks' in their sixties while others run marathons in their eighties. Nevertheless, you have to have great respect for advanced age. The older the patient, the more limited will be his physiological reserves — not only to withstand your operation but also (even more) to tolerate and survive any potential complication. **Like a house of cards, aged folks maintain a fragile system quite well... until it gets disturbed**. So ignore all those retrospective series, published from time to time in surgical journals, boasting of "a hundred pancreatic resections (or hepatectomies) in *octogenarians* with no mortality". You can be sure that a few deaths occurred immediately before and after the declared period of the study and were thus excluded. And anyway, it is highly unlikely that you will be able to match those over-optimistic outcomes. Don't be gullible, be skeptical.

Predicted longevity

Use your judgment or *actuarial life tables* (readily available online) to calculate the life expectancy of aging patients. You will see that your 90-year-old female patient, even if she is in excellent health, is expected to live around 4-5 years. Do you still want to proceed with a laparoscopic repair of the ventral hernia which bothers her minimally? **But remember that people are not statistics** and don't underestimate the value of even a few months at the end of life (e.g. relieving an intestinal obstruction in abdominal carcinomatosis is sometimes possible). They might be the most important months. Talk to the patient. Old people in particular often have surprisingly clear views of what they want and expect from you and from life in general.

Comorbidities

Be aware of any associated comorbidity, especially if major or advanced. You surely know that elective operations should be performed very rarely in patients with grade IV chronic obstructive lung disease (COPD), uncontrolled congestive heart failure (CHF), advanced (Child's C) cirrhosis or uncontrolled diabetes.

Medications

There is no need to remind you that patients taking steroids or other immunosuppressants are susceptible to poor wound healing and infections. And in this day and age we hardly see an aging patient who is not consuming a 'blood-thinning' agent such as aspirin, clopidogrel (Plavix®) or warfarin (Coumadin®) which could increase the risk of intra- or postoperative bleeding (⮂ Chapter 3).

Obesity

Hippocrates said more than 2000 years ago: "Patients who are naturally very fat are apt to die earlier than those who are slender." And he was dead right. Any operation in the very obese is more difficult and more prone to complications than in the thin. This is even truer when it comes to management of complications. Repairing an umbilical hernia with mesh in the morbidly obese may seem to you not a great deal. But then try to manage the abdominal wall defect obscured under the huge hanging apron of fat when your repair gets infected and the mesh has to come out! However, being too thin (BMI <18.5) is also a significant risk factor for peri-operative M&M. **As with anything in life: too much or too little of anything is not good**.

Nutritional status

In our ('developed') part of the world over-nutrition rather than malnutrition is the problem. This is not the case elsewhere. Any disease process interfering with the mechanisms of eating and/or digestion could result in inadequate nutritional status, with its well-documented adverse effect on healing. **Indeed, the serum level of albumin offers an excellent prognostic tool**: not only does it reflect the nutritional status but also the severity of the acute or acute-on-chronic disease. The lower the albumin level, the higher the predicted M&M. When operating, for example, on someone with albumin levels of 1.5g/dL or less you know that you have to do the minimum (e.g. avoid intestinal suture lines if possible) and expect trouble after the operation. On the other hand: albumin levels of >3.5g/dL are reassuring. **Measure albumin prior to any major operation**; avoid or delay elective surgery in malnourished patients. You know how to optimize their nutrition.

Performance status

The patient's ability to function in daily life is a reflection of his physiological status and reserves and thus predicts his ability to withstand the planned operation. Grading systems to score functional capacity are available (the **Karnofsky performance status** seems to be the best known), but as you know, or will soon discover, the main value of all such scoring systems is in research — in practice they add nothing beyond decorating patients' charts to the satisfaction of administrators and politicians. On the other hand, a few questions to the patient and/or members of his household concerning the patient's daily activities are all that you need. An elderly gentleman who can shovel his driveway clear of snow is a promising candidate for any operation; the one who gets short of breath climbing onto the examination couch is *unfit for a haircut under local anesthesia* (we exaggerate only slightly).

The walk/climb test

Occasionally, evaluation of risk by history is doubtful. In that case — take your patient by the hand and *schlep* him for a walk. Stride as fast as he seems to tolerate along a corridor of your hospital or clinic, and climb him up the stairs one or two floors. Any patient able to endure such a physical challenge has a cardiorespiratory system which would withstand any major surgery. If your patient proves reasonably fit then there is no need for further fancy and expensive evaluation such as lung function tests or thallium stress tests.

Eyeballing the patient (the 'end-of-the-bed' test)

Essentially, applying the above steps, you would not need more than 25-30 minutes to 'eyeball' the patient — "the gleam in his eye and the strength of the grip." Of course, if your 'eyeballing' discloses potential problems or uncertainties, and if it suggests that a certain organ (e.g. heart) could be further improved before the operation — or the decision to proceed with it — then by all means **refer the patient to a specialist** (e.g. cardiologist, endocrinologist) for further evaluation.

Patients' risk stratification with grading/scoring systems

An increasing number of these systems have been introduced, and are continuously being modified and 'revised', with the aim of adding objectivity to pre-operative assessment (and the CV of their authors). Another purpose of these systems is to provide a 'common language'; rather than say: "this patient was very ill", you would be able to be more accurate and meaningful: "this patient was grade IV!" The risk classification system proposed by the **American Association of Anesthesiologists (ASA)** is simple enough to achieve wide usage around the world (■ Table 2.1). However, it has numerous limitations: first, it is so vague that the same patients get classified differently by different doctors; second, the term "systemic" is confusing — for example, is myocardial infarction, or advanced COPD, a local or systemic disease?; third, 'local' diseases (e.g. intestinal infarction) can be life-threatening but are ignored by the system; fourth, it ignores chronic health status. Therefore, let us leave the ASA to our *gas passers*; it does not have much use for us. **A much more accurate risk stratification system is the APACHE II** (Acute Physiology and Chronic Health Evaluation) which captures the severity of the patient's **acute disease** — either medical (pneumonia) or surgical (peritonitis) — along with his **chronic health** and **age**. The accuracy of the APACHE II has been validated for a wide range of ACUTE medical and surgical conditions, in

Table 2.1. American Society of Anesthesiologists (ASA) classification system.	
ASA grade	Description
1	A normal healthy patient
2	A patient with mild systemic disease
3	A patient with severe systemic disease
4	A patient with severe systemic disease that is a constant threat to life
5	A moribund patient who is not expected to survive without the operation
6	A declared brain-dead patient whose organs are being removed for donor purposes

and outside the critical care environment. In general it stratifies the patients into three risk groups:

- **Low** (scores <10) where postoperative outcome is predicted to be excellent.
- **High** (scores >20) denoting critical disease and thus predicting poor outcome and complications.
- **Intermediate** (scores 11-20) where "anything can happen".

But again, while useful in comparing groups of patients between studies and hospitals and in facilitating audit, such scores do not have much value in the individual patient: you will treat them the same whether their APACHE II Score is 7 or 25, right? Tools to calculate APACHE II are available online (http://www.mdcalc.com/apache-ii-score-for-icu-mortality). In Europe mainly, the P-POSSUM scoring system has been specifically designed to estimate M&M in general surgical patients. Particularly in low-risk patients this system tends to overestimate morbidity. The more 'risky' the procedure the more accurate is the predicted risk. A calculator is available online (http://www.riskprediction.org.uk/pp-index.php).

Cardiac risk stratifications
Various protocols are used by cardiologists to estimate the risk of cardiac complications in non-cardiac surgical patients; the most popular is that described by Goldman and Detsky — (http://medcalc3000.com/CardiacRisk_G.htm).

After all the complex evaluation and grading by consultants **you have to eyeball the patient again**. Remember that 'one-system doctors', like the cardiologist for example, who may be satisfied that there is "no active myocardial ischemia" and that "the cardiac ejection fraction is adequate", occasionally tend to paint old wrecks with fresh paint — like in an auto body shop. But when an accident occurs, when major disaster strikes, the paint cracks and the car wreck is exposed. So a patient with a history of congestive heart failure, an old MI and compensated COPD may be "cleared" (as "low risk") for major vascular surgery, but when and if excessive intra-abdominal bleeding occurs, his sick heart won't compensate. **BEWARE!**

Additional considerations in the individual patient

Occasionally the patient has an indication for operation and is assessed as being fit for it but **an operation is inadvisable**. A few examples:

- **Remote source of infection**. You do not want to proceed with a non-emergency operation in a patient harboring any infective process — regardless of magnitude. The minor folliculitis observed at the pubic hairlines may infect the mesh placed to repair an upper abdominal hernia. A transient bacteremia caused by urinary tract infection may seed your hip prosthesis. **First treat the infection, eradicate it, and only then can you proceed with the planned operation**.
- **Hostile operative field**. Some patients clearly need an operation which they could withstand but are simply **inoperable** because of **local-anatomical constraints**. For example: a large recurrent incisional hernia after multiple repairs, with pieces of old mesh expected to adhere to the abdominal wall and viscera. Surely you do not want to operate unless the hernia is **strangulated**. Similarly, you have to think twice before deciding to operate for **small bowel obstruction associated with peritoneal carcinomatosis** or **radiation enteritis**.
- **Expected futility**. A morbidly obese patient may have a painful ventral hernia which you could repair. But as long as he is grossly obese the chances of the hernia recurring are high. Let him first lose weight or undergo a bariatric operation.

When faced with specific constraints your options are: cancel the operation, postpone it, choose a different one or use an alternative access.

The selection of a specific procedure

A few aphorisms express it all:

- Everything in surgery is patient selection — the chief determinant of mortality and morbidity.
- The punishment (operation) has to fit the crime (indication).
- There is nothing like a major operation to make someone show their real age.
- High-risk diseases should have low-risk operations.
- In the kingdom of surgery: Biology is King, Selection is Queen, Technical maneuver is the Prince.

In summary: selection means choosing the right patient for the operation and the right operation for the patient. The sicker the patient — the more compromised his physiology — the lesser the magnitude of the operation should be.

Before embarking on any operation you should estimate the RISK/BENEFIT ratio, which should be well below 1 — the lower, the better. Always ask yourself: if successful, how much will the operation benefit my patient? What are the risks? Should I go ahead? If this were my wife or father — would I operate on them? If it were me, would I want to undergo the operation? Studies show that surgeons and their families are much less likely to undergo surgery in comparison to others.

Time and again we see patients failing to recover from the poorly selected operations to which they were subjected, whether an aorto-bi-femoral bypass for intermittent claudication when an endovascular procedure (or no procedure at all!) would suffice, or a futile Whipple operation for locally advanced pancreatic cancer.

Obtaining a road map for the operation

Modern imaging modalities offer operative road maps which often help us:

- **To select (or abort) a specific operation**. For example, a CT showing liver metastases would advise against resection of the pancreatic mass.
- **To choose access and incision**: when you know exactly where the problem is you do not need a long 'exploratory' midline abdominal incision. (Follow the rule of the Finnish surgeon, Hannu Paimela: "Surgery is easier when the incision is placed over the organ to be removed.")

- **To avoid intra-operative pitfalls**. For example, a CT before aorto-bi-femoral bypass would warn you about an abnormal ('retro-aortic') location of the left renal vein, thus avoiding potential intra-operative disaster.

Therefore: **before any operation, elective or emergency, always review personally all available images**. Make it a habit to look at them **together with the radiologist**. Often, your presence and the additional clinical information you provide, allow the radiologist to focus better on the area of interest and to come up with additional insights. **A surgeon relying only on a written radiology report is like a seaman sailing out without scrutinizing the maps**. And there is nothing wrong in having the CT scan available in the OR while operating; you don't have to memorize it!

When to operate — timing?

So you have the indication, you've figured out which operation to do and you know that the patient is fit for it. Should you now proceed to the operating room? Not so fast! Is the timing right?

Consider this:

- **In general, elective and semi-elective operations are less morbid than the emergency ones**. Operating during the day, when the surgeon is well rested and the operative team is at its optimal capacity and quality, is safer than rushing to it at night. Thus, for example, most appendectomies can wait for the morning (⮑ Chapter 17).
- Certain surgical emergencies are best **cooled down** before an operation. For example, it is not advisable to hurry with a laparoscopic cholecystectomy on an acute gallbladder presenting after 3-4 days of symptoms (⮑ Chapter16).
- In some patients you will need to **postpone** the operation in order to make it safer (e.g. improve nutritional status, stop smoking, lose weight, and cease taking 'blood thinners').
- Even in an emergency situation you will have to **optimize** your patient's physiology before proceeding (see below).

So do not rush! (The only indication to really "rush to the OR" is the need to control an exsanguinating hemorrhage.) Not even if your list tomorrow or next week is empty. And: "Never admit for operation elective cases straight from the outpatient department."

Of course, to avoid 'legal complications' you should not proceed before taking a detailed informed consent following a discussion with the patient and family (⮑ Chapter 10).

Final questions

Are you sure that you are the best person for the job?
Francis D. Moore

This is what you have to ask yourself before any operation. Are you qualified to do what you intend to do? Frankly, isn't there anyone in your own environment, your town or geographic area, who can do it better and safer? If so: can you get him to assist you? And if not — shouldn't you refer out? **Be your own devil's advocate! Beware of surgical ego, work in a team!**

Avoid **funktionslust**. Over and over again we have seen how even great surgeons got into deep trouble by succumbing to *funktionslust*. This lengthy quotation describes it well:

> *Funktionslust is the desire to perform a technical procedure because we perform it well... it refers to the joy and pride from performing a skill well. The accomplished musician, the skilled athlete, the ballerina, and the skilled surgeon are all justifiably proud of their skills and usually have a love for practicing their art. But funktionslust can also be a curse. It can be a temptation to do a larger procedure, where a smaller simpler procedure would suffice. Funktionslust may prevent a surgeon from learning a new technique that appears to be less satisfying in terms of the pure joy of operating. Funktionslust may be a factor in a surgeon's failure to refer a patient to another specialist: for nonsurgical treatment or for a different surgical procedure.*
> **Roger S. Forster**

Is your hospital the right choice for the planned operation?
Even if you are confident of your surgical powers to execute the operation, should it be done in your hospital? In other words: if you were the patient, would you want to undergo such an operation in your own hospital — that is, if you could find locally a surgeon as talented as you are? ☺

This is an opportunity to get acquainted with the term **"failure to rescue"** **(FTR)**.

The mortality rates after major surgery and trauma differ among hospitals: there are 'low-mortality hospitals' and 'high-mortality hospitals'. The spectrum is wide; for example, (in the USA) the mortality rate after pancreatic resection can be 13 times as high in high-mortality hospitals as opposed to the low-mortality ones.

Significantly (and perhaps surprisingly), the **rate of postoperative complications is similar at the** *worst* **and** *best* **hospitals** and is more dependent on patients' characteristics (e.g. age, comorbidities, nature of the operation) than the nature of the hospital. On the other hand, **mortality rate does depend on the characteristics of the hospital** — its facilities and overall experience with the specific procedure. Why is this so? **Because high-mortality hospitals are poorer at recognition and management of complications once they occur** — **they fail to rescue (FTR) the complicated patients!**

So even if you are a graduate of a fellowship in oncological surgery, do you really wish to proceed with a pancreatectomy in your new district hospital which lacks a modern ICU? Or do you want to perform a total cystectomy in a private clinic lacking in-house intensivists or a CT scanner? The question is not only whether you can successfully complete the operation, but **will you be able to rescue the patient if he develops major complications?** These are crucial considerations!

Pre-operative optimization-preparation

That patients taken for an *elective* operation should be in the best shape possible is obvious. You can, and must, spend as many days or weeks as needed to optimize their chances of harmlessly sailing through the planned procedure. But also patients needing *emergency* surgery have to be optimized. In larger hospitals with sufficient day-time emergency surgery capacity (dedicated ORs), some of the emergency operations (but not for active bleeding, end-organ ischemia or severe sepsis) can and should be performed in day time, with fresh eyes and hands. Again, the necessity to rush a patient directly to the OR is extremely rare and limited to dire situations requiring **immediate hemostasis** (e.g. vascular injuries, free rupture of an aneurysm). **Otherwise, in the vast majority of patients you have to spend at least three hours optimizing their physiology to better tolerate the anesthesia and operation**.

For a simplified version of 'why and how' of pre-op optimization we recommend Chapter 6 in *Schein's Common Sense Emergency Abdominal Surgery* (Springer Verlag 2010) — in this book we strictly avoid the 'copy/paste' of anything from our previous writings. But here are a few words: **The chief goal is to improve the delivery of oxygen to the cells**, as cellular hypoxia translates to subsequent cellular dysfunction, systemic inflammatory response syndrome (SIRS), organ failure and adverse outcome. You want to improve oxygen delivery to the tissues by increasing arterial oxygenation and tissue perfusion. We bet that you know how to achieve these goals: "Principles of optimization: air goes in and out; blood goes round and round; oxygen is good."

Intra-operative considerations

So now your patient is brought to the operating room. **Even before the nurse has placed the scalpel in your hand there are plenty of opportunities to prevent mishaps and complications**.

Let us assume that your well organized and disciplined nursing staff has already marked the 'correct side' of the inguinal hernia or the specific limb to be amputated. (Our proactive nurses even mark the assumed site of the gallbladder prior to cholecystectomy, in case we forget on which side gallbladders lie.) Believe it or not, and despite recent intense efforts to **prevent wrong-site surgery**, adverse events "that should never happen" occur about 40 times a week nationwide (in the USA). Therefore, **trust nobody! Do it yourself**. Always talk to the patient before the anesthetists start putting him to sleep — let him verbalize what operation he is going to undergo and on which side.

This is an opportunity to stress that arriving in the OR after the patient has been anesthetized is a dismal scene. Rushing into the room to find the patient asleep and covered with drapes opens the door to errors. The optimal scenario is for you to encounter the patient prior to his transfer to the OR: here you can at leisure repeat to him and his family the final points of the operative plans. Here you can meet (and *schmooze*) additional members of the family — yet another effort at 'risk management'! (⊃ Chapter 10).

Check lists

There is no need to reproduce here any of the Surgical Safety check lists which most probably are already in use in your OR ("sign in, time out, sign out") and are being promoted globally by the WHO. You can even download the app (free from the Apple store) for such a check list to your smart phone. Nor are we going to deal with the safety of anesthesia and its potential complications as we decided against dedicating a chapter to matters of anesthesia. Instead, we will summarize our **pre-incisional complication-reducing** maneuvers prior to the incision as "the 13 Ps" (■ Table 2.2).

Table 2.2. The 13 pre-incisional Ps to prevent postoperative complications.

PACS (picture archiving and communication system)	Review (again) the images: think about where to place the incision
Prophylaxis	Antibiotics to prevent (mainly) wound infection and measures to prevent deep vein thrombosis (whatever is your hospital policy)
Place a Foley catheter (or nasogastric tube)	To monitor urine output in prolonged and/or major operations or avoid injury to the bladder in pelvic surgery (in the absence of a distended stomach the NG tube can wait until the patient's asleep)
Prevent Pyrexia (and hypothermia)	By this we mean warming the patient to prevent hypothermia, which is known to contribute to postoperative infections
Placement and Position Padding	It is your job to help the nurses place the patient on the table in an optimal position and pad any potential pressure points to prevent damage to the skin and peripheral nerves or even a compartment syndrome
Palpate	Now it is your last chance to re-examine the operative field
Prepare	You can let the nurses prepare the operative field after pointing what (additional) areas you want them to include
Plan	While you scrub think again about what you are going to do: go through your plan in your mind. Did you forget anything? Remember: "many lives have been saved by a moment of reflection at the scrub sink." [**Neal R. Reisman**]
Pray	Give a little prayer for the success of your operation even if you are not 'a believer', for who knows it may help. "Pray before surgery, but remember God will not alter a faulty incision." [**Arthur H. Keeney**]
Professor	Calling the professor for approval, advice or help is optional ☺

The operation

As this is not a text on operative surgery and specific intra-operative considerations are dealt with later, in the various chapters, we'll touch only on a few unifying principles well described here:

> *A good operation depends on conservatism, consistent with efficiency; simplicity of technique; operative skill, which includes gentleness, dexterity, and careful speed; and maximal benefit from minimal interference.*
>
> **Charles F.M. Saint**

During the early days of your internship you started realizing that the key points of any operation, whether excision of a sebaceous cyst or a hemi-corporectomy, are: **exposure, hemostasis and repair**. You become a self-reliant surgeon only if you can: **expose the operative field, handle the tissues well, remove whatever indicated, avoid contamination, stop all bleeding, repair intestine and blood vessels and close up**. The more adroit you become in achieving these tasks, the more successful will be the operation and the better the outcome.

Be a 4-D surgeon and master at Decision-making (yes, this patient needs an operation), **Determination** (waiting does not make the problem easier to solve or go away), **Dissection** (through normal tissue planes when knowledge of anatomy is crucial, and through tissues destroyed by inflammation or previous operations, where restoring original anatomy is the key for good exposure), and **Detailed** reconstruction (every stitch has to be placed optimally, don't rush).

Complexity

Earlier in this chapter we mentioned complexity as one of the chief determinants of postoperative M&M. Let us dwell a little on what makes an operation complex and what we can do to make it less so.

The term "minor" is imprecise and we are familiar with the adages that "a minor operation is what the other person has" or "a minor complication is one that happens to somebody else". But even patients know that some operations are very *simple* or *minor*, for example, most office procedures under local anesthesia; that some are a little more *complex* or *bigger* (e.g. repair of inguinal hernia), and some even more so (e.g. cholecystectomy). Many patients also know that some operations are *complex* or *major*, like colonic resections, or resection of the pancreas, liver or esophagus which are considered *really major* procedures.

In 1965, Small and Witt [1] — based on a national questionnaire of surgeons — used the following variables to devise a scale weighing how minor or major an operation is, or was (Table 2.3).

Table 2.3. The Small and Witt scale.

Expected mortality	Elective vs. emergency	Legal risk
Potential morbidity	Usual duration of operation	Postop difficulties
Amount of trauma	Required OR facilities	Special training needed
Extent of dissection	Type of anesthesia	
Condition of patient	Requirement for assistants	

But Lewis S. Pilcher, the Editor of the *Annals of Surgery*, said it all more than 100 years ago. Responding to a question about the definition of major and minor surgery he wrote:

> *I would say that major surgery includes all work requiring a general anesthetic; all operations which involve openings into the great cavities of the body; all operations in the course of which hazards of severe hemorrhage are possible; all conditions in which the life of the patient is at stake; all conditions which require for their relief manipulations, for the proper performance of which special anatomic knowledge and manipulative skill are essential...You will see that there is still left an abundant field for the practitioner of minor surgery.*

Pilcher understood that the deeper we go, the more we cut, the more tissue we remove or crush or destroy, the more blood we lose and replace, the more we have to fix and repair, the more risks we take, the longer we take doing all of the above — the more complex the operation becomes and, consequently,

[1] Small RG, Witt RE. Major and minor surgery. *JAMA* 1965; 91: 114-6.

the greater its rate of complications. Unlike anesthesiology, which is like **flying** (it's the takeoff and landing that count, the rest is just cruising, unless something goes wrong), surgery is like **diving**: you start descending carefully, hoping to find what you are looking for. Once you are at your target, you start ascending being watchful to do that in an orderly fashion to avoid complications. You can only relax after you have reached the surface.

There will always be minor and major operations and, accordingly, a wide spectrum of complexity; but in order to reduce the risk of complications and improve outcomes **we can strive to reduce the complexity of any operation we perform**. The disease or condition that your operation tries to cure, or alleviate, demands that you do an operation of a certain complexity. But even then you can try and reduce it — here are a few key points:

- **Choose the simplest operation** to fit the specific indication, situation and patient. **There are many ways to skin a cat — the simplest is usually the best**.
- **Do not escalate the procedure**. It is ever so tempting to 'do more', but wise surgeons know how to suppress their natural tendency to 'muck around'. The more you do, the more harm you can create — do only what is absolutely necessary.
- **Avoid bleeding**. The amount of blood lost during the procedure correlates directly with postoperative M&M. This is true for any operation. Remember: **the best clotting factor is the surgeon!** Don't hesitate to use factor 14 (suture).
- **Avoid unnecessary transfusions**. The use of even minimal amounts of blood products increases mortality, wound and pulmonary complications and length of stay. Unless your patient is bleeding rapidly and in shock it is best not to transfuse blood products during the operation (⟳ Chapter 3). Old blood is bad for your health.
- **Avoid intra-operative contamination** as much as possible.
- **Respect the tissues**. The rate of wound complications after 'clean' operations (e.g. repair of hernias) varies greatly between individual surgeons. Why? Because rough surgeons create more tissue trauma — making the operation more complex. Treat the tissues gently!
- **Access**. Choose the most direct and least traumatic access possible. It is best to use *minimal access*, whether open or laparoscopic, if deemed adequate and safe, rather than placing big incisions.
- **Duration**. The more complex the operation, the longer it takes to execute. And excessive duration is associated with a long list of anesthetic and surgical complications such as pneumonia, deep vein thrombosis, hypothermia and wound infection. On the other hand, rashness and haste may lead to impulsiveness and carelessness. **You**

have to find a balance. Let us quote Danny Rosin: "There is slow and there is slow. It can result from slow, continuous, confident and accurate movements, or from unnecessary repetitive, inaccurate and ineffective movements. I accept the first option to be fully legitimate; the second is not to be praised."

All the above measures aim to reduce local and systemic inflammation thus minimizing the systemic inflammatory response syndrome (SIRS) and multiple organ dysfunction (MOD) which are the big killers of the surgical patient. Your motto in conducting any operation should be: **KISS (keep it simple, stupid! ☺)**.

The end of the operation

Are you happy?

Most experienced surgeons — deep in their hearts — can predict the postoperative course at the end of the operation. If they walk out of the OR with a smile, happy like a clam, it means, usually, that everything went according to expectations, that they are satisfied with what they did and that the postoperative course, most likely, will be uneventful. On the other hand, if they are unhappy, if on the drive home they mutter "hell, I should have…" or "why didn't I?", and if they wake up in the middle of the first postoperative night thinking about the anastomosis — then one has to expect complications. There is no doubt that the happiness of the surgeon or the lack of it correlates with outcome. **Thus, you have to ensure your happiness before the end of the operation — before it is too late!**

To do so you will have to go through the following '**end of operation' check list**. Only the instrument and sponge count will be prompted by your OR staff — the rest is up to you.

Instrument and sponge count

This is standard in any operating room. Always listen to your nurses: if they say something is missing then look for it. The missing sponge may be on the floor, under the drapes, or lost in the pelvis — dig for it. The count may be wrong — repeat it. If you cannot find what is missing, bring in the image intensifier (if you do not have one get a plain X-ray) and image the operative field. Leaving behind an instrument or sponge, or anything else, is never 'acceptable', not even following a dire emergency. It will always lead to non-defendable litigation. On occasions when you have to leave behind a sponge or instrument intentionally (e.g. to tamponade a bleeding liver) you should document it in the operative report.

Now, in your head, continue with the check list, which obviously would be different for each surgical specialty.

Here is our 'pre-closure' check list following abdominal surgery:

- Is hemostasis perfect? ✓
- Source control achieved? ✓
- Peritoneal 'toilet' completed? All fluid sucked out? ✓
- Anastomosis: Water tight? Viable? Not under tension, well positioned? ✓
- Potential sites for internal herniation dealt with? ✓
- Small bowel comfortably placed below the transverse colon? ✓
- Omentum placed between intestine and incision? ✓
- All additional fascial defects (e.g. trocar sites) closed? ✓
- Nasogastric tube in position? (if needed) ✓
- Drains (only if indicated!) in place? ✓
- Need a feeding jejunostomy? ✓
- Should I close the abdomen at all? Or leave it open? ✓

Remember: one of the most important aphorisms in abdominal surgery: **"When the abdomen is open you control it, when closed it controls you!"**

The operation is not finished after the anastomosis has been completed; nor has it been concluded when the fascia has been closed. **The operation is terminated only when the patient is wheeled out of the operating room**. Negligent skin closure by an inexperienced junior resident may lead to a wound infection complicating your otherwise surgical *tour de force*. Even the dressing of the wound is prone to complication: skin tape applied too tightly may injure the surrounding skin. So supervise everything until the end including the placement of abdominal binder (after laparotomy) or scrotal support (after repair of inguinal hernia) or the elevation of the lower limb after foot surgery. **No amount of genius can overcome a preoccupation with detail**.

Postoperative considerations

There are **three main tasks** that you have to complete immediately after the operation, before rushing to your office for that so desired cup of coffee (plus a 'power nap' if you are lucky) or to one of the not so desired useless meetings which you are forced to attend:

- **First, go out and talk with the family**. They are your best allies. Invest in them. They are waiting anxiously to hear what you did and how their loved one has fared. Do not keep them waiting. By the way, during lengthy procedures you should have communicated with the family through the nursing staff, sending them updates from time to time (⮌ Chapter 10).
- **Write postoperative orders**. If you did it already before the operation you may need to change or add to it based on intra-operative findings and events: More fluids? Longer course of antibiotics? Send patient to the Intensive Care Unit?
- **Dictate or write an operative report**. Do it now — do not postpone — while operative details are fresh in your mind. A solid operative note is a valuable weapon against any review process, or should the case become legal. **What has not been written does not exist!** A month or year after everything has been forgotten, what is left is the document; how it looks reflects on you and your practice (⮌ Chapter 10).

Should the patient be discharged?

Many procedures are performed these days on an 'ambulatory' (outpatient) basis. The impetus for sending patients home as soon as possible is mainly financial — to contain costs and further enrich insurance companies. But some patients would prefer to spend a night in the hospital, enjoying a few doses of morphine, rather than crawl into the car, and up the stairs, into their bedroom. **Remember: the fact that the patient has been scheduled for an ambulatory operation does not mean that he has to go home immediately after the operation**; instead, you have the right and obligation to keep him in the hospital if you believe that it is medically (or socially) necessary.

Even if the operation was uneventful and you think the patient should be discharged immediately after recovering from whichever anesthesia was used, **make it routine to see him personally prior to discharge**. Are his vital signs OK? Is the patient fully awake? Are dressings well applied and clean? Is the patient up and about and has he voided? Is his abdomen soft? Now — when he is fully awake — talk to him on what has been done, dwell on details of discharge instructions (e.g. diet, physical activities, shower...), warn him about potential complications and provide information on whom to call with further questions or where to go with urgent problems. A printed information sheet with all such information, including the management of the wound and contact numbers, is most valuable. And of course, this is another opportunity to touch the patient and be nice to his family — showing them that you care. Not only could it prevent medical and legal complications but it adds to your reputation.

Remember: if you are 'unhappy' with the patient, consider keeping him overnight in the hospital. **In the USA and other countries "unplanned readmissions" to the hospital are considered complications**. They are flagged by the 'system' and discussed by the quality assurance bodies. You do not want the lap chole discharged in the afternoon to return to the ER at night, in hypovolemic shock. The tachycardia at discharge should have warned you that not everything is *kosher*.

The postoperative course

It is not our intention to reproduce here a manual of intensive care or a treatise on postoperative care. But obviously, many complications can be prevented by optimal postoperative treatment. The following is a list of **principles** to be expanded elsewhere in this book:

- **You are personally responsible for everything**. Once you operate on a patient he or she is yours! Shared responsibility means that no one is responsible! Personal postoperative care, including the minutest details, avoids mishaps. Watch your patients like a hawk (even in the ICU!).
- **Oxygen is good!** Optimal supply of oxygen is crucial to each and every cell of the postoperative patient. See to it that he gets it. The image of patients wheeled out the recovery room without an oxygen mask or tube on their face or nose makes our blood boil. It does not matter that the O_2 saturation at room air is adequate as this may change in a few minutes. *Hypoxia not only stops the motor, it wrecks the engine*.
- **Bring the oxygen to the tissues. "Oxygenate, perfuse, and piss is all that it is about!"** Maintain adequate blood volume by judicious fluid management. Avoid flooding the patient with too much water and salt, resulting in obligatory weight gain and swelling of tissues. Over-hydrated patients are prone to numerous medical and surgical complications including congestive heart failure, respiratory distress, delayed wound and anastomotic healing and abdominal compartment

syndrome. All your patient needs is enough water to replace insensible losses (500-1000ml) and to produce urinary flow of 0.5ml/kg per hour (30cc per hour in the average person). Additional losses (e.g. NG tube) should be replaced selectively on an ad hoc basis but writing an order for 150ml/hour of saline and going to sleep will result in a swollen patient. Accurately measuring INPUT and OUTPUT is crucial. **A Foley catheter is the best monitoring device to assess the adequacy of resuscitation and perfusion!**

- **Avoid unnecessary blood transfusion** (see above and ⟳ Chapter 3) also in the postoperative phase. For most patients, a hematocrit of 30% is more than satisfactory. We would rarely transfuse a postoperative patient with a hemoglobin above 7g/dL unless he is critically ill or suffers from an underlying cardiorespiratory disease. **Consider transfused blood a potential poison**.

- **Control pain!** Hippocrates said it thousands of years ago: "…for since the person being cut usually suffers pain, this suffering should last for the least time possible…", but even today many randomly questioned postoperative patients complain that they are under-treated for pain. Poorly controlled pain delays recovery and contributes to complications (e.g. atelectasis, pneumonia, bedsores). It makes patients and their families unhappy and anxious. Consider pain the 'fifth vital sign' and routinely and repeatedly ensure that your patient does not suffer unnecessarily. Narcotics are, however, a potential double-edged sword — learn to use them safely.

- **Keep the alveoli open**, encourage bottle-breathing exercises!

- **Out of bed!** The sooner you kick the patient out of bed and get him walking about, the faster he will go home. Patients confined to bed are prone to a long list of complications such as atelectasis/pneumonia, deep vein thrombosis, decubitus ulcers, prolonged paralytic ileus and more. See to it personally — do not leave it to the nurses — that your patient is out of bed as soon as possible, preferably a few hours after the operation, any operation!

- **Get rid of lines and tubes!** All the tubes and lines we use to manage and monitor postoperative patients tie them to the bed and inhibit mobilization. Each tube and line is associated with potential iatrogenic complications. Thus, consider removing the nasogastric (NG) tube, indwelling venous or arterial lines and urinary catheters as soon as they are not needed. Some were not indicated at all anyway.

- **Use nasogastric tubes selectively**. The credence that the NG tube 'protects' a distally-placed bowel anastomosis is ridiculous as liters of juices are secreted each day below the decompressed stomach. Nasogastric tubes are extremely irritating to the patient, interfere with breathing, cause esophageal erosions and promote gastroesophageal reflux. Most post-laparotomy patients do not need NG decompression — not even following major *elective* upper gastrointestinal procedures. NG drainage is indicated, however, following emergency abdominal operations, in mechanically ventilated patients, in obtunded patients, and after operations for intestinal obstruction. Consider removing the NG tube on the morning after surgery or as soon as its output diminishes and ileus subsides. If in doubt you may want to cap or clamp the tube for 12 hours before removing it and observe how this is tolerated by the patient. A small percentage of patients will need the tube to be reinserted because of early postoperative small bowel obstruction or persistent ileus (⊃ Chapter 8).

- **Let your patients eat**. Do not starve or over feed them. Use the enteral route whenever possible — it is safer and cheaper. Ask what and how your patient would like to eat, they know best. The old rituals of gradually increasing the permitted volume and consistency of oral fluids are passé. When enteral feeding is impossible, total parenteral nutrition is rarely necessary unless the starvation period extends beyond 7-10 days or if the patient has been malnourished prior to the operation.

- **Prevent constipation**. "**The moment patients can eat, fart and crap they forget the operation and who their surgeon was**." Constipation can develop also after operations which do not produce ileus, due to bed rest, use of opiates and the incisional pain generated by the defecating process. After anal surgery (e.g. hemorrhoidectomy) it can be devastating. Pre-emptive measures should be taken on discharge, if not already *before* the operation.

- **Do not treat fever**. "The real danger in fever is not the pyrexia but the poison causing it" [Augustus Charles Bernays]. **Temperature is not a disease — do not treat it as such**. Postoperative fever reflects the patient's inflammatory response (SIRS) to different insults including infection as well as surgical trauma, atelectasis, transfusion and others. SIRS does not always mean sepsis (sepsis = SIRS + infection). "Fever is not a disease caused by lack of antibiotics." Fever should not be treated reflexively with antibiotics; it should not be stifled with antipyretics as the febrile response has been shown to be beneficial to the host's defenses. However, fever is a potential warning sign: more on it in ⊃ Chapter 4. **Beware: when a very high temperature develops during or after general anesthesia, always consider the possibility of malignant hyperthermia!** (Unexplained fever >40°C [105°F], muscle pain and rigidity…). It is very rare and most of us have never seen it. But ignoring it, and delaying treatment often leads to unfortunate outcomes, even death! **If hyperpyrexia is associated with delirium think about neuroleptic malignant syndrome**.

- **Realize that the problem usually lies at the operative site**. Fever and tachycardia on day five after intestinal surgery is not 'pneumonia'; antibiotics cannot block the hole in your anastomotic suture line.
- **Continue preventing DVT** (see above).
- **Use postoperative antibiotics appropriately**. Unnecessarily prolonged administration is not harmless (➲ Chapter 4).
- **Remove drains as soon as they are deemed unnecessary** — often they were redundant anyway (➲ Chapter 4).
- **Always worry and continue worrying**. Trust only yourself and do not count on anyone doing the worrying for you. Reserve optimism until the day after discharge, or even better, until the first postop office visit. Until then, plan for the next worst potential problem.

A man who doesn't worry at all doesn't care a whole lot. I should not want a man who did not care a whole lot operating on me.

J. Chalmers Da Costa

The system

Already in the previous chapter we grumbled about the so called SYSTEM(S): the ever-growing monsters, commonly controlled by politically-motivated, often medically uninformed and for profit individuals, which increasingly dictate how we practice medicine and surgery. In many instances complications and poor outcomes can be attributed to a dysfunctional system — at all levels — rather than to any individual surgeon. When you have to perform a Cesarean section at 3 a.m., on a morbidly obese patient, with the only assistance provided to you by a minimally trained nurse, is it a wonder that you have inadvertently entered the urinary bladder? Sure, but so what? That it is not your fault does not matter. You cannot complain against that nurse and you cannot moan against the system — if you do, you will be lynched or squashed like a cockroach. The system has the money; it has an army of lawyers at its disposition — it always wins. Unfortunately, we have to adapt to our local system, find proactive ways to protect patients from its harms. To survive we have to take responsibility even if there is no doubt that it was the system's fault. **Remember**: the system never apologizes; instead it finds ways to blame you. The system is never accused or put on trial. We are!

Excellent results don't just happen — they are earned!

Chapter 3

Hemostasis and bleeding

Samir Johna and Moshe Schein

The only weapon with which the unconscious patient can immediately retaliate upon the incompetent surgeon is hemorrhage.

William Stewart Halsted

The entire message of this chapter can be summarized in just a few statements:

- The volume of blood lost during any operation correlates directly with its outcome.
- The need for transfusion of blood and blood products during any operation has a major impact on subsequent morbidity and mortality (in cancer operations it also adversely affects long-term outcome).
- The more blood you lose, the more blood you need to give — the higher the risks of postoperative infection and organ system dysfunction!
- A good surgeon is a **hemostatic surgeon**!
- A wise surgeon knows when to transfuse — how much and which products — and, as importantly, when *not* to transfuse.

How to be such a hemostatic and wise surgeon, avoiding blood loss and transfusion, is the crux of this chapter. This is not a manual of hematology nor a guidebook to the blood bank — if you need a refresher course on the clotting cascade, or wish to learn about emerging experimental hemostatic agents, you need to look elsewhere. Here we'll stick to basics, discussing what you can (nay, must) do before the operation, during the operation and after it, to save blood and to treat bleeding complications. **For as careful as you may be, only those who don't operate never experience unexpected hemorrhage**.

Pre-operative considerations

We know that "an ounce of prevention is worth a pound of cure". So, what can you do *before* the operation to assure optimal intra-operative hemostasis?

The time-**honored history and physical examination** remain the most reliable way to **identify bleeding tendencies**: the lack of any history of abnormal bleeding during or after surgical procedure such as circumcision, dental extraction or trivial trauma (e.g. shaving) is reassuring, and should be documented in the medical records.

In our increasingly aging population, it is now difficult to find a patient who is not on some **blood thinners** — in our practice almost every other patient regularly takes aspirin or clopidogrel (Plavix®); many are on chronic warfarin (Coumadin®) treatment for various reasons (■ Figure 3.1). Remember that non-steroidal anti-inflammatory drugs (NSAIDs) may increase the risk of bleeding. Many patients do not know that some over-the-counter medications interfere with hemostasis and won't report taking them unless specifically asked. A while ago we repaired an inguinal hernia in a teenager who did not stop oozing during the operation. After the operation he admitted: "yesterday I took a few aspirins for headache…" Always inquire about ALL medications the patient consumes and act as described below.

Numerous studies have shown that *routine* **pre-operative laboratory clotting tests** are of value *only* in patients with a history of a bleeding diathesis or who take anticoagulants. Despite this, some anesthetists still demand to see the platelet count, the INR and the PTT before putting a patient to sleep for a major operation. Some radiologists won't insert even a PICC line without having the results of such tests. These are sad symptoms of 'defensive' medicine — we all have to fight this in our own environment (usually without much success). Of course, specific clotting tests are indicated for specific indications (e.g. INR in the patient on warfarin).

What to do with all those 'blood thinners'?

It clearly depends on the specific circumstances. **How urgent is the procedure?** For example, elective cholecystectomy vs. penetrating abdominal trauma — you know that some cases are extreme emergencies, others are only urgent, and some 'emergencies' can be cooled off (e.g. acute cholecystitis). It also depends on the **magnitude** of the procedure: while we

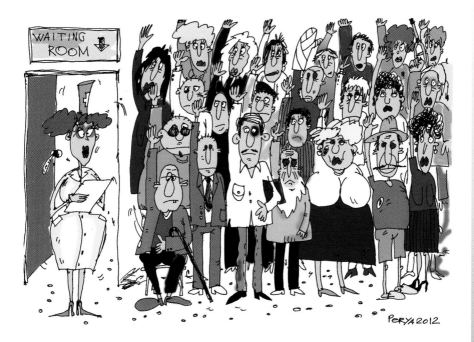

Figure 3.1. "Who is taking aspirin or clopidogrel?"

don't mind excising a sebaceous cyst in a patient receiving aspirin and clopidogrel, we would want those agents stopped well before, say, a laparoscopic colectomy. The literature and internet are saturated with detailed guidelines on the peri-operative management of antiplatelet agents and anticoagulants. **Here we offer a simplified version of our daily practice — you will see that in essence it all depends on the nature of the surgical disease and the indications for the antiplatelet agents or anticoagulation.**

Elective procedures

Antiplatelet agents

In general terms these should be stopped before the operation; some talk about ten days, others would be happy with five — but let us agree on a week, OK? As always you have to apply some common sense (this is why you're reading this book, right?): in our experience minor procedures on the surface of the body (e.g excision of skin cancer) can be performed safely in patients taking a full dose of aspirin and/or clopidogrel. Careful hemostasis with sutures and/or diathermy and a few minutes of **pressure** are all that's needed. Otherwise, insist on stopping these agents — what's the rush to operate! Having said that, if a patient is scheduled for, say, an elective hernia repair, has been a little confused and took his last dose of aspirin four days before the planned procedure — it is not the end of the world. Proceed, insist on extra-careful hemostasis and everything will be OK. Use your judgment and don't be dogmatic; we hate dogmas! However, be aware that **there are some patients in whom stopping antiplatelet agents can be dangerous**. For example, you don't want to stop clopidogrel in patients with a 'fresh' or not so fresh coronary stent without talking to the cardiologist — in many such patients elective surgery should be postponed (for six weeks to six months, depending on the nature of the stent) until the antiplatelet agents can safely be discontinued.

Warfarin

A huge number of our patients are maintained, for various indications, on chronic anticoagulation with this troublesome agent. In some, the indication is solid (e.g. a recent deep vein thrombosis) but in others it's flimsy — the patient's physician decided that it would be 'safer' to continue anticoagulation for life only because he thinks so (don't laugh, this situation is not uncommon). **There is no question that warfarin has to be stopped — the recommended time is five days — before most operations** (except for minor cutaneous procedures which can be done safely even if the INR is prolonged). The main question is **who are the patients who should receive 'bridging therapy' with unfractionated heparin, or low-molecular-weight heparin (LMWH) on those five days during which their INR is being normalized?**

Bridging therapy should be considered in patients with **mechanical heart valves, a history of DVT or atrial fibrillation (AF)**. We bet that your hospital has an established 'bridging protocol' but here is a short version of what we do.

It depends on the risk in the individual patient of developing thrombotic complications. Patients belonging to the 'high-risk' group need 'bridging'; those in a 'low-risk' group do not. **Who are the 'low-risk' patients?:**

- Patients with those types of **artificial heart valves** which are less prone to thrombus formation and with no other risk factors for stroke (e.g. diabetes, hypertension, advanced age). Always let the patient's cardiologist or personal internist decide!
- **Atrial fibrillation** patients with a **low (0-2) CHAD score** and no prior history of stroke or transient ischemic attacks (TIA). (You don't know what a CHAD score is? Here it is: prior stroke/TIA - 2 points, congestive heart failure - 1 point, hypertension - 1 point, diabetes - 1 point, age >75 - 1 point.)
- **Patients with a history of DVT/pulmonary emboli** more than 12 months previously, the last such episode being without 'active' thromboembolic risk factors (cancer, cardiomyopathy or thrombophilia).

Patients who do not belong to the low-risk group are routinely bridged — the vast majority with subcutaneous LMWH (enoxaparin), which is stopped 12-24 hours before the operation. A minority, considered extremely high risk are bridged with an unfractionated heparin infusion which is stopped 4-6 hours prior to the operation and restarted postop.

Please familiarize yourself with the methodology of bridging **but never take the decision on whom NOT to bridge alone**. A few months ago we did a straightforward right hemicolectomy for cecal cancer in a lady suffering from chronic AF who, according to her physician, didn't need bridging as her CHAD score was 1. On postoperative day three she developed a major stroke and died! No scoring system is 'perfect' in the individual patient. We were devastated but, at least, it was not our decision *not* to bridge… And of course the stroke may have had nothing to do with the chronic AF in the first place.

Emergency procedures

What to do with patients on 'blood thinners' who need an emergency procedure?

Antiplatelet agents

The operative hemorrhagic risk for aspirin alone is increased by an average factor of 1.5. When clopidogrel is added to aspirin, the bleeding risk is higher. But, if the operation cannot be postponed then you have no choice but to proceed — as the Arabs would say: "*Allah Yerhamo!*" (God has mercy…) — our surgical existence involves constant risk-taking and we assess the risk/benefit ratio of everything we do. But if you can wait, if you can safely cool off the emergency into a semi-emergency, then please wait; the longer — the better. Please note that the serum half-life of clopidogrel is very long and transfused platelets will be rapidly inactivated by any residual circulating drug. **The value of platelet transfusion in this situation is very doubtful but since we cannot be certain (ever) of compliance with medication a trial of platelet administration may be worthwhile, particularly if the patient is bleeding and therefore eliminating circulating clopidogrel**. One unit of aphoresis platelets (single donor) should increase the platelet count by 30,000-60,000/µl in a 70kg adult. Therefore, two units should be adequate for hemostasis. (If your center still uses the 'old' conventional units, then each is supposed to raise the count by 5000; giving 6-8 units is the rule…).

Warfarin

Most surgeons are not comfortable operating if the INR is higher than 1.5. So, if the operation cannot be deferred until the drug is metabolized or the patient is bridged, then you will have to **reverse the anticoagulation**. In dire emergencies use **FFP (fresh frozen plasma)**: each unit of FFP raises the level of clotting factors in an adult by 3-5%. The recommended dose is 10-20ml/kg body weight which corresponds to 4-6 units in a 70kg adult. If you can wait longer then consider giving **Vitamin K**: a single oral dose of 2.5mg, which, however, may take 24-36 hours to work. (It can also be injected intravenously in a single dose of 1.5mg and this is expected to work within 6-8 hours, but is associated with a very small risk of an anaphylactic reaction.)

A new landmine!

Another inceasingly used medication to prevent strokes in those with atrial fibrillation due to causes other than heart valve disease, and at least one additional risk factor for stroke (congestive heart failure, hypertension, age, diabetes, and prior stroke), and to prevent deep venous thrombosis is dabigatran (Pradaxa®). Dabigatran is a direct thrombin inhibitor. It must also be stopped at least 24 hours prior to low-risk surgeries for bleeding, otherwise it is better to be stopped 2-4 days prior to surgery. Neuroaxial anesthesia should be avoided. There is no known antidote to this drug which has now been linked to numerous deaths following trauma and/or emergency surgery. Even the *New York Times* described it as "A promising drug with a flaw…" citing a surgeon who said, "you feel helpless…" Others call it "the cardiologist's darling, the intensivist's headache, and the trauma surgeon's nightmare!" Yet another glorious chapter of modern medicine…

Intra-operative considerations

Bleeding in the belly is like fire on a ship — you run towards it.
Jeffery Young

As you well know some operations are bloodier than others; it all depends on the site, extent and indication for the operation. Surgeons, each within his/her specialty, should know which specific operation may be associated with significant blood loss and, accordingly, cross-matched blood should be available. **But the magnitude of blood loss and the need for transfusion are also surgeon-dependent**. During your training years, or while assisting other surgeons, you must have been exposed to **different 'attitudes' to surgical hemostasis**. At one end of the spectrum you had to watch (with great suffering and self-restraint) those super-pedantic, obsessive compulsive individuals, who chase each red blood cell, suture ligate every capillary, roast the fat with diathermy and fulgurate a dry liver bed (after cholecystectomy) with the argon beam coagulator (ABC). At the other end of the spectrum you probably had the delight to watch the 'butcher' type surgeons — those who enjoy operating in a pool of fresh blood. They, who often consider themselves *macho*, proceed boldly with little regard to the blood being shed. Their motto is "all bleeding stops eventually". Often they are right, because most patients have robust clotting mechanisms, but the patient will pay the price of blood lost with complications. We are sure that you, well familiar with both of these attitudes, choose to practice somewhere in the middle of the spectrum — you know how important it is to work in a dry field, you understand which bleeder can be left alone and which has to be controlled and how. Below are a few general points:

- **Surgical or medical bleeding?** In most cases the bleeding is *surgical* (technical), but occasionally you will encounter the so called *medical* bleeding due to **coagulopathy**. Serious *surgical* bleeding **requiring** massive blood transfusion may eventually lead to *coagulopathy*.
- Generalized oozing inside and outside the surgical field indicates a missed congenital or acquired *coagulopathy*. Difficult to localize and fast pooling of blood in the surgical field is generally caused by **venous injury**. On the other hand, when bright red blood hits the ceiling in spurts, you must look for **arterial injury**.
- **The best clotting factor is the surgeon!** Meticulous dissection is the key to good hemostasis. Knowledge of anatomy and utilization of the correct tissue planes minimize bleeding. Once you know how to dissect properly during elective, non-hurried surgery, you can do it rapidly when needed; it just takes knowledge of anatomy and a little practice. The 'third' stage of dissection involves going to areas where normal, virginal anatomy is destroyed by inflammation or previous surgery. The key here is to find the tissue planes (they are still there — your fingers are the safest dissecting instrument!) and restore previous anatomy before attempting reconstruction. **You must check the wound repeatedly to control bleeders. Even minute 'pumpers' can cause significant blood loss if you have been operating for several hours**. Do not brush off the anesthetist's estimate of your blood loss even if it hurts your ego. Remember that partially severed small vessels will not contract as expected during the initial phases of hemostasis. Do not let the assistant *wipe* the wound with a sponge since this may strip away the initial platelet plug — he must only *dab* at bleeders.
- When you operate for major bleeding or have caused it, stem it with whatever temporary measures seem appropriate to the situation. Do not lose your cool. Apply direct pressure with your finger or a sponge (a 'sponge on a stick' can control even a hole in the inferior vena cava!). **Stay calm**: surgeons who panic and attempt hemostasis in a chaotic manner lose their patients. A relevant aphorism: "Whenever you encounter massive bleeding, the first thing to remember is that it is not your blood…" [Raphael Adar].
- **Communicate with the anesthetist and the surgical team**. Allow the anesthetic team to catch up with blood loss and order appropriate blood products. Ask for better lighting (e.g. head light), an extra

suction and summon additional experienced hands if available. **Share with all present your war plan**. Only then go ahead and try to fix what's hemorrhaging. How often have we seen surgeons persisting hysterically in a futile chase after the source of bleeding, while the patient slides into the **triangle of death** (acidosis, hypothermia, coagulopathy)? **Old martial art *sensei's* advice: The more blood there is, the calmer the surgeon must be. Take control of the situation!**

● Most probably **the source of the blood is where you expected it to be**. If this is not the case, **search elsewhere**: pulling on the omentum during colectomy may tear the capsule of the spleen; retracting on the liver to expose the duodenum may have damaged it. You may need proximal and distal vascular control in named-vessel injury — whether to repair or ligate the bleeding vessel and how exactly to do it depends on the specific situation and is out of the scope of this brief text. In most instances, a ligature, a suture or a clip (plus/minus diathermy) will do the job. You can use more **advanced energy emitting devices** (e.g. harmonic scalpel, Argon beam coagulator) if available. **Adjuvant local hemostatic agents** (e.g. gelatin foams, cellulose pads, collagen fleece, topical thrombin, or fibrin/synthetic sealants) are sometimes beneficial.

● **You should familiarize yourself with special blood-saving maneuvers specific to the operations you perform**. These may be adopted routinely or selectively according to the situation. **For example**: preliminary control of the renal pedicle prior to nephrectomy, the *Pringle maneuver* before dividing hepatic parenchyma or **subtotal cholecystectomy** (or cholecystostomy) rather than cholecystectomy in cirrhotic patients who are likely to bleed from the gallbladder bed. Consider also what your anesthetist can do to minimize blood loss — for instance, keeping the patient 'dry' during major hepatectomies (aiming at a central venous pressure [CVP] of zero) has been shown to decrease blood loss significantly! We do not wish to dwell on autotransfusion and 'cell savers'...

● **Careful inspection before closing** the wound eliminates the possibility of missing delayed bleeders that have been in spasm during surgery. It is not a bad idea that you release the retractors to look at the wounds, and deflate the pneumoperitoneum every now and then in laparoscopic surgery to look for subtle bleeding. During operations involving large surfaces in the subcutaneous area (e.g. when doing 'component separation'), we use *hydrogen peroxide* irrigation. This stops some oozing and makes it easier to see the small bleeders that need coagulation. (Remember, however, that the use of hydrogen peroxide irrigation of closed cavities has been associated with adverse effects, possibly due to *venous gas embolism*.)

- **Whatever you do, do not forget the principles of 'damage control' that have become the standard of care in the management of complex surgical or trauma cases.** Do not hesitate to **pack** stubborn surface ooze or venous bleeding and come back to fight another day.
- Be aware that the **source of bleeding (and/or shock) may be remote from your actual operative field.** We remember repairing a stabbed femoral artery in the groin, while the anesthetist continued moaning that the patient is hypotensive. *Well, let him moan…* and we continued with the vascular anastomosis until the patient arrested. After failed resuscitation, when we turned him around, we discovered a tiny stab wound in the upper back — the patient had been oozing to death into the chest while we obsessed with the finicky arterial reconstruction. **Always think outside the box and listen to what others have to say!** In other cases the 'remote' cause of shock could be pericardial tamponade or tension pneumothorax. **In general, from time to time you have to stop focusing on the narrow surgical field and consider the whole picture.**
- **Remember the 14 Ps of hemostasis:** see ■ Table 3.1.

Table 3.1. The 14 Ps of surgical hemostasis: what to do if the patient is still bleeding? *Developed by Ahmad Assalia, modified from Schein's Common Sense Emergency Abdominal Surgery, 3rd Edition. Springer Verlag, © 2010.*

First	Then consider
Apply PRESSURE	PLATELETS
with PACKS or PADS	fresh frozen PLASMA
have PATIENCE	PROTAMINE (to reverse heparin)
suture with PROLENE® (or whatever)	and PACKED cells (if still bleeding)
	call the PROFESSOR for help
	add PPI (proton pump inhibitors) for UGI bleeding…
	use PASG (pneumatic anti-shock garment) for bleeding from broken pelvis
	Finally, PRAY so that your patient does not arrive at the POST-MORTEM

> *I do know that it is harder to control bleeding from the back
> side of the portal vein than it is to land a 737 with an engine
> on fire.*
>
> **Richard C. Karl**

Postoperative considerations

Postoperative bleeding

"But *it was dry when I closed...*" How often have we heard, or uttered, that cliché! It is always the same: whenever we have to drain a wound hematoma or to re-explore for intraperitoneal bleeding we automatically exclaim: "S###. It was dry when I closed!" Well, in many cases it was not as 'dry' as we think it was; but it doesn't matter whether it was dry or not — now we have to face up to the complication.

Postoperative bleeding can be *visible* (rare) or *hidden* (more common). The *visible* bleeding is into the wound or through the drain — take notice: **bleeding through the drain can be misleading; what comes out of the drain is often only the tip of the iceberg** (see below). Visible bleeding is a no-brainer; depending on the amount and rate of bleeding you may need to re-explore, to find and control the source.

Hidden **bleeding into the cavities** (abdomen, retroperitoneum, chest, etc.) is, however, **treacherous**. Signs often are 'soft' and vague; diagnosis and decision-making can be clouded by the 'surgical ego' with its inherent difficulty to acknowledge failures. From our experience at morbidity and mortality conferences, and with 'legal' cases, we could write an entire chapter with case reports of patients who **bled to death** after an operation, but were denied timely reoperation by their surgeons. The story of each such tragic patient is different, but the lessons learned are relatively simple and must be emphasized time and time again:

Semper fatigo, et suspicantur! (Always worry and suspect!).

A recent case of ours is outlined over the page.

You don't want us to bore you with the signs and grades of hypovolemic shock — that orthostatic hypotension is an early feature as is a mild tachycardia (if the patient is not receiving beta-blockers), that urine output reflects the volume status and that the level of hemoglobin/hematocrit lags

A lady underwent a straightforward laparoscopic cholecystectomy for acute cholecystitis. A few hours after the operation we called the nurse in charge to ask about the patient.

"Oh Doc, she is doing well, her vitals are OK and she has been drinking. No pain at all."

"Did she void?" we asked.

"Yes. But she became dizzy on the way to the bathroom, almost fainted. Blood pressure dropped to 90/60. I gave her a bolus of Ringer's... I wonder whether I should restart her blood pressure medications; you know she's on beta-blockers?"

"What's coming out of the drain?"

"Last time I emptied it... when she returned from the OR, there was 25cc. I didn't check it since..."

"OK, I'll be there in ten minutes!"

We found the patient lying in bed and smiling. Her heart rate was 100/minute. We lifted the blanket to look at the drain: the bulb was half full with fresh blood. We took her back to the OR — her tummy was full of fresh blood. As often is the case, we did not find any 'major' active bleeding; she had been oozing from the gallbladder bed and omental adhesions; the pre-operative dose of enoxaparin was probably a contributing factor.

hours behind the blood loss (unless it is massive). But we will advise you again not to be fooled by low-output drains — fresh clots may occlude the drains which therefore may not reflect true blood loss.

The decision on what to do when suspecting *hidden* bleeding is not easy. Some tips:

- **Try a fluid challenge**; say a liter bolus of crystalloids, to see whether it corrects the early signs of hypovolemia. If this is not enough then the patient is losing volume somewhere.
- **Reassess the patient's past medical history**. For example, a prior inferior myocardial infarction or beta-blockade may prevent tachycardia. **Remember that hypotension after surgery is not always related to blood loss**: persisting effects of anesthetics, whether general or epidural, and narcotics may cause hypotension. In

patients on chronic steroids, acute adrenal insufficiency (Addisonian crisis) may provoke hypotension, which generally responds to corticosteroids.

- Profound shock and full blown abdominal compartment syndrome caused by an expanding hemoperitoneum is easily recognized! **You should rush to the OR and open the abdomen**. Less dramatic presentations (like the post-LC patient we described above) and when the patient is hemodynamically stable, should be managed on an individual basis. In selected cases, CT imaging will show the amount of free blood in the cavity — if not significant then re-exploration can be avoided.
- Think about the possibility of **coagulopathy** (see below).

Remember: the suspicion that your patient is bleeding 'somewhere' should be always in your mind. You cannot manage such patients over the phone. Taking the correct decision, whether to re-explore or wait, requires you to be at the patient's bedside. Recruit your colleague for an unbiased opinion since your emotional attachment and ego may prevent you from making the right decision. There is almost nothing worse in surgery than losing your patient to postoperative bleeding — **your threshold to reoperation should be appropriately low!**

When to resume antithrombotic drugs?

Antiplatelet drugs (aspirin and/or clopidogrel) can be restarted immediately after the operation, particularly in patients at high risk of thromboembolic events (e.g. coronary stent *in situ*). Bridging therapy should be restarted within 24 hours (at the evening after the operation or the next morning) and continued until the warfarin (which is restarted — if oral intake is possible) achieves a therapeutic level. After operations that carry a higher risk of postoperative bleeding (e.g. cardiac, major oncological, hepatic, etc.), or when you are worried about the adequacy of hemostasis, wait 48-72 hours before restarting the heparin. Such recommendations are not written in stone and much is left to your judgment — the science of a gray area...

What about bleeding in trauma? (see also ➲ Chapter 24)

Bleeding in trauma patients is a different animal! Unlike elective procedures, trauma patients are additionally disadvantaged by risk factors that can make bleeding worse. We often wait eagerly at the trauma bay to milk as much information from the paramedics as possible about the circumstances of the events.

"Was he restrained?"

"How long was the extrication time?"

"Was he ejected?"

"Was there a large pool of blood at the scene?"

It is not unusual for many trauma patients to be inebriated. Alcohol causes peripheral vasodilatation, and with prolonged exposure to the ambient temperature, hypothermia sets in. With hypotension and hypothermia, acidosis soon follows creating the perfect storm — the death triangle.

Despite improvements in trauma care, uncontrolled bleeding contributes to one-third of trauma-related deaths and is the leading cause of **potentially preventable early in-hospital deaths**. Therefore, it doesn't take a genius to figure out that successful resuscitation of the trauma patient with uncontrolled bleeding requires the early identification of potential bleeding sources followed by prompt action to achieve three essential goals:

- Minimize blood loss.
- Restore tissue perfusion.
- Achieve hemodynamic stability.

Bear in mind the need for early assessment of comorbidity and any history of pre-existing medication that may prolong bleeding.

So how can you become a better trauma surgeon?

It is probably a good idea to start with a better appreciation of the '**golden hour**'. If you do not want your patient to succumb, you must complete your evaluation, assess the magnitude of bleeding, identify the source of bleeding, decide if you need to intervene, and execute the whole plan within the golden hour. We suggest you refer to the **American College of Surgeons Advanced Trauma Life Support Classification** for guidance on the clinical assessment of hemorrhage severity. Unless early resuscitative efforts are fruitful, all trauma patients in shock with an identified source of bleeding should be subjected to urgent intervention to stop the bleeding. Stable patients can be evaluated clinically to rule out major bleeding into the chest, or for the presence of an unstable pelvic fracture. Focused abdominal sonography for trauma (**FAST**) is an excellent tool in the search for intra-abdominal bleeding and can be done quickly at the trauma bay if you have appropriate experience in the use of ultrasound. Some patients may still require CT scan evaluation. The new generation CT scanners (64 slice scanners) can perform whole-body CT in less than 30 seconds! Make sure that your patient is stable before you send him to the CT scanner, particularly when the CT scanner is not within the ER department. Having witnessed the chaos many times we know that the CT suite is not a good place to resuscitate a crashed patient. Don't let it become necessary in your patient!

You have determined that your patient does not need an intervention — for the time being. Now what?

Ideally, patients are admitted for serial physical examinations and laboratory evaluations. **The reality is that many of these trauma patients are admitted only to be subsequently ignored**. The admitting doctors are often busy and may forget to perform the prescribed serial examinations and as a result marked deterioration in the clinical condition of the patient is completely missed! Sometimes reliance is placed on serial hematocrit measurements to monitor progress. A major limitation of this approach is the confounding influence of resuscitative measures; changes in hematocrit are difficult to interpret in the context of administration of intravenous fluids and red blood cell concentrates. Therefore, serial hematocrit measurements as an *isolated* marker for bleeding should not be used. Serum lactate estimation may be useful, and measurement of the base deficit, derived from arterial gas analysis, is an indirect measurement of global acidosis secondary to impaired tissue perfusion.

What if you face a need for a rapid control of bleeding?

> *It is usually a bad sign if the anesthesiologist is asking you if you are losing a lot of blood during a case, especially when you are not.*
>
> **Michael Hoffman**

The source of bleeding, when identified, dictates the proper course of action. For pelvic ring disruption and hemorrhagic shock, immediate immobilization of the broken pelvis is imperative. You do not have to be a skilled orthopedic surgeon to save a life here. A makeshift immobilizing device can be fashioned by tying the bed sheet (placed transversely on the gurney on which the patient is lying) across the pelvic rim, thus closing the open-book pelvic fracture. This technique is often enough to arrest or slow down the bleeding while you organize definitive therapy. Call your interventional radiologist to mobilize his team for possible angiographic embolization. If you practice in the land of nowhere — or in the case of an *open* **bleeding pelvic fracture** — then exploration with direct surgical control of the bleeding should be exercised whenever possible. Occasionally, we find ourselves in a swamp of blood at a time when the patient is facing the above mentioned 'triangle of death'. Then you must exercise 'damage control' where **pelvic packing** may bail you out and save your patient's life. Do not forget to stabilize the pelvic ring. You can use pelvic binder or a C-clamp with or without the help of an orthopedic surgeon.

How should you manage non-surgical bleeding and coagulation in trauma?

Blood and blood products

> Unless your patient is actively bleeding to death, it is simply best not to transfuse any blood product... (but) of course, if the patient is bleeding rapidly and is in shock, then RBCs, plasma, and platelets are required.
>
> **John B. Holcomb**

Remember, transfuse only when absolutely necessary. With all blood and blood products always consider transfusion risks such as transfusion reactions, allergies, hemolysis, transmission of infection, lowering of immunity, worsening of cancer outcome, congestive heart failure, and transfusion-related acute lung injury (TRALI). There is a huge body of evidence to show how potentially damaging blood administration is to the patient. For example, studies show that Jehovah's Witnesses undergoing cardiac surgery (and refusing blood) have better outcomes. Think about each and every unit of blood you transfuse.

It is still debatable **at what level of hemoglobin one should consider transfusion**. RBCs play an important role in coagulation in addition to their role in oxygen transport. A target hemoglobin level of 7-9g/dL is considered adequate for most trauma patients. Some believe, however, that while such a low threshold is reasonable for ICU patients it should be higher— ~10g/dL in acutely bleeding trauma patients or surgical (e.g. GI bleeding) patients.

In patients with massive bleeding or significant bleeding complicated by coagulopathy (prolonged PT, aPTT more than 1.5 times normal), or in patients already on oral anticoagulants (vitamin K antagonists), you should consider transfusing prothrombin complex concentrate (PCC). When not available, you should transfuse thawed FFP at an initial dose of 10-15ml/kg body weight. This can be repeated as needed.

As for **platelets**, you should not consider transfusion if the platelet count is $50 \times 10^9/L$ or above, except in patients with massive bleeding, disseminated intravascular coagulation, or hyperfibrinolysis when a platelet level of $75 \times 10^9/L$ or above is recommended. In patients with severe head injury and intracranial bleeding, a platelet level of $100 \times 10^9/L$ or above is recommended. You can start with 4-8 units of platelet concentrates or one apheresis pack. It can be repeated as needed.

You should also consider transfusion of cryoprecipitate or fibrinogen concentrate when there is inherited or acquired hypofibrinogenemia (less than 1g/L). You can start with 3-4g that can be repeated as needed.

Massive blood loss

> It is usually a bad sign if there are three or more anesthesiologists in the operating room at the same time and none of them is reading the newspaper.
>
> **Michael Hoffman**

When the patient loses his entire volume of blood (approximately 5L) in a few hours, he is said to have suffered massive blood loss. The patient is obviously in trouble, and consequently needs a similarly massive transfusion (10 U or more of RBCs over 24 hours).

The aim of resuscitation ideally is to achieve tissue perfusion and resolution of shock without causing complications of hypervolemia like pulmonary edema, congestive heart failure, abdominal compartment syndrome, dilution coagulopathy, or, rarely, even compartment syndrome of encapsulated organs, particularly the kidneys.

Recent experience, particularly from the US military in Iraq and Afghanistan, has shown that transfusion with whole blood leads to better outcomes than RBCs in trauma settings. **The policy now is to use fresh whole blood (FWB) when available, or alternatively use the '1:1:1 ratio' — equal parts RBCs, FFP, and platelets** — in the battlefield MASH units and military hospitals. Among its other advantages the use of this ratio decreases the volume of other resuscitation fluid, therefore decreasing the complications of massive crystalloid use. Crystalloids have neither oxygen-carrying capacity nor clotting factors. This policy is gradually permeating into civilian trauma practice.

Epilogue

Now that you have learned about hemostasis and bleeding, we'd like to emphasize that while acquisition of knowledge and skills is imperative in the adequate management of hemostasis and bleeding, they are simply not enough. You must show a positive attitude towards what you have learned and commit to act accordingly. Learned knowledge and skills will get you nowhere if you do not translate them into positive behavior. **Let us illustrate**: we were on call at the hospital when a 'code blue' was called. By the time we arrived at the location, we could see a dozen professionals including internists, hospitalists, anesthetists, and surgery residents. They were all staring at a patient who had undergone a total thyroidectomy earlier that day. Apparently she had bled and developed a huge neck hematoma. She turned blue right in front of them while they struggled to intubate. At least half of them knew what needed to be done, and a few of them were actually trained to act in such circumstances. They had the knowledge and the skills to quickly open the wound and evacuate the hematoma, but no one had the nerve to act. So what good did all the knowledge and the skills do? It took us only a few seconds to save her life!

> "Be strong and of a good courage, fear not, nor be afraid..."
>
> **Deuteronomy 31:6**

Chapter 4

Postoperative infections

Moshe Schein

Every operation in surgery is an experiment in bacteriology.
Berkeley Moynihan

Sepsis is a slight upon surgical virility.
John Alexander-Williams

Prior to the 19th century, before Louis Pasteur and Joseph Lister radically modified the face of surgery by recognizing the importance of bacteriology and asepsis, the lethal shadow of infection was cast over each and every operation. In those days the practice of surgery was the practice of producing pus! Indeed, Hippocrates believed pus formation to be beneficial: "The wound should be treated in such a way as to produce suppuration as quickly as possible." Even today postoperative infections still threaten the outcome of any operation we perform and, furthermore, surgeons continue to treat a huge spectrum of conditions caused by infection with micro-organisms (mainly bacteria).

Postoperative infections are associated not only with increased mortality and morbidity but also huge financial consequences. In the USA in 2009, the in-hospital cost of treating (only) surgical site infections (SSI) was estimated to be over 1.2 billion dollars! Infections that develop after any operation stain our reputation: a patient with an infected mesh following a hernia repair, who has to undergo a reoperation to remove the mesh, and is then left with the original hernia, possibly even larger, after two costly operations, is rarely satisfied with the explanation that "s**t happens…"

The term "surgical infection" is considered to include any infection that should or could be managed surgically and any infection (*medical* or *surgical*) that develops after an operation. Obviously, a chapter like this cannot encompass the entire topic of surgical infections to which whole textbooks have been dedicated. Therefore, in this chapter we will try to provide you with the principles only — a framework to better understand the prevention and treatment of postoperative infections. In subsequent chapters you will read about infective complications relevant to the main theme of that chapter — here we'll focus on the big picture.

Fundamentals, truisms

Let's begin with some background information which we believe is crucial to the understanding of postoperative infections:

- **Local inflammation is not always infection!** It is imperative to understand that symptoms and signs of local inflammation after the operation do not immediately imply the presence of local infection, although clinically the entities may be difficult to distinguish: for example, *sterile superficial thrombophlebitis* at the site of an i.v. line vs. *septic thrombophlebitis* caused by *Staphylococcus aureus*. Similarly, not every angry-looking wound should be diagnosed immediately as *wound infection* (oops, we forgot that the term "wound infection" is outdated, now replaced by SSI...). **What makes local inflammation an infection is the presence of micro-organisms — usually bacteria!**
- **SIRS (systemic inflammatory response syndrome)** is not equivalent to sepsis! Amazingly, more than 20 years after the late Dr. Roger C. Bone pioneered the definition of these entities, people still confuse systemic inflammation (SIRS) with sepsis. We still read expert opinions by distinguished professors of surgery, claiming, for example, that a patient dying from multiple organ failure (MOF) a day or two after massive hemorrhage did so because of *septic shock*, i.e. infection. This, of course, is nonsense. **To diagnose septic shock one needs to demonstrate a source of infection.** In fact such a patient will have died from SIRS, induced by shock, leading to progressive multiple organ dysfunction (MOD), and then multiple organ failure (MOF). **You have to understand the difference between sterile inflammation, whether local or systemic, and infection or sepsis; otherwise you should not be a surgeon (nor a malpractice lawyer ☺).**

So here are the (simplified) definitions:

- **SIRS: fever (>38°C), tachycardia (>90), tachypnea (>20), leukocytosis (>12,000)**. Such criteria are so non-specific and all inclusive that it has been said that even the engagement in vigorous sex can produce SIRS ☺! Be that as it may, the modern surgeon (you!) has to view surgical patients as being INFLAMED by inflammatory mediators, generated by an acute disease process, either inflammatory, infectious or traumatic. The greater the inflammation, the sicker the patient, and the higher the expected mortality and morbidity. Do realize that some therapeutic steps taken in an attempt to halt your patient's inflammation may in fact contribute to it — adding fuel to the inflammatory fire: e.g. excessive surgery, inappropriately performed, or too late, just contributes to SIRS.
- **Sepsis: the systemic inflammatory response to infection — i.e. SIRS + a documented source of infection**.
- **Severe sepsis: as above associated with organ dysfunction** or hypoperfusion (e.g. made manifest by lactic acidosis, oliguria, or hypotension — when hypotension coexists we call it **septic shock**).
- **Multiple organ dysfunction syndrome (MODS): altered organ function** in an acutely ill or injured patient (e.g. respiratory distress, renal dysfunction, etc.).

So what has all this to do with our postoperative patients? Why do we have to stress those definitions? Because it helps us to understand that *not* every patient manifesting symptoms and signs of infection is actually infected, and thus not all need be treated as such — with antibiotics for instance.

For example:

- The trauma of surgery can produce significant SIRS — see below about postoperative fever.
- Atelectasis produces SIRS but (usually) it is not pneumonia.
- Any massive trauma can result in severe SIRS and MODS, but unless there is a documented source of infection it is not SEPSIS.
- Severe postoperative pancreatitis can manifest as severe systemic *sepsis*, but usually it is a STERILE process — not sepsis!

Capisce? ☺

Do think about those definitions all the time. By all means, consider the possibility of infection in your postoperative patient and try to exclude it. But do not cry wolf!

Before we carry on let us remember that many of the general principles of avoiding complications discussed above (⊃ Chapter 2) are as important, if not more so, in the prevention of postoperative infection as what we are going to say here. Now let's dwell on the prevention and treatment of infective complications before, during and after the operation, using an abdominal procedure as a key example.

Pre-operative considerations

> *If you operate on infection you get infections.*
>
> *In peritonitis, operating on a poorly resuscitated patient is like throwing both ends of the rope to a drowning man.*

Already in ⊃ Chapter 2 we advised you to avoid elective operations unless sites of remote infections are well controlled, as you do not want to contaminate, or seed your operative field with bacteria residing elsewhere. And of course the better the general condition of the patient, including his nutritional status, the more robust will be his immune system and hence the resistance to infections. **Also remember: the importance of optimal control of diabetes mellitus before, during and after the operation: inadequate control of sugar contributes to infection and poor wound healing!** Finally, **cessation of smoking** as early as possible before the operation should diminish the risk of infections and improve healing. Good luck with implementing this advice in clinical practice!

There is no point in reprinting here a manual of *asepsis* as we are convinced that the OR nurses in your hospital, scrutinized by the 'infection control police', are doing whatever they can to keep the OR environment clean, and operative procedures 'aseptic', in order to minimize the incidence of infection so that the hospital looks good (at least on paper) when it is inspected by credentialing bodies — if something like this exists in your country.

Common sense dictates that malodorous patients should not stink (or stink less) on the morning of their operation. Repairing a hernia in a moist groin, obscured by an apron of fat, where the skin is rarely exposed to fresh breeze or sunshine — an ideal site for cultivating of mushrooms — is a recipe for a wound infection. See to it that such patients take a good bath prior to coming to the hospital, or arrange for a good clean up by the nurses on the morning of surgery. A pre-operative shower with *chlorhexidine gluconate* has been shown to reduce wound infections.

These days everybody knows that **shaving** of the operative field at home is counter-productive as it digs up bacteria from the hair follicles onto the surface of the skin — increasing the likelihood of wound infection. Instead, shaving, preferably using a disposable electrical clipper, has to take place in the operating room, just before preparing the skin. A thorough surgeon does the hair clipping himself — it can be irritating to have long tufts of hair in the operative field, but this often happens if you let others 'shave, prep and drape' for you.

We will skip the topic of **pre-operative bowel preparation** (which is still somewhat controversial) and leave it for our colorectal guru in the relevant chapter (⊃ Chapter 14). The remaining pre-operative measure to discuss here is the matter of **prophylactic antibiotics**.

Prophylactic antibiotics

The best prophylactic antibiotic agent is the skilled surgeon. But still, judicious usage of prophylactic antibiotics has drastically reduced the incidence of peri-operative infections. Please note that while antibiotic prophylaxis has been proven of great value in decreasing the rate of **wound infection** (SSI), its benefits are much less obvious concerning the prevention of postoperative **intra-abdominal infection**. (The incidence of the latter is relatively low — so the power of antibiotic studies is insufficient to detect any significant benefits of prophylactic antibiotics.)

Naturally, the **higher the risk of infection the greater the indication for prophylactic antibiotics**. Where and when such risk is negligible in absolutely 'clean' cases (e.g. breast lumpectomy, varicose vein surgery) the value of prophylactic antibiotics is less obvious. However, in 'contaminated' cases (e.g. colon surgery), the predicted risk of infection is higher and consequently antibiotics are indicated. By definition, 'dirty' cases (e.g. perforated appendicitis) are... dirty and this means **infection**; in such cases antibiotics are not only *prophylactic* — preventative — but also **THERAPEUTIC!** The literature tends to distinguish between 'clean-contaminated' and 'contaminated' cases but we find this arbitrary, inaccurate and unusable. In the following chapter on "The wound" (⊃ Chapter 5), we will explain further and expand on this classification and remind you that prophylaxis is valuable in all contaminated cases and **selected clean** ones.

Protocols of prophylactic peri-operative antibiotics exist in most institutions.

But here is a reminder:

- **Target** the agent against the predicted bacterial flora at the site of operation (e.g. *E. coli* in colorectal surgery, *Staphylococcus* in a hernia operation).
- Use the **cheapest agent with the narrowest spectrum** possible (e.g. a first-generation cephalosporin rather than a fancy-expensive X-generation one).
- Aim at achieving the **highest blood and tissue level** at the time of the incision — this is when the wound is most susceptible to infection. Thus, administer the drug on the OR table, do not let it hang up hours before surgery.
- **Higher doses** are required to achieve adequate tissue levels in obese patients and in those who are shocked or bleeding.
- **Maintain drug levels during the operation**. If prolonged, and the drug short-acting, you have to repeat the dose.
- **Do not extend prophylaxis**. Many studies have showed that a single dose is adequate in most instances. We won't argue if you wish to add one or two postoperative doses, but anything beyond this is futile and not indicated. **The fate of the wound is sealed during the operation, not after it**. Remember the risks of *prolonged prophylaxis* such as *C. difficile* colitis and the emergence of antibiotic-resistant bacteria.

Ronald L. Nichols has summarized this aptly: "Historically, the most common errors in usage include the widespread use of antibiotic prophylaxis in clean surgery and the faulty timing of administration. The most common error today is continuation of the agents beyond the time necessary for maximal benefit." And Owen H. Wangensteen, the great surgeon of Minnesota, said it many years ago: "Prophylactic antibiotics will turn a third class surgeon into a second class but will never turn a second class surgeon into the first class one." We concur.

Contamination versus infection

Before moving back into the OR we should highlight a crucial concept: **the difference between *contamination* and *infection*** — which is not recognized or is ignored by many docs — and which influences the postoperative course, treatment and outcome.

Contamination consists merely of the presence of micro-organisms within the tissue, before an inflammatory response has taken place. For example, soiling of the peritoneal cavity by a fluid rich in bacteria, as in the immediate aftermath of a penetrating intestinal injury; peritoneal contamination occurs commonly in the course of routine elective surgery of the gastrointestinal tract. The presence of bacteria-laden matter within the injured soft tissue represents contamination — only when cellulitis develops can it be called infection. Likewise, during appendectomy when a few drops of fecal material drop into the pelvis, this is contamination — not infection. Contamination is treated by mechanically cleaning the involved tissues and leaving the rest to **mother nature** — the natural defense mechanisms; perioperative administration of prophylactic antibiotics will suffice. There is no need for prolonged administration!

Infection is the continuum of contamination: both the presence of micro-organisms (and their toxins) as well as the **inflammatory response** of the involved tissues (e.g. peritonitis, pus formation). Obviously, avoiding contamination prevents infection.

Intra-operative considerations

We are sure you do not want us to teach you how (long) to scrub your hands and which solution to use to prepare the operative field. That the true role of the face mask is to protect you from the patient's blood and fluids rather than protect him from your mouth's bacteria is well established. So what else can you do to prevent infections *during* the operation?

It all depends on what type of operation you are doing. If it is a '**clean**' operation (e.g. ventral hernia repair), the key consideration is to **avoid contamination** at all costs. If the procedure is '**contaminated**' (e.g. colectomy) your key concern is to **minimize contamination**. But if you operate on an already infected — '**dirty**' — case the vital step in curing the infection, and preventing its continuation or recurrence, is SOURCE CONTROL (see below).

Of course, there are other intra-operative factors common to all procedures which should be considered with the aim of minimizing postoperative infection:

- **Tissue perfusion and oxygenation** should be optimized during the operation. Bacteria thrive in ischemic tissues where antibiotics fail to penetrate.

- **Duration of operation**. The longer the operation, the more exposed the tissues — the higher the risk of infection. You should be meticulous but not slow like a turtle.
- **Hypothermia**. Low core body temperature raises the incidence of infection. Maintain the patient's temperature by covering and heating exposed parts and warming i.v. fluids. Naturally, excessive duration of the operation contributes to hypothermia.
- **Blood loss and hemostasis**. We know that blood loss and the subsequent need for transfusion correlates with postoperative infection. Careful hemostasis and the evacuation of shed blood prevent hematomas which are an ideal culture for the growth of bacteria. Remember the Spanish proverb: *la mierda y la sangre no ligan!* (S**t doesn't mix [well] with blood).
- **Optimal handling of tissues**. Excepting the magnitude of contamination/infection (or the lack of it) the **surgeon is surely the most important factor in avoiding (or causing) infection**. Even within the same department some surgeons have significantly less infective complication than others. To be among the former group you have to know what you are doing and do it well — briefly, create less tissue trauma by careful dissection along anatomic planes — they are there to help surgeons. Be gentle! Achieve hemostasis (no need to turn everything to coal), use (sparingly) modern suture material (no silk!), avoid drains unless absolutely necessary (usually they are not!).
- **Environment**. Where exactly the operation takes place does matter. The rate of infection tends to be higher in teaching hospitals than in say, private non-teaching institutions. Just enter the OR in any large University Hospital and you will understand why: people walking in and out of the OR all the time, students and observers standing on high stools leaning over the table, residents doing the operations or consultants taking their time to teach. No wonder that a single experienced surgeon doing the same operation with the same nurse in a small, peaceful OR can achieve lower rates of infection.
- **Other rituals**. Many other rituals — mostly scientifically unproven — are being used by surgeons in the continuing struggle to avoid infection. For example: changing gloves during the procedure, adhesive drapes to cover the skin, wound protectors, and of course, irrigation-lavage… (see below).

As with many things in surgery and medicine it is often impossible to assess the importance and benefits of any of the above steps in *isolation*, but *bundled together* they prevent infection and represent what one would call "good practice".

Now let us focus on the **operative principles of eradicating infection: source control and toilet**.

Source control

Source control implies controlling the origin of contamination-infection. **Eliminating the source is the key step and this is true for any type of surgical infection**. To cure the infected diabetic foot you have to get rid of the infected bone (osteomyelitis); to remedy an infection affecting any synthetic graft (mesh, prosthesis) you have to remove the graft; to arrest the spread of necrotizing soft tissue infection you have to excise all the devitalized, necrotic tissue; to resolve any abscess you have to drain the pus — *ubi pus, ibi evacua!*

Source control is of course vital in the management of intra-abdominal infections, to interrupt the delivery of bacteria and adjuvants of infection (bile, blood, fecal matter, barium) into the peritoneal cavity. It may require a relatively simple procedure such as appendectomy for acute appendicitis. Sometimes, a major resection to remove the infective focus is indicated, such as colectomy for perforated diverticulitis. Generally, the choice of the procedure, and whether the ends of resected bowel are anastomosed or exteriorized (creation of a stoma), depends on the anatomical source of infection, the degree of peritoneal inflammation and SIRS, and the patient's pre-morbid reserves. Occasionally, the source cannot be eradicated as the expected price to pay for its removal is deemed too high. Less radical options may then be used, such as diversion (e.g. colostomy proximal to a rectal injury) or drainage (of a leaking duodenum).

Toilet

Once the source of infection is eradicated, cleaning the tissues has to be performed to minimize the bacterial load and remove the adjuvants of infection. The basic methodology to achieve these is unchanged over decades and is based on two main maneuvers: **"remove/debride all crap"** and **"dilution (irrigation) is the solution to pollution."** The prevailing dogma — oh, so difficult if not impossible to prove scientifically — is to wash-irrigate *everything* at the end of the operation, be it clean, contaminated or dirty. The volume of lavage depends on local circumstances and the individual surgeon's obsessiveness-compulsiveness, ranging from a few cc of saline to many liters — not stopping until the surgeon's underwear is wet. Some would add antibiotics to the lavage; others would add even antiseptic agents. **Pressure irrigation** of contaminated soft tissues has been advocated by orthopedic surgeons and others.

Toilet measures have been more extensively scrutinized in contaminated or dirty abdominal operations than other conditions. Liquid contaminants and infected exudates should be aspirated and particulate matter removed by swabbing or mopping the peritoneal surfaces with moist laparotomy pads. Although cosmetically appealing and extremely popular with surgeons, there is no scientific evidence that intra-operative peritoneal lavage reduces mortality or infectious complications in patients receiving adequate systemic antibiotics. Similarly, peritoneal irrigation with antibiotics is not advantageous, and the addition of antiseptics may produce local toxic effects. So irrigate copiously (to use a term popular among American surgeons) if you wish but know that it will not accomplish much. **Your own eyes are your best guides: what looks clean is probably clean enough.** Try to confine the irrigation to the contaminated area — to avoid spreading s**t all around — and do remember to suck out all the lavage fluid as there is good evidence that leaving irrigation fluids behind interferes with peritoneal defenses by *diluting the macrophages.* **Bacteria swim perhaps better than macrophages!** Be it as it may, even a 'symbolic irrigation' would make your nurses happy, reflecting (when documented in our operative notes) that you made efforts to prevent infection. [A while ago I was sued by a patient who had developed septic arthritis after the repair of a soft tissue laceration near the elbow. In court 'my' expert witnesses, citing the operative notes, emphasized how carefully I cleaned and irrigated the wound... the plaintiff was unsuccessful!]

What about drains?

Should you leave one or more at the end of the operation to prevent infection or hasten its resolution? Well, it depends... on the specific pathology and its location. The following chapters will mention drainage when relevant to the discussion but here are some basic tenets.

Drains are either prophylactic or therapeutic.

Prophylactic drains are employed:

- To prevent **infection** by evacuating residual serum, blood, debris from the site of surgery and from any *dead space* left behind (e.g. after draining a large soft tissue hematoma).
- **To control *potential* or *expected* leakage from a suture line with the aim of establishing a controlled external fistula** (e.g. drainage of a colonic anastomosis).
- **To alert about complications** (e.g. allowing early diagnosis of gastric leak following bariatric surgery).

Therapeutic drains are employed:

- **To achieve source control which cannot be achieved by other means** (e.g. draining a leaking duodenal suture line to create a controlled external fistula).
- **To drain an established abscess or infected fluid collection** (e.g. soft tissue abscess, pancreatic abscess, hepatic abscess).

One has to realize that the rationale and need for drainage are drastically different when the **peritoneal cavity** is concerned, as opposed to other locations. **Unlike soft tissues the peritoneal cavity possesses excellent local defense mechanisms which render drains (except in selective circumstances — see below) obsolete**. This is not true in soft tissues: here the chief role of drainage is to keep the abscess cavity, or dead space, empty allowing its collapse and healing from inside out. Essentially, drains prevent the closure of skin on top of the still contaminated/infected cavity, thus preventing persistence/recurrence of infection.

Indications for drainage in abdominal operations [1]

The following is a brief summary.

Prophylactic drainage:

- **High probability of a leakage of bile or pancreatic juice**. A drain placed for biliary or pancreatic leak may be lifesaving and curative, such as near the **pancreatojejunal anastomosis after a Whipple procedure**.
- **High-risk suture lines — for example: duodenal suture lines** (e.g leak-prone **duodenal stump** after Billroth II gastrectomy). The **retroperitoneal duodenum** is more susceptible to leakage and thus draining it would make sense, as after duodenotomy to control post-ERCP hemorrhage. **Esophageal suture lines** are relatively high risk for leakage, thus its drainage is advocated. **Urological suture lines** are also prone to leakage of urine and deserve to be drained (e.g. partial nephrectomy).

What about prophylactic abdominal drainage for expected intra-abdominal bleeding to alert the surgeon and prevent hematomas? It has been said: "If you have to use drains to take care of postoperative hemorrhage

---

[1]   *Schein's Common Sense Emergency Abdominal Surgery*, 3rd Ed. Springer Verlag, © 2010: Chapter 42.

then you did not finish the operation", and… "Drainage is a confession of imperfect surgery." [Howard Kelly].

In most cases in which you leave drains for bleeding or oozing, they are unnecessary and produce little; they also produce little even when severe bleeding develops — showing only the 'tip of the iceberg' or becoming completely clogged. Having said that, leaving a suction drain for a day or two, to prevent accumulation of blood or serum in a confined space, such as the gallbladder bed (after a 'difficult cholecystectomy') or the pelvis after anterior resection of the rectum, could prevent infective complications in selected cases — but even this notion is controversial.

Remember the old dictum:

Drainage of the general peritoneal cavity is a physical and physiological impossibility.

Yates JL, ~1905

Therapeutic drainage (in abdominal operations):

- **As a source control measure: this is the chief indication!** As we stressed above drains should be used to establish a controlled fistula when the source of contamination/infection cannot be eradicated due to anatomical or technical constraints.
- **Drainage of an *established abscess*.** Many surgeons still believe that a well-formed collection of pus deserves a drain, especially when the abscess is *non-collapsible* or has *thick walls*. **However, we believe that within the peritoneal cavity (as opposed to abscesses within parenchymatous organs such as the liver) such abscesses are extremely rare.** In most cases after you drain the pus (e.g. a peri-appendicular abscess associated with perforated appendicitis), the adjacent tissues fill up the drained space, and the infection is cured by the source control (appendectomy) and peri-operative antibiotics. The drain accomplishes nothing!

Despite the dictum that it is impossible to effectively drain the free peritoneal cavity, drains are still commonly (mis)used. During our international (surgical) travels we are often exposed to abdomens (after operations for peritonitis) that look like porcupines: a drain sticking out of each quadrant. It seems that there are surgeons who still believe that *wide abdominal drainage* accomplishes something. But it accomplishes nothing! Drains left within the free peritoneal cavity are rapidly walled off by adhesions. Very soon they are contaminated by skin flora and their scanty output comes from the infected drain tract — if left longer than a day or two they function only to drain their own tract! For the long list of potential complications caused by drains see ■ Table 4.1.

Table 4.1. Potential complications of drains.
✓ Increase rate of wound infection (in wounds adjacent to drains)
✓ Drain tract infection
✓ Drain *fever*
✓ Drain tract hernia
✓ Drain tract bleeding
✓ Intestinal obstruction
✓ Erosion of bowel
✓ Erosion of vessels
✓ Failure to retrieve (caught by fascial sutures or torn or knotted)
✓ 'Lost' drain: migration into the abdomen or breakage
✓ Contamination of sterile tissues
✓ Prevention of healing of fistulas (drain abutting on the intestinal defect)

No drainage is better than the ignorant employment of it.
William Stewart Halsted

Closure of the abdomen and wound

A common dilemma at the end of a laparotomy for abdominal infections: "to close or not to close" the infected abdomen? For details about which complications are **prevented and created** by avoiding closure of the abdomen consult our previous book [2]. About leaving the wound open at the end of the operation see the next chapter (◔ Chapter 5).

Postoperative considerations

You want to:

● **Prevent** postoperative infection.
● **Treat** existing infection.
● Diagnose and treat **recurrent and persisting infections** and *new* infective complications.

---

[2] *Schein's Common Sense Emergency Abdominal Surgery,* 3rd Ed. Springer Verlag, © 2010: Chapter 52

Preventing postoperative infection

The principles of prevention outlined in ⊃ Chapter 2 apply here as well:

- Early mobilization and timely removal of nasogastric tubes reduces the risk of atelectasis and pneumonia; timely removal of i.v. lines and urinary catheters will lessen thrombophlebitis and urinary tract infection (UTI), respectively. **In brief: get rid of the plastic load ASAP!**
- Don't be mad with us if we repeat: optimal oxygenation, tissue perfusion, control of blood sugar levels and avoidance of (unnecessary) blood transfusion prevent infections!
- Adequate postoperative nutrition is important. **Use the enteral route whenever possible because it enhances immunity and is associated with a lower rate of infection (and is cheaper) when compared to the parenteral route.** Of course, the enteral route can and should be used also in patients who cannot be fed by mouth. In such situations consider feeding them directly into the small bowel through transanastomotic feeding tubes or feeding jejunostomies placed preferably intra-operatively — you have to think about it already during the operation! **Remember that patients with adequate baseline nutritional status tolerate 7-10 days of postoperative starvation and do not need anything beyond the salt, sugar and electrolytes in the i.v. *maintenance* fluids.** Consider adding parenteral nutrition (peripheral or central) if the enteral route is not available beyond the first postoperative week due to prolonged ileus, external GI fistulas, a need for reoperation or other complications.
- **Antibiotics.** *Prophylactic* antibiotics prevent infection when given *before* and *during* the operation — not *after*! A single pre-operative dose suffices! However, we won't argue with any worried surgeon who feels better with 'extended prophylaxis', adding a few doses, for a day, in selective *high-risk cases* — for example: a diabetic patient after an arterial bypass with a synthetic graft, or an immune-depressed patient undergoing repair of a hernia with mesh. Having said that, **prolonged** antibiotic prophylaxis after an elective 'clean' (e.g. mastectomy) or a 'contaminated' (e.g. colonic resection) operation should be strongly condemned. It does nothing except increase bacterial resistance, cost and the incidence of other complications (e.g. *C. diff* colitis, drug fever). Yes, we have said it before.

Treating existing infection

You already know that the *source control* you have just accomplished was the most important step in eradicating the infection. Now you should continue providing optimal supportive care, administer *therapeutic* antibiotics — aimed at eradicating *residual* bacteria at the operative site — and watch your patient like a hawk (see below).

A few words about **postoperative therapeutic antibiotics**: again, antibiotics are useless if the source of infection is not controlled, or if recurrent/persistent infection is not diagnosed and drained. **Antibiotics should be continued after the operation (beyond the *prophylactic* peri-operative administration) if the operative findings suggest the presence of *infection* rather than *contamination*.**

The **duration** of postoperative administration remains relatively controversial, but the old dogma of prolonged administration (e.g. for 7 or 10 days) is passé. The duration should be decided on an individual basis based on the findings at operation and the condition of the patient:

- If source control seems totally to eradicate the infection — we like to call it "**resectable infection**" (e.g. necrotizing cholecystitis, gangrene of bowel) — and no infection (pus!) has been observed outside the resected source — a day or two of postoperative administration would suffice.
- If, however, infection has been found outside the source (e.g. perforated viscus, local or diffuse peritonitis), a longer course of antibiotics is indicated.
- **For intra-abdominal infections, courses of more than five days are rarely indicated,** unless there is evidence of persisting infection, or concern that the source has not been properly dealt with.
- Traditional dogma maintains that antibiotics should be continued until fever subsides and white blood cell count normalizes. Such a policy often leads to excessive administration as SIRS can persist after infection has been eradicated. Thus, a little spike of fever or persistent leukocytosis should not deter you from stopping the antibiotics. Stop and watch! (see below).
- When the patient can eat, the **i.v. antibiotics can be switched to oral**, continued at home if indicated.

What is the role of microbiological cultures?

The truth is that most cultures surgeons take represent a huge waste of resources because the results rarely influence the actual management of our patients and outcomes. This is because the microbiology of surgical infections is mostly **predictable**. So is the bacteriology of secondary peritonitis which responds readily to an empiric broad-spectrum antibiotic regimen, initiated pre-operatively, that includes agents effective against Gram-negative bacteria (e.g. *E. coli*) and anaerobes (*Bacteroides fragilis*). And anyway, in most cases culture results become available only well after the completion of the antibiotic course. Did you ever see a case of diffuse peritonitis due to a perforated viscus where results of intra-operative cultures influenced the choice of postoperative antibiotics? We haven't.

However, peritoneal cultures are useful in the following scenarios:

- **Primary peritonitis** where there is no intra-abdominal source of infection; the fluid contains an organism that has migrated from somewhere else.
- **Secondary peritonitis** developing in hospitalized patients — a typical example would be postoperative peritonitis, which often involves *opportunistic* infections.
- Peritonitis in **immunocompromised** patients (e.g. AIDS) and those already on antibiotics.

In **soft tissue infections** the rationale for obtaining cultures is stronger; the main impetus is to identify resistant bacteria such as MRSA (methicillin-resistant *Staphylococcus aureus*) which might require specific antibiotic therapy.

Diagnose and treat recurrent and persisting infections and *new* infective complications

> *As long as the abdomen is open you control it. Once closed it controls you.*

This, we believe, is one of the most important maxims in abdominal surgery. Nay, it applies to surgery in general. For once you have closed the wound whatever has been left inside becomes a 'black box', and this is as true in the era of CT and MRI (at least during the first few postoperative days) as it was before. Hence, you have to be ever vigilant, maintain a high index of suspicion — oh, how we hate that cliché — in order to detect any infectious complication simmering deep within the operative field. **An innocent, perfect looking, operative wound means nothing, for well below it the abscess, the leak, the phlegmon may lurk like a time bomb**.

So how do we know that infection persists or redevelops?

- Suspect problems when that **patient does not recover from the operation as expected**: the laparoscopic cholecystectomy patient has to be at home, up and about, eating and passing wind, almost pain free, the latest by the second postoperative day (POD). The colectomy patient should be smiling and happy around POD five, if not before. If recovery is sluggish, you have to start worrying! In brief: "If the patient having undergone major abdominal surgery does not start looking better on postoperative day four than before the operation, something is wrong." [Ari]

- **The continuation of SIRS** beyond POD one or two should make you a little anxious! Persisting tachycardia suggests that things are not *kosher*! Obviously, there are non-surgical reasons for the patient's heart to race (e.g. hypovolemia, hypoxia, anemia, high fever...), but think also about a looming surgical calamity such as undrained pus or ischemia/necrosis of something.

- Traditionally, **postoperative fever** has been a key element used by surgeons to identify postoperative complications. The common causes of postoperative fever are outlined in ■ Table 4.2. But the pattern of fever matters as well. Unfortunately, gone are the glorious days — most of you are probably too young to have experienced them — of temperature charts hanging on the wall behind each bed. You could immediately appreciate the TREND: be reassured that everything is well (an almost flat line of normal temperature) or becoming fretful

Table 4.2. Causes of fever (SIRS) after the operation.

Postop day	Cause
1-3 (early)	Physiologic: SIRS due to the operative trauma Atelectasis
4-6 (intermediate)	Pneumonia, UTI, thrombophlebitis (i.v. site) *Early* wound infection due to *Strep. pyogenes* — spreading (rare!) 'Brewing' or 'simmering' **surgical complication** (see below) Deep vein thrombosis #
7-10 (late)	**Wound infection** (suppurative and contained) **Deep-seated infections** (e.g. infected collections, abscesses, anastomotic leaks)

This item is mentioned in numerous sources. However, I never saw postop DVT presenting with fever...

noting the steep valleys/peaks of the *septic* pattern. **Early low-grade** pyrexia is usually *physiologic*, representing residual SIRS due to the operative trauma or the local inflammatory sequelae (absorption of blood; the drainage of pus by itself may result in pyrexia!). **Intermediate low-grade pyrexia** often hints that an infection is simmering and boiling *somewhere* — you do not know exactly what and where, but in a day or two you will see the wound infection or diagnose the anastomotic leak. Or — God is Great — it will subside and everything will be OK. **Late spiking of temperature** usually hints at the presence of undrained pus!

- **Leukocytosis.** An elevated white blood cell (WBC) count is part of the inflammatory response. Do not consider it in isolation but together with the whole clinical picture. Again, it may hint at an infection but in many cases it will subside spontaneously. Do not chase it frantically or treat it with antibiotics, if the patient is doing well otherwise. Often we would discharge a patient with a significantly elevated WBC count — on follow-up a week later it proves to be normal. However, you should worry about a very low WBC count that could be a sign of developing sepsis.

- **The complete picture is more important than fever and a WBC count!** When the patient "feels well", his ileus subsiding, appetite returning, wounds healing and clinical exam negative, a few spikes in temperature and an elevated WBC count are not too worrying. When the ladies put the lipstick on and the men start to shave (or think about sex) you can relax!

The diagnosis and treatment of **specific postoperative infections** will be discussed in the following chapters. For now we will stress only this: the key is to be concerned — **expect the worst case scenario and be relieved when your nightmares do not materialize.** Observe, and reassess your patients as often as you can, make a little detour to the hospital on Sunday morning, on your way to the fishing grounds or golf course; some would prefer the church. Rather than flooding them with antibiotics use your clinical judgment to target additional imaging studies — reassuring if negative; if positive they lead to appropriate management (■ Figure 4.1).

So, yes, you should consider and rule out pneumonia, UTI and other *non-surgical* causes of stubbornly persisting postoperative SIRS. However, you have to remind yourself again and again that the **Problem Usually Lies at the Operative Site!**

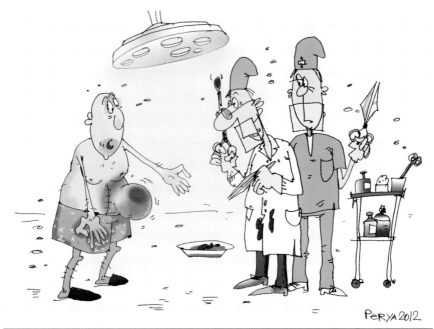

Figure 4.1. Assistant: "It is an abscess Sir!" Surgeon: "I do not understand it — we gave him an appropriate dose of antibiotics…"

The cause of fever or *septic state* in the surgical patient is usually at the primary site of operation unless proven otherwise. Most surgeons are aware of this fact but not a few prefer to *deny* it. We hear about such cases at the M&M meetings and in legal depositions — cases not only from some third rate hospitals but also from 'ivory towers'. The story is typical and repeats itself *ad nauseum*: a postoperative patient developing SIRS and progressive organ failure… leading to death while the surgeon lives in denial and fails to address the real problem. Some call it the **ostrich syndrome**.

Mark M. Ravitch said: "The last man to see the necessity for reoperation is the man who performed the operation." This is often true. Unfortunately, in many cases there is no one around willing to take over the case or at least influence the responsible surgeon to see the light and do the right thing.

But now, we hope that you, dear reader, will be more assertive when dealing with postoperative disasters (not only your own) — now you know to **"look for pneumonia in the wound!"** And if it's not there, suspect a suture line leak…

Postoperative intra-abdominal infections are one of the main reasons why general surgeons do not sleep well at night. However, as we do not like to copy/paste what we wrote recently elsewhere, and because we would like to keep this book short, we would like to refer you instead to Chapters 12 and 52 of our other book[3].

> Meanwhile close your eyes, raise your hands and repeat: **"I should always look for the source of the problem at the site of my operation, I am not an ostrich! I should always look..."**

---

[3] *Schein's Common Sense Emergency Abdominal Surgery*, 3rd Ed. Springer Verlag, © 2010.

Chapter 5

The wound, the wound...

Moshe Schein, Paul N. Rogers, Ari Leppäniemi and Danny Rosin

Surgeons who have extremely low rates of SSI suffer from 'selective forgetfulness'.

Hiram C. Polk

The surgical wound is the only remnant of your operation the patient can actually see. His family or girlfriend cannot look at the healing anastomosis but they are likely to be impressed by a good looking wound (■ Figure 5.1). We remember a patient dying of a stroke that developed a week after undergoing a colectomy; his wife looked at his exposed abdominal wound and said: "Doc, you did such a good job!" (Meaning: "the operation succeeded but the patient is dying..."). To look good the wound has to undergo almost perfect healing. But you and we know that most postoperative wounds are not perfect. Everybody talks about wound infections but the postoperative wound is prone to a wide array of complications, all of which are aberrations of the normal healing process.

The current focus on **wound infection rate** as a measure of quality of care has generated a huge body of 'authoritative' reviews and guidelines, in print and online, dedicated to the topic of **SSI**: this is the term they want us to use: "**surgical site infection**". You now have a choice: either go and read one of those lengthy documents — here is a well-written online document: "Guideline for Prevention of Surgical Site Infection", 1999 [1] — or stay with us for a simplified version.

---

[1] http://www.cdc.gov/hicpac/pdf/guidelines/SSI_1999.pdf.

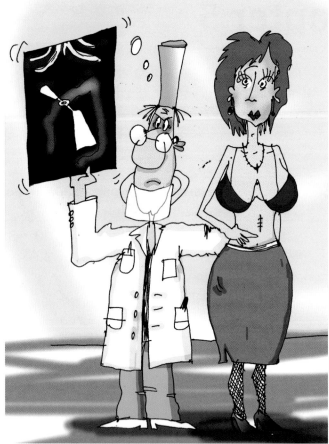

Figure 5.1. Patient to surgeon: "The scar looks lovely. I'm very happy with you... going to recommend you to everyone!"

Before proceeding to practical matters let us remind ourselves of a few definitions coined by the 'infection control' policy makers:

- **Superficial incisional SSI**: this is the typical wound infection we see. It involves the skin and subcutaneous tissue — often essentially a **wound abscess**.
- **Deep incisional SSI**: infection involving deep soft tissue (e.g. fascia and muscle layers of the incision). This of course is a rare scenario. This entity includes what clinical surgeons like us would rather call "necrotizing soft tissue infection" and treat it accordingly with debridement, wide drainage and antibiotics.

- **Organ/space SSI.** Only God knows why we need such a term (?). Shouldn't we call the baby its name: peritonitis, empyema — for "space SSI"; liver abscess, anastomotic phlegmon — for "organ SSI"?

In the previous chapter we promised to expand on the classification of operative wounds and the risk of infection: here it is in ■ Table 5.1. Now you'll fathom that distinguishing between 'clean-contaminated' and 'contaminated' cases is rather arbitrary if not subjective and has little practical rationale. Also do realize that the figures (%) for the risk of infections and the actual rates of infections, cited by various researchers are of little relevance to your individual patients. **In practice** what matters is that clean operations should be associated with a *minimal* risk of infection and dirty ones with a *high* rate. In between lie the contaminated cases — the more contaminated, the higher the risk of infection.

Table 5.1. Classification of operative wounds and risk of infection.

Classification of procedures	Criteria	Examples	Risk of infection
Clean	Usually elective, potential sources of contamination are <u>not</u> present (respiratory, biliary, gastrointestinal and urogenital tracts not violated)	Repair of hernia Mastectomy Vascular procedures	<2%
Clean-contaminated	(Elective) operations with opening of the respiratory, biliary, gastrointestinal and urogenital tracts with minimal spillage	Cholecystectomy Colectomy Cesarean section	<10%
Contaminated	Gross spillage from the gastrointestinal tract, presence of infected bile or urine, *early* penetrating trauma	Resection of bowel for intestinal obstruction, cholecystectomy for empyema, appendectomy	~20%
Dirty	All operations for established infection, *late* penetrating trauma	Perforated appendicitis... bacterial peritonitis of any cause	~40%

Here we allow ourselves a (rare) cynical comment: we do not trust too much the published figures of wound infection. To be credible, audits of surgical wounds have to be conducted by trained *independent* observers using strict and accurate criteria — not by the surgeons or their disciples. All wounds have to be directly and periodically assessed — chart reviews and questionnaires are extremely inaccurate. In addition: citing the overall rate of wound infections, without stratifying them according to the type of patients (their risk factors for infection) and the specific operations they underwent, means nothing. Even within a subspecialty the incidence of SSI varies according to the specific procedure. For example, in colorectal surgery, rectal operations are more prone to infections than say, elective sigmoidectomies for diverticular disease. Wounds on the head or neck, where the blood supply is excellent, are less prone to infection than wounds on the abdomen or lower limbs. Also, the method of operation has to be considered: laparoscopic operations (fewer infections) vs. open ones. **In brief: the crude overall rate of SSI cannot serve as an accurate measure of quality of care**. Finally, these days, when the vast majority of patients are discharged within a few days, wound complications appear at home and not in the hospital, and are diagnosed and treated (and left unreported) by surgeons at follow-up in their offices. Do you know many surgeons who would report each and every infection or advertise them in public?

Pre-operative considerations

About what you can do before the operation to prevent SSI we have told you in the previous chapters (e.g. control diabetes, stop smoking and so forth). However, at the risk of repeating ourselves, we will list here (■ Table 5.2) the known risk factors for SSI, which, in addition to the classification of the wound (■ Table 5.1) should influence your decision on whether to administer prophylactic antibiotics in the individual patient.

Prophylactic antibiotics

The principles were discussed in ⤵ Chapter 4 and now here is our practical advice. As we already have said: prophylactic antibiotics are not necessary where the risk of infection is negligible — you cannot improve on perfect results. So when are they indicated? Obviously, in any case which is not considered 'clean' (■ Table 5.1).

Table 5.2. Factors known to add to the risk of SSI.

Local factors	Systemic factors
Insertion of **foreign bodies** (mesh, graft, prosthesis)	Obesity
Irradiated operative field	**Immunosuppression** (corticosteroid use, HIV, chemotherapy for cancer, massive transfusions)
Adjacent potential **source of contamination** (colostomy)	**Poor nutritional status**
Poor hygiene of operative site (deep moist skin fold where you could cultivate champignons ☺)	ASA class >2 (American Society of Anesthesiologists classification system; ⮌ Chapter 2)
Use of **drains**	**Diabetes mellitus**
	Recent surgery
	Extreme age

But what about the clean cases?

- Prophylaxis is beneficial in mastectomy and repair of incisional hernia.
- It is advisable in cases where the punishment of infective complications is extreme — vascular and neurosurgical procedures.
- It is advisable when infection-prone synthetic materials (mesh, prosthesis) are inserted.
- It is advisable when other specific (systemic or local; ■ Table 5.2) risk factors are present.

Which agent?

We talked about this already in ⮌ Chapter 4. You have to target the presumed contaminants in the operative field. In a clean operation this usually implies a resident of the skin, the *Staphylococcus* species — which is also a common cause of SSI after contaminated operations, rather than the bacteria which colonize the operated viscus.

For **clean operations a single dose of a first-generation cephalosporin** is the preferred prophylaxis. This is also true for other procedures but we won't put you before the firing squad… if you decide to add a dose or two after the operation (as long as you remember to discontinue it the next day — latest). Consult your hospital policy!

Now you realize that in practice most surgical procedures deserve antibiotic prophylaxis or that prophylaxis is at least 'optional' in most — don't we use mesh for the majority of hernias? Aren't our patients increasingly obese and diabetic? — except some 'perfectly clean' operations (e.g. varicose veins or removal of soft tissue tumors) in low-risk patients. However, **there are always exceptions and controversies**. For example, some studies have shown that prophylaxis is not necessary in laparoscopic cholecystectomy (although it is considered a 'clean-contaminated' operation), as the postoperative incidence of SSI is negligible. What to do? As you wish — it is optional.

There is no harm in a single-dose prophylaxis: apply your judgment — if you believe that the patient is at risk of SSI, use prophylaxis!

Remember to give it just before the incision is made!

Intra-operative considerations

The likelihood of wound infections has been determined by the time the last stitch is inserted in the wound.

Mark Ravitch

There is much you can do during the operation to prevent wound complications:

- Avoid contamination of the wound. Steps towards such a goal may include — especially during contaminated/dirty procedures — protecting the skin and using a fresh 'closing tray of instruments' for closure of fascia and skin. Changing contaminated gloves, after completing the anastomosis, is advisable!
- Operate efficiently and carefully — don't 'abuse' the tissues.
- Dissection is the key to any operation, and knowledge of anatomy is the key to atraumatic dissection — the (mostly) avascular tissue planes are there to help the surgeon!
- Do not chargrill the skin and underlying tissues with excessive use of diathermy.
- Avoid/obliterate dead spaces if possible. Use subcutaneous stitches in obese patients.

- Drains increase the risk of SSI; use them only when absolutely necessary.
- The way you close the skin matters. Closure with monofilament sutures — subcuticular if possible and avoiding noxious silk — leads to better results than using skin staples. Spend the extra few minutes on meticulous skin closure. Do it yourself, it will pay off.
- Do not place contaminating colostomies in the main abdominal wound (is anyone still stupid enough to do this?). It's good to have at least 5-10cm between the wound and the colostomy.
- The longer the incision you place, the higher the risk for wound complications. This is a no-brainer. A long midline incision for perforated appendicitis is at much higher risk for complications than a transverse RLQ incision.
- Instillation of an antibiotic agent (in the form of powder or solution) into the incision before its closure is another *optional* preventive measure. It ensures a high level of the drug exactly at the site where it is needed. Some surgeons use it in clean procedures (e.g. hernioplasty) in lieu of systemic administration. Any effort to reduce the concentration of micro-organism in the wound makes sense!

Non-closure or delayed closure of the wound?

As you surely know, wounds which are closed heal by *primary intention*; those left open to heal/scar down spontaneously heal by *secondary intention*. Wounds left open and later, within a few days, closed surgically heal by *tertiary intention* (also termed "delayed primary closure"). **Per definition, open wounds do not get infected**. You can rub feces on them and fail to produce infection! Therefore, for generations surgeons have been avoiding closure of high-risk wounds (mostly after 'dirty' procedures) to prevent infection. Is such a practice advisable and beneficial?

Well, it is, but mostly to you, the surgeon, much less so to the patient. Of course, if you leave all wounds open your SSI rate will be zero. But this will expose the patient to the morbidity of open wounds plus the need for local care and the inferior cosmetic results — that is if you decide not to do a delayed closure, which of course is an additional procedure under local anesthesia... with its own wound complications.

Rather than subjecting patients to the morbidity of open wounds we close all wounds in contaminated cases. In **grossly dirty cases** the first author uses wound WICKS: I suture the skin with interrupted nylon sutures and insert wicks cut out of *Telfa®* between the sutures all the way down to the level of the fascia. A bulky gauze dressing is applied over the wound. The wicks, which are removed after 72 hours, serve to drain the subcutaneous layer. Using this method the first author forgot when he last saw an SSI after open appendectomy for perforated appendicitis. He highly recommends this method!

Furthermore, even if SSI develops after an isolated dirty case, it is not the end of the world — see below.

Postoperative considerations

Uncomplicated wounds are sutured wounds that heal uneventfully by primary intention. All others are **complicated wounds** — those are common if and when obsessively assessed by independent observers. However, when 'reported' by surgeons they become "rare" or "minor" due to our natural tendency to suppress or ignore adverse outcomes. As with anything in surgery there are minor or major problems:

- **Minor wound complications** are those irritating aberrations in healing that do not impede the primary healing of the wound: a hematoma, a seroma, a little erythema, some serous discharge, minimal necrosis of the skin edges. The distinction between an infectious and non-infectious process is difficult and also unnecessary as the vast majority resolve spontaneously or with minimal local care. (**Suture abscesses** belong to this group: these are small *pustulas* developing at the site of suture insertion; there may be some surrounding erythema. They resolve readily when the sutures are removed. Antibiotics are unnecessary.)
- **Major wound complications** are those that interfere with the process of primary healing and require an intervention: a large hematoma needing evacuation or a wound abscess (yes, we mean superficial SSI) in need of drainage.

Can wound infections be prevented *after* the operation?

> *A closed surgical wound is immune within a few hours even to the smearing of feces. But let that wound discharge blood or serum or lymph or bile or pancreatic juice and it can... trap those airborne and hand-borne bacteria.*
>
> **Allan Pollock**

So, while intact wounds become impervious to the environment within a few hours — you can leave them exposed (or covered if you wish) and shower them with impunity — some postoperative wounds remain susceptible to *secondary infection* within the hospital. The latter can be prevented by adhering to basic infection control methods. Most important: washing your hands and early discharge from the bacterial-laden hospital (**Ari's rule: "a hospital is a bad place for a healthy patient!"**).

The management of wound complications

The punishment should fit the crime. Minor complications should be observed — the majority will resolve spontaneously. Starting antibiotics because a wound is a little erythematous or 'weeps' a tiny bit of serous discharge is not going to change anything: if the wound is destined to develop an infection it will, with or without antibiotics.

So unless you diagnose **early streptococcal infection** of the wound — mentioned in all books but extremely rare (always suspect when the patient develops significant pyrexia and/or excessive wound pain during the first few postoperative days) or early development of **necrotizing soft tissue infection** arising in the wound (i.e. deep incisional SSI), which is also very rare, there is nothing you have to or should do with the wound until postoperative day 5-7: this is when wound infections present and are ready to be drained (see below).

Having said that we should emphasize that early infection with *Streptococcus pyogenes* often leads to rapidly developing necrotizing fasciitis, multi-organ failure and death — if not promptly diagnosed and treated. Early diagnosis, however, may be difficult because the necrotic process is hidden under the skin — all that you notice is a reddish wound with some serous discharge. So this is what we recommend:

- Always suspect early infection with *Streptococcus pyogenes* when postoperative SIRS and incisional pain seem inappropriately exaggerated.
- Expose the wound — look under the dressings even if this is only postoperative day 2-3!
- Against the background of such a scenario, if the wound appears angry, open it. Take a sample of fluid for a Gram stain: if your diagnosis is correct it will show the typical chains of *Strep. pyogenes*.
- If so: radically open the wound. Excise any necrotic subcutaneous tissue. Administer appropriate antibiotics. Re-explore and re-debride as many times as necessary. **Procrastination is lethal!**

Wound seromas and **hematomas** should be drained unless minor and asymptomatic. Left untreated they may become infected. **Expectant management of large wound hematomas is inadvisable.** While clots (old blood) tend to be lysed and reabsorbed rapidly from serous cavities (e.g. peritoneum), the reabsorption process within soft tissues is slow. The technique of evacuation of hematomas depends on size (imaging with US is helpful) and location, and whether they are liquefied — thus amenable to needle aspiration (needle aspiration through the healing incision is virtually painless) — or contain clots. The latter can be removed (under local anesthesia) through small incisions or by reopening the wound. A short-term drain is left in the drained cavity if necessary.

[This is perhaps an opportunity to add a sentence about **post-traumatic hematomas of the extremities,** so common after falls and blunt trauma. Physicians often recommend an expectant approach believing that the hematomas will reabsorb. But often they do not: instead, the hematoma gradually renders the overlying skin ischemic. **To avoid infected skin ulcers and delayed healing we recommend early evacuation of any post-traumatic hematoma of significant size (i.e. >3-4cm).**]

How to manage wound infections

Superficial incisional SSI

This is the variant we most frequently see. It represents a 'walled-off' wound abscess, with minimal involvement of adjacent soft tissues. Commonly, the wound abscess starts simmering 2-3 days after the operation, with low-level spikes of fever and erythema of the wound. Do not rush to poke in or open the wound — disturbing a wound which may not progress to pus formation. Be patient, wait a day or two, let the infection mature and declare itself. Starting on postoperative day 5-7, when the wound is 'hot' and tender, this is the time to drain it.

A prevalent misconception is that the whole length of the wound should be laid open. This is usually unnecessary: removing a few skin sutures or staples from the segment of the wound which appears most involved and draining the pus usually suffices. Of course, if infection persists the rest of the wound can be opened a day or two later.

The **aftercare** should be as simple as possible with the aim of letting the drained wound heal from within out — like any abscess cavity. Open, shallow wounds are covered with dry gauze and cleaned once or twice daily with water and soap. Deeper wounds we would pack very gently with gauze to afford drainage and prevent premature closure of the superficial layers (a common error by novices is to pack the wounds too tight thus delaying closure) and change the packing every day; repacking is rarely needed beyond a week or so. **There is nothing better for an open wound than a shower or bath** (and a little fresh air in between, as long as the wound does not dry).

Local care and problem wounds

This is what is needed for most wound infections. However, some infected wounds are 'problematic' — extensive, deep and stubborn. Nurses and the so called 'wound experts' from 'wound clinics' promote elaborate and expensive wound care methods in order to justify their continued involvement (and billing...). Local application of solutions or ointments of antiseptics or antibiotics destroy micro-organisms and human cells alike, induce allergy and encourage bacterial resistance. The industry is aggressively promoting various devices for vacuum wound therapy, claiming that the application of negative pressure has beneficial effects on the healing of wounds. Obviously, vacuum devices facilitate treatment of deep wounds buried within layers of fat, or 'productive' wounds (e.g. intestinal fistula in the middle of an abdominal wall defect), but applying an expensive vacuum device on minor wounds is ridiculous.

Honey — simple and cheap honey from the supermarket, not the expensive 'medical honey' — is the *only wound care agent* used, for many years by the first author for all 'problem' wounds (postoperative and otherwise). For more details look at the brochure given to patients treated with honey in ■ Table 5.3.

Antibiotics for superficial incisional SSI?

What is true for any simple subcutaneous abscess treated with incision and drainage holds good also for superficial incisional SSI: **antibiotics are not necessary**. A short course of antimicrobials is indicated only when surrounding cellulitis is present and, obviously, in cases of deep incisional SSI. However, in some countries (the USA for example), surgeons are more likely to prescribe antibiotics even for simple SSI. The reasons for this are poorly defined but must include 'defensive medicine' and patients' expectations ("Doctor, don't I need antibiotics?").

Wound swabs? Wound cultures? Gram stains?

If the humble wound abscess does not need antibiotics why should we culture it? Don't we know which bacteria are usually responsible? And how sure are we that the isolated micro-organism is actually the one responsible for the infection and not one of the insignificant contaminants residing on your neck tie or on any surface in the hospital? **The truth is that most wound cultures obtained are useless and do not contribute anything to management**. But again, wounds are being swabbed and cultured because

Table 5.3. Use of topical honey on wounds.

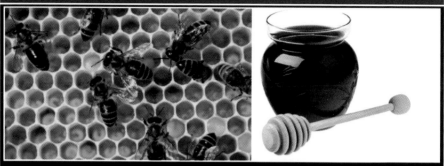

For thousands of years HONEY has been known and used for its healing properties when applied on infected and 'problem' wounds. The advantages of HONEY over many of the 'modern' commercial products are:

- HONEY kills the bacteria which contaminate open wounds and cause infection.
- HONEY, being hyperosmolar, 'sucks' out pus and fluids from the wound, thus cleaning it and reducing swelling.
- HONEY does not damage the patient's own tissues and thus does not interfere with the healing which takes place. It promotes healing. It is absolutely safe!
- HONEY is much cheaper and more affordable than alternative commercial products.

Practical considerations for the clinical use of honey

- The amount of honey required on the wound relates to the amount of fluid exuding from the wound diluting it. The frequency of dressing changes required will depend on how rapidly the honey is being diluted by exudate. In most patients a once-a-day change of dressing suffices.
- The honey should be applied to an absorbent dressing prior to application. If applied directly to the wound, the honey tends to run off before a secondary dressing is applied to hold it in place. Cover the honey with a few 4 x 4 gauze; use tape or bandage to keep the dressing in place.
- Each day remove the dressing, wash the wound directly under the shower until clean (the old honey is washed away) and apply a new dressing. Do not rub the wound directly so as not to damage the healing process.
- The HONEY should not be applied to the normal (not involved) skin beyond the edges of the wound.
- Any depressions or cavities in the wound bed need to be filled with HONEY to ensure the antibacterial components of the honey diffuse into the wound tissues.
- Some patients will complain of local stinging or 'burning' immediately after application of the honey. This should subside within 10-15 minutes. A Tylenol may help.

of prevailing dogma and a defensive attitude ("Doc, why didn't you obtain a culture from that wound?", the malpractice lawyer will ask...) and let us not forget that the microbiological laboratory needs to support itself...

We have to stress however that MRSA (methicillin-resistant *Staphylococcus aureus*) is currently endemic in the United States (and elsewhere) and is increasingly responsible for postoperative wound infections. The prevailing dogma maintains that hospital SSI caused by MRSA should be treated with bug-specific antibiotics. Therefore, if you practice in a MRSA-endemic area (i.e. where in general antimicrobial drugs are misused and over used...), you had better culture the infected wound. But again: there is no need to treat MRSA cultured in an open but *non-infected* wound.

Other forms of SSI

As we mentioned above, the **deep incisional SSI** involving the fascia is much more than a 'wound infection'. **It occurs rarely in isolation but mostly reflects the tip of the (infected) iceberg** — with deeper sources of infection (in the abdomen, for example) infecting the fascia, which is often dehisced. Management is based on imaging, source control, aggressive debridement, extensive drainage and broad-spectrum antibiotics, according to the principles outlined in ⊃ Chapter 4.

Organ/space SSI has nothing to do with the wound...

In the 15th century Ambroise Paré said: **"I dressed him and God healed him." This is as true today as then. So let God do the job and do not interfere too much!**

Chapter 6

Leaking gastrointestinal anastomoses

John Hunter, Wen-hao Tang, Moshe Schein, Mark Cheetham, Caitlin W. Hicks, Jonathan E. Efron

---

This chapter has been subdivided into the following five sections:

1. Basic considerations.
2. The esophagus.
3. Stomach and duodenum.
4. Small intestine.
5. Large bowel and rectum.

---

1 Basic considerations [1]
Moshe Schein

Somebody's leak is a curiosity — one's own leak is a calamity.

The gastrointestinal anastomosis is to the surgeon what the parachute is to the parachutist. Both can fail with disastrous consequences — but there are a few differences:

- It is extremely rare for a parachute not to open — it is not so uncommon for the anastomosis to fail.
- Packing and maintenance of parachutes is a uniform act while there are many variants of anastomoses.

---

[1] Anastomotic obstructions will be briefly discussed at the end of this section.

- Opening a parachute is a simple, standardized undertaking — fashioning an anastomosis is a little more complex.
- Surgeons often lose sleep worrying about the fate of the anastomosis they have just constructed (I do! See ■ Figure 6.1). But when the parachute fails no one is left to worry. Fortunately, for us surgeons, when an anastomosis fails it's not our life that's in mortal danger.
- When the parachutist dies there is no one to remember but his family, but the surgeon will remember the anastomotic leak and its consequences — unless he is a psychopath. And if he doesn't manage the leak satisfactorily he may be reminded about it in court!

With the exception of exsanguinating postoperative hemorrhage there is nothing that the surgeon fears more than a leaking anastomosis. When a patient succumbs to a postoperative myocardial infarction it can be described as an "act of God"; but when he bleeds to death because of faulty hemostasis

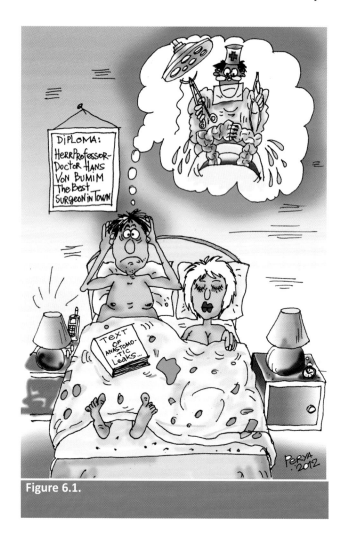

Figure 6.1.

(⟳ Chapter 3), or develops an anastomotic leak with its horrendous consequences, then all fingers point at the responsible surgeon. For these reasons, the topic of anastomotic leaks is rather emotional to most surgeons.

Not only do anastomotic leaks more than triple the mortality and early morbidity rates of surgery but they also impact heavily on **late results**:

- By causing stricture formation at the anastomotic site.
- By significantly decreasing (oncological) survival rates after cancer operations.
- By condemning patients to live with (often permanent) stomas.
- And finally by hugely increasing the cost of care.

Anastomotic leaks present a tremendous challenge to the surgeon due to their wide clinical spectrum and **unpredictability**. I remember a patient who leaked from a duodenal suture line and expired within 24 hours; I recall patients with few local manifestations but an abdomen full of bowel content, who were 'well' but gradually developed irreversible multi-organ failure — when the reoperation came too late.

In this chapter a group of contributors will discuss anastomotic leaks and their management along the **entire GI tract** — from the esophagus (where the incidence of leak is the highest), through the small bowel where it is the lowest, down to the low rectum where the probability of leakage is again high. **I will start by discussing a few unifying concepts relevant to any suture line joining two hollow conduits (i.e. an anastomosis) created within the human body**.

Pre-operative considerations

The integrity of any anastomosis created at any site along the gut depends on four main factors: the patient, the bowel, the surrounding *milieu* and the surgeon. All factors are important but there is no doubt that the last one — YOU, the surgeon — towers above all the rest! Of course your technical ability to perform a secure anastomosis is crucial to the outcome; but, as we will see, even more important is your ability to judge **when an anastomosis should be avoided!** ■ Table 6.1 expands on those four main factors and will be used as a framework for the following discussion.

Patient-related issues must be addressed before the operation. **Think like this**: anything which depresses the repair mechanisms of the patient's tissues will put his anastomosis at risk — what is true for the wound and fascia, discussed in previous chapters, is true for the intestinal anastomosis.

Table 6.1. Common factors influencing anastomotic healing (or leaking).

Patient	Bowel	Milieu	Surgeon
Nutrition (albumin level)	**Edematous?** (e.g. after massive fluid resuscitation; decreased venous outflow)	Infection of the space where anastomosis lies (e.g. peritonitis, empyema)	**Too much tension on anastomosis** (i.e. poor surgical judgment!)
Cardiovascular stability (shock)			
Respiratory status (hypoxemia)	**Inflamed?** (e.g. inflammatory bowel disease)	Severe inflammation adjacent to the anastomosis (e.g. acute necrotizing pancreatitis)	**Anastomosis not watertight/airtight** (i.e. faulty technique!)
Uremia	**Poorly perfused?** (e.g. vasculitis)		**Stapler dysfunction — due to faulty device or improper use...**
Chronic steroid intake		No parietal cover leading to exposed anastomosis (loss of abdominal wall, laparostomy)	
Cytotoxic drugs			
Non-steroidal anti-inflammatory drugs (NSAID) intake		Abdominal compartment syndrome (decreasing mesenteric perfusion)	
Uncontrolled diabetes			
Smoking			

I will now bore you again with the principles outlined in ⟳ Chapter 2. We hope that by now you understand that:

- Attempting any anastomosis (even small bowel!) in a debilitated patient, with a **serum albumin** level 'on the floor', is like using a parachute with a large hole in its canopy! **Nutritional status has to be improved if possible!**

- The **factors associated with poor wound** healing mentioned above in ■ Table 6.1 (anemia, hypoxia, uremia, malignancy, steroids, cytotoxic drugs, uncontrolled diabetes) do not help in the healing of the anastomosis. Non-steroidal anti-inflammatory drugs (**NSAIDs**), especially the COX-2 selective agents, are known to interfere with anastomotic healing. Don't use them before or *after* the operation.

- The **ends of the anastomosed bowel have to be well perfused**. **Shock** (hypotension!) regardless of cause, **mesenteric arterial disease** (including vasculitis due to polyarteritis nodosa or other collagen diseases), **uncontrolled hypertension** producing arteriolar spasm, postoperative **intra-abdominal hypertension** reducing cardiac output and mesenteric arterial flow — can all hamper healing of the anastomosis.

- **Nicotine** is a vasoconstrictor: have your patient stop smoking for as long as possible prior to the planned operation and anastomosis.

- **Anything which swells the intestine endangers the anastomosis** — the tissues to be sutured or stapled together must be healthy (you cannot suture together two blocks of butter). **Think this way: anything which swells the patient's tissues swells the intestine as well** — for example: systemic inflammatory response syndrome (SIRS), sepsis, aggressive fluid resuscitation (e.g. after trauma and hemorrhage), reperfusion syndrome (e.g. after restoration of perfusion to the ischemic gut). The **hypoalbuminemia** just mentioned causes generalized tissue edema — including the gut. There are also **local factors which could swell the bowel** — for instance: mesenteric vein thrombosis, portal hypertension, Budd Chiari syndrome or kinking of the mesentery.

Unfortunately, we cannot provide a formula or a computer model which weights the importance of any of the above factors in the healing of an anastomosis and/or predicts its leaking risk in the individual patient. Obviously, not all of these factors can be corrected but **it is your duty to try and optimize your patients to the best of your ability** *before* **any operation during which an intestinal anastomosis is being planned, so that the anastomosis has the best chance of healing**. Naturally, in **emergency situations** you don't have the luxury of prolonged pre-operative assessment and optimization. Here you must consider all the factors provided in ■ Table 6.1 and act accordingly.

Intra-operative considerations

As ye sew, so shall ye reap. Anastomoses 7:42.

David Dent

The parachute must be in perfect condition and packed meticulously, ready to deploy — the anastomosis must be perfect as well. **Here are a few principles which are as important for an esophageal anastomosis as for a rectal one.**

To be perfect the following **cardinal principles** must be obeyed:

- **Perfusion. The blood supply to the anastomosed bowel has to be perfect.** Whatever segment of bowel is used to construct the anastomosis you have to ensure that its blood supply is meticulously preserved. **Use your eyes**: Is the bowel pink? Are the arterial branches supplying it pulsatile? Is there brisk bleeding from the divided ends of mesentery or bowel? If the answer to any of these questions is negative then you have a potential problem.
- Only **healthy bowel ends** should be joined: not inflamed, not denuded, not covered with fat.
- **Tension. Excessive tension on the anastomosis is a recipe for a leak.** After the operation, as bowel swelling and distension increase due to local inflammation and ileus, the tension will further increase and pull the anastomosis apart. Before creating the anastomosis make sure that both ends come together comfortably, not as a straight bowstring but as a loose segment of cooked spaghetti.
- **Watertight/airtight**. The anastomosis has to provide a seal against liquid and gas and it will do so if properly constructed.

Which is the best anastomotic technique?

The ideal anastomosis doesn't leak and doesn't obstruct — allowing normal function of the intestine as soon as possible. There are many ways to skin this particular cat and every experienced surgeon believes that his anastomotic technique — adopted from his local gurus, perhaps with a touch of personal genius — is the 'best'. Obviously, different anatomical locations within the intestinal tract call for different techniques. But in general there are many ingredients to choose from: you can use staplers or sutures (sutures can be mono-filament, braided, absorbable or non-absorbable); you can construct the anastomosis in a single layer or a double one; you can place interrupted sutures or use a continuous one. Many additional (novel or reinvented) anastomotic devices are promoted by medical equipment manufacturers (e.g. sutureless compression ring) but let us not get carried away.

So which of the ingredients and in what combination are the safest?

Answer: as long as you adhere to the previously stated **cardinal principles** you can use any of the above — since all methods, if correctly performed, are safe. Nobody can fault you for using the anastomotic method with which you are most familiar and comfortable. **But let us add a few caveats** below— with which not everybody will agree (isn't almost everything in surgery controversial?).

Narrowing/obstruction
A single-layer anastomosis is less prone to this complication than a multi-layered one. Strictures are also more frequently found following an end-to-end anastomosis performed with the circular stapler (especially when the smaller sizes are used).

Technical misadventures
Technical misadventures seem to be more common with staplers unless you use them routinely. There is a learning curve with any new device. Unpacking the most recent model of stapler and firing it for the first time, while your assistant reads from the attached leaflet, puts the anastomosis at risk.

Staplers vs. sutures
This controversy has been almost solved. Both methods are great if well performed. And let us face it: the 'modern', younger generation of surgeons prefers staplers in any situation they can be employed. However, we should remember that even the stapler aficionado has to use a needle holder and suture when the device misfires, or cannot be employed because of specific anatomic constraints. Thus, surgeons need to be equally dexterous in hand-sewn and stapled anastomotic techniques. Do you still remember how to suture small bowel to small bowel?

The swollen or thick-walled intestine
There is some evidence (level V) that, in trauma patients, stapled intestinal anastomoses are more prone to leak than the hand-sewn ones. This has been attributed to post-resuscitation bowel edema — the staplers cannot 'fine-tune' to the edema of the bowel but the surgeon's suturing hands can. In my own experience, a continuous, monolayer anastomosis occasionally fails in edematous bowel. It seems that as the bowel edema subsides, the suture becomes loose. Therefore, now when suturing edematous bowel I prefer to use a closely placed single layer of interrupted sutures — individually tied 'not too tight, not too loose' — in order to avoid cutting through the bowel wall, and obviate the risk of loosening when the edema subsides. "The safety and efficacy of hand-sewn and stapled anastomoses are equal, except when they are not..." [Thomas M. Haizlip].

Testing the anastomosis

A well-performed anastomosis should be airtight and watertight and thus leak-proof. There is no need to test routinely easily constructed anastomoses such as those placed within the small bowel or the intraperitoneal colon. However, most surgeons opt to test potentially 'problematic' anastomoses (e.g. in the lower rectum, esophagus, or following gastric bariatric procedures). The **air leak test** is popular for rectal anastomoses: the bowel above the anastomosis is clamped, the pelvis is filled with saline and air is injected into the rectum. If air bubbles are observed leaking, an attempt to identify and correct the defect is indicated — if unsuccessful or doubtful, a proximal diverting stoma is necessary. In other locations (esophagus, stomach), anastomoses are usually tested with **blue dye**, diluted and injected through a tube into the esophagus or the stomach. This gives the anesthetist some occupation, beyond reading the *Wall Street Journal* or the *Times of India*...

Covering the anastomosis

Regardless of the level of evidence many surgeons believe (me included) that wrapping the anastomosis with healthy-vascular adjacent tissue — mainly the **omentum** — is beneficial. Common sense dictates that such maneuvers help to seal and abort leaks in evolution.

Drains

The use of *prophylactic* drains in specific locations will be discussed in the individual sections but here are a few general points:

- The main rationale of drains is to 'control' the leak (see below) and avoid the need for reoperation.
- Drains are much more effective in 'controlling' leaks of fluid (e.g. duodenal content) than leaks of semi-solids from the colon.
- Drains provide a false sense of security — the fact that the drain is dry means little!

Avoiding the anastomosis?

In general and especially in the practice of surgery, it is easier to decide to 'do something' rather than 'do nothing'. The decision *not* to anastomose is particularly grueling because it condemns the patient to having a stoma! But when the alternative to a stoma is a leak — with all its potential complications — then the decision not to anastomose becomes lifesaving. The section above and ■ Table 6.1 list factors that influence anastomotic healing or leaking — remember them and incorporate them into your decision-making. **Again**: neither formula nor proven algorithm is available to guide you and you have to use your common sense, based on experience; and if you have no significant experience you have to rely on your local mentors who, as you know, commonly tend to be enslaved to their own dogmas. **So think about the condition of the patient, the bowel and the milieu**. That you are a top knife we have no doubt at all… yes, occasionally you may get away with a risky anastomosis but… often not.

> *If you do a colostomy there will be always someone to ask you why not primary anastomosis? If you do a primary anastomosis there will be always someone to say why not colostomy? Only being a presidential candidate is worse in this regard.*

Postoperative considerations

Is there anything we can do after the operation to prevent anastomotic leaks? Not much beyond optimizing postop care. The fate of the anastomosis has been decided once the abdomen is closed; now what is left for you is to provide optimal postoperative care, see that tissue perfusion and oxygenation are OK — obviously, a hypovolemic, shocked patient won't heal his anastomosis as well as the stable one — and wait for the pleasing sounds of flatus to proclaim that healing is on its way. Hurrah!

"There is no way a patient is going to eat a hole in the anastomosis." [P.O. Nyström]. This is true: prolonged nil per mouth periods and elaborate feeding rituals (clear, soft, solid…) do not prevent leakage. The same is true for the routine use of nasogastric (NG) tubes — even in upper gastrointestinal procedures. However, one has to use common sense and treat each patient individually depending on the site of the anastomosis: for example, acute gastric dilatation could endanger a fresh gastric suture line.

Last thing: remember that studies suggest that **postoperative use of NSAIDs (e.g. diclofenac) is associated with an increased risk of anastomotic leaks**. Take this into consideration!

The diagnosis and treatment of a leak

The diagnosis of an anastomotic leak is a tremendous blow to the surgical overdeveloped ego. The possible repercussions for the patient and the surgeon are so threatening that the surgeon's natural inclination is to adopt **defense mechanisms** like denial, repression or rationalization. Again and again I see (or have observed) in clinical practice, at morbidity and mortality meetings, or when reviewing legal cases, patients with obvious signs of anastomotic leak sliding into sepsis and multi-organ system failure, with their surgeons simply looking away — their diagnostic skills and perception of reality blocked by the fear of confronting the obvious and dealing with it — whatever efforts and pride this entails. Sometimes I even had the impression that the responsible surgeon would prefer the patient to succumb to the leak as fast as possible: better to let him die from the alleged pneumonia than admit that the anastomosis has leaked!

But you won't look away. Instead you will live by this rule: if the patient is not progressing as expected after the operation, if he fails to meet the normal milestones of recovery — always suspect a leak, unless proven otherwise.

What is the meaning of "the patient is not progressing as expected"?

Let's consider for example a patient undergoing a right hemicolectomy for cecal cancer, with an ileo-transverse stapled anastomosis. Within a few days (3-5) you expect him to be afebrile, with normal vital signs, weaned off opiates, up and about, tolerating diet and *farting* or even starting to move his bowels. A wonderful hint that "everything is healing" as expected and that the ileus is resolving, is the recovery of appetite ("I wish I could have bacon and eggs for breakfast…") or the 'lipstick sign' in ladies.

The opposite of uneventful recovery is continuing pain, clinical and laboratory evidence of SIRS/infection and persistent ileus.

The **diagnosis of an anastomotic leak needs vigilance!** Unless you actually observe bowel content emerging from the drain, or pouring through the incision (i.e. a 'leak you can see' — as described below) you can only *suspect* it. **The symptoms and signs of leaks are non-specific** (e.g. there are many potential sources for fever and ileus) and they are masked by incisional pain, analgesia, antibiotics and the patient's comorbidities. This is why you have no choice but always to suspect a leak based on any constellation of **vague signs**. And again: **in most patients the signs of anastomotic leaks are soft!** The abdominal wound may look perfect while the inside is FOS (full of s**t!).

When reviewing charts of patients dying of an anastomotic leak (small bowel, colon, UGI), I notice a recurrent pattern: the patient does not recover 'as expected': there are numerous 'soft signs' such as fever, tachycardia, demand for opiates, persistent ileus, elevated white cell count or other manifestation of inflammation/infection 'somewhere'. The patient is examined by the surgeon and his residents (registrars) who dutifully write in the chart "no peritoneal signs"; and if (useless) drains were inserted at operation they enter:

"drains not productive". Legions of consultants are then summoned (infectious diseases, cardiologists, nephrologists and so forth) to provide additional opinions; they too scribble obediently: "no evidence of peritonitis"; and order bizarre tests. **And meanwhile, the patient's abdomen is awash with bowel contents and/or pus and he is slowly dying.** For even when the intestinal leak is uncontrolled, it often does not immediately kill patients who are well supported and receive broad-spectrum antibiotics — often prescribed by the anxious clinician either empirically or for the alleged 'pneumonia'. But gradually the septic state worsens, various organs start to dysfunction and then fail — and it all ends in another mortality which is rapidly forgotten or excluded from the 'retrospective' or allegedly 'prospective' series.

I am sure that you have had the opportunity to observe similar scenarios in your immediate environment — perhaps even one of the cases of your own boss. I hope that by now you understand, so let us recap briefly:

- **Most patients with an anastomotic leak do not manifest an 'acute abdomen' or 'peritonitis'.**
- **In most patients with an anastomotic leak, when drains are *in situ*, the drains do not produce s**t or bowel contents.**
- **In most patients with an anastomotic leak the diagnosis of leak is not written on the patient's forehead.**
- **The symptoms and signs of a leak are usually 'soft'. Always suspect!**
- **If you review, in *retrospect*, cases of leaks, you will discover that there were almost always some *heralding signs*: spikes in temperature, residual ileus, persistent leukocytosis, etc. All were overlooked or ignored.**

If these points are the only message you take home after reading this chapter I will be satisfied! (But wait, another important message is awaiting you below!).

The clinical spectrum of anastomotic leaks

It should be clear by now that anastomotic leaks do not present in a uniform manner. I now wish to consider some examples of their heterogeneity.

Early vs. late

- Some leaks appear '**early**', within 2-3 days after the creation of the anastomosis. Such leaks are *rare* and are usually attributed to **technical mishaps** — the anastomosis was inadequate from the start. Either it was not watertight/airtight or the sutures/staples were inserted in tissue resembling peanut butter. The presentation tends to be more dramatic than usual: in the early postoperative phase there are no adherent surrounding structures to 'contain' the leak which therefore tends to be diffuse — producing peritonitis and clinical sepsis.

- **'Late'** leaks, also *rare*, presenting beyond the tenth day after the operation. By that time the patient is usually assumed to have recovered from the operation — out of the woods (and the hospital) or nearly there. We assume that the anastomosis was initially sound but gradually the tissues give away perhaps due to relative ischemia or depressed healing mechanisms (e.g. steroids, previous radiation therapy). By this stage local adhesions have already formed to 'contain' the leak and the clinical picture is consequently relatively silent. A common outcome is a peri-anastomotic collection or abscess. A typical example of a 'late' leak would be that occurring after low anterior resection of the rectum.
- **The classic timing** for the appearance of leaks is neither early nor late — but around a week after the operation. The vast majority of leaks present between days five and eight postop. But, as stressed above, **they may have started to 'simmer' a few days earlier!** Some talk about the "**fifth day tachycardia rule**": tachycardia on the fifth day after bowel anastomosis in an otherwise healthy patient may be the first sign of a leak!

Visible vs. concealed

- This is easy! You see the leak — bowel contents pouring out of the drain (rare); or you are horrified by bile or feces soaking or staining the wound and dressing (not so rare). In these cases, the patient would usually have shown some worrisome symptoms and signs which you chose to 'watch' or ignore. A **visible** leak, although alarming and depressing to the patient and his surgeon, might actually be considered 'good news': first — the diagnosis has been established by itself; second — such leaks are often 'controlled' (see below).
- On the other hand, if the leak is **concealed**... the story continues... you have to diagnose it first.

Controlled vs. uncontrolled

- A leak which has found its way to the outside of the skin, through a drain or the surgical wound (i.e. the **visible** leak just mentioned), with *all* intestinal effluents being effectively eliminated by this route, and not constantly contaminating the surrounding spaces, is defined as **controlled**. Such leaks, if not immediately treated with an operation (usually they should not!), become **external controlled fistulas**.
- When, however, only a portion of the leaking effluent gushes to the surface of the skin (or none if the leak is **concealed**), then the leak is **uncontrolled** — implying continuing contamination of the neighboring spaces. **An untreated uncontrolled leak is a death sentence and the**

surgeon's role is to eliminate it (i.e. stop the leakage if possible) or control it (i.e. drain it better). This will be discussed below.

- The **distance of the anastomosis from the skin matters**. An esophagogastric anastomosis in the neck tends to '**control**' itself through the nearby cervical incision. Conversely, a similar anastomosis placed deep in the chest needs to be **controlled** by you, which — as you will find in the next section — is far from easy.

Contained vs. free

The extent of contamination from an anastomotic leak varies greatly and this has huge implications for the clinical picture, the choice of treatment and the prognosis. The spectrum is wide, even within each of the following categories:

- **Free leak**: the anastomosis is disrupted. Intestinal juices/feces gush out and spread all around in the abdomen or chest. **If not immediately controlled the prognosis is grim**.
- **Contained leak**: here the leak is contained by early adhesions and adjacent tissues (omentum, viscera, and abdominal wall) and the natural local defense mechanisms. The range of possibilities is sizable and also the clinical scenarios and outcomes. A walled-off collection or a well-formed abscess (e.g. pericolic) can develop, and this may drain spontaneously back into the bowel lumen. In many instances the only treatment required is CT-guided drainage or even just conservative treatment with antibiotics.
- An extreme example of a **contained** leak is the **mini-leak** — an entity hardly mentioned in the literature, for surgeons prefer not to utter the term "leak" if the actual leak is not obvious. This is a 'tiny' anastomotic leak, usually occurring late after the operation when the anastomosis has been already well sealed off. Abdominal symptoms are limited and the patient is relatively well — some local pain and tenderness and a mild SIRS. A mini-leak could represent a 'peri-anastomositis' — an inflammatory phlegmon (visualized by CT) around the anastomosis. This entity commonly responds to antibiotics. It can result in early **anastomotic obstruction** (see below).

Diagnostic steps

The choice of diagnostic steps when a leak is obvious or suspected depends on the anatomical site of the anastomosis and will be discussed in the individual sections to follow. Here is a brief outline of **diagnostic principles**.

Visible leaks

- When the leak is **visible**, the patient systemically 'ill' with obvious peritonitis (after an abdominal operation), further imaging is usually unnecessary — the diagnosis is clear and so is the treatment — **an operation!**

- When the leak is visible but there are no immediate indications for **reoperation** you need to image the patient to define the extent of the leak (**free? contained?**) and to decide whether it is **controlled** (to be managed non-operatively?) or **not controlled** (CT-guided treatment or reoperation?).

Concealed leaks

When you suspect a leak, but do not see it, you'd better diagnose and delineate it, before deciding how to proceed. Rushing to the operating room with a *suspected* leak, when the leak may not exist — while sometimes necessary (e.g. after bariatric procedures — ⮑ Chapter 23) — is not such a good idea. The choice of imaging lies mainly between a **contrast GI study** and a **contrast CT** to be discussed below in the individual sections.

Whatever imaging you choose to obtain please **remember**:

- Use **water-soluble** contrast — not **barium**! Having said this, occasionally 'thin barium' may demonstrate a leak not apparent with Gastrografin®.
- To diagnose a leak you do not have to see contrast flowing out through the hole in the anastomosis; in fact, **in many cases you won't be able to demonstrate the actual leak**. You will have to rely on **softer findings** (e.g. peri-anastomotic bubbles of air, fluid collections) and correlate these with the clinical picture in order to establish the diagnosis.

Treatment of anastomotic leaks

The following are only a few broad principles as the management of leaks at specific sites will be detailed below. In general, the approach to any anastomotic leak should be selected based on the:

- **Anatomical location** (each one with its specific technical constraints).
- **Condition of the patient** (systemic and local repercussions).
- **Nature of the leak** (contained vs. free, controlled vs. uncontrolled).

Mingling the above variables leads to a large number of clinical scenarios which should be approached on an individual basis but broadly fall into the following categories:

- **An emergency reoperation**: for non-contained and uncontrolled leaks with systemic repercussions.

- **Attempts at conservative treatment +/- image-guided percutaneous drainage**: for **contained leaks** in stable patients.
- **Conservative treatment**: for well-controlled leaks — established external fistulas.

What to do during the reoperation will be detailed below. In general the aim is '**source control**' of the leak either by resecting the leaking anastomosis or by improving its drainage. Much will be detailed in the specific sections: however, at this point I wish to emphasize that **new suture or staple lines in the setting of a leaking anastomosis are going to fail! Any reanastomosis is going to leak again! Suturing a hole in a leaking suture or staple line is going to lead to another leak! And patients who leak again get sicker and many of them die! Don't feel sorry for the patient and try to spare them a stoma when it's necessary. The most important reoperation is the first reoperation!** Below we are going to stress again and again the futility of trying to 'fix' the leaking intestinal holes — if this is the only message that stays with the readers of this chapter then it has accomplished something! (Do you still remember the other message mentioned above?).

For the principles of the management of controlled fistulas see below in the section on small bowel.

Remember: leaks can happen — this is an integral part of any operation. It is the delayed or missed diagnosis and inadequate treatment which kills the patients and/or leads to successful litigation.

Early postoperative anastomotic obstruction

This chapter wouldn't be complete without mentioning the topic of (early) postoperative obstruction of the anastomosis — a less dramatic and morbid situation than leakage but still a frustrating complication. A few observations:

- This problem affects mostly **upper gastrointestinal** (after esophageal, bariatric or gastroduodenal procedures) and **colorectal anastomoses**. Small bowel or colo-colic anastomoses are much less likely to develop obstruction or narrowing.
- **The incidence** is higher in stapled (EEA) and multi-layered anastomoses than sutured, single-layer ones.
- **The etiology** and predisposing factors are faulty technique, poor perfusion of anastomosed bowel or irradiated tissues interfering with normal healing processes; a 'mini-leak' often develops leading to an excessive local inflammatory response — edema/swelling which obstructs the lumen.

- **The clinical picture** is obvious: absent or delayed transit through the anastomosis, and so the diagnosis — by contrast studies (use Gastrografin®!) and/or endoscopy — is readily made.
- **The treatment should be conservative in almost all cases. Very rarely you have to reoperate for early postoperative anastomotic obstruction — to do so implies that you are impatient or stupid!** For with time — it may take a week, or a few weeks — local inflammation will resolve and the anastomosis will open up. Sometimes a stricture develops which in most cases will be amenable to endoscopic dilatation.
- **After partial gastrectomy** *delayed gastric emptying* is often confused with anastomotic obstruction: in both situations the instilled contrast sits in the stomach and doesn't move distally. Endoscopy will provide the diagnosis; and anyway both conditions will resolve within a few weeks. I have seen surgeons rushing to reoperate with disastrous consequences. **Remember**: delayed gastric emptying after partial gastrectomy can last for weeks! **The key word is patience**.

2 The esophagus
John Hunter

Esophagus: as a result of the muscle being loosely knit, anastomosis implies suturing the unsuturable...

Ivor Lewis

The esophageal anastomotic leak is one of the most feared complications in surgery. It is a common condition, occurring in 5-25% of all esophageal anastomoses. It is frequently lethal, causing death in 20-30% of patients who have an intrathoracic leak, but rarely causing mortality when the leak is in the cervical region. Historically, the anastomotic leak rate was higher in the neck than in the chest, but in the laparoscopic era the rate of esophageal anastomotic leaks in the neck and the chest are now equivalent. This introduction brings us to the first question: **how do you prevent an anastomotic leak?**

Pre-operative considerations

Prevention

Prevention of esophageal anastomotic leak starts with an understanding of the major factors contributing to leak. Far and away, the most common reason for leak is **poor blood flow and/or tissue oxygenation of the gastric conduit. Secondary issues include excessive tension on the anastomosis,**

and anastomotic technical errors. Causes farther down the list include poor wound healing as a result of malnutrition and drugs (i.e. chemotherapy or glucocorticoids).

Inadequate tissue perfusion

The most common reasons for an inadequate supply of oxygenated blood to the anastomosis include cigarette smoking, diabetes, cardiovascular disease, *postoperative* hypotension and *postoperative* sepsis. **When the first three features are present pre-operatively, we will often perform 'ischemic preconditioning' by taking down the fundic blood supply (short gastric and posterior gastric arteries) and clipping the left gastric artery anywhere from 2-12 weeks before esophagectomy**. While it may seem extreme to wait 12 weeks to perform esophagectomy after the diagnosis of esophageal cancer is made, patients undergoing induction (neoadjuvant) chemoradiotherapy will often need a *jejunostomy* tube (J-tube) placed prior to the initiation of therapy. At the time of laparoscopic jejunostomy, the gastric fundus is devascularized, and a clip is placed on the left gastric artery if there is no tumor involvement of the left gastric pedicle. Experimental and clinical data provide evidence for the benefit of ischemic preconditioning in improving blood flow and reducing anastomotic leakage [2]. Esophagectomy with gastric pull-up is then performed 6-8 weeks after completion of a six-week course of neoadjuvant chemoradiation.

Postoperative hypotension is to be avoided at all costs. Frequently, minor postoperative hypotensive episodes will be treated with large amounts of fluid by a well-meaning intensivist, only to the detriment of the lungs and the heart, increasing the likelihood of postoperative atrial fibrillation. Instead, we are inclined to use a balanced approach to postoperative fluids, and are not adverse to **low-dose norepinephrine** to maintain mean arterial pressures at 60 or above. Research from our lab demonstrates that norepinephrine actually improves blood flow to the conduit, decreasing the amount of ischemia. **Tissue hypoxia also contributes to anastomotic leak**. It is very important to keep the arterial O_2 saturation above 90 postoperatively, and avoid other vasoconstrictors, the most prominent of which is nicotine. A mandatory program of smoking cessation prior to esophagectomy can be a very helpful adjunct in the prevention of anastomotic leak. **We will rarely perform this operation if a patient has not been willing to quit smoking for at least one month pre-operatively**.

---

[2] Reavis KM, Chang EY, Hunter JG, Jobe BA. Utilization of the delay phenomenon improves blood flow and reduces collagen deposition in esophagogastric anastomoses. *Ann Surg* 2005; 241: 736-45.
Perry KA, Enestvedt CK, Pham TH, Dolan JP, Hunter JG. Esophageal replacement following gastric devascularization is safe, feasible, and may decrease anastomotic complications. *J Gastrointest Surg* 2010; 14: 1069-73.

Intra-operative considerations

Tissue tension

If the gastric conduit is too short, the esophago-anastomosis will be under tension. As in all surgery, excessive tension is a great risk factor for dehiscence. We have found two factors that help reduce the likelihood of tissue tension. **The first of these is adequate mobilization of the duodenum and pylorus**. The duodenal mobilization is fairly straightforward with a thorough *Kocher maneuver* starting at the common bile duct and running around the second portion of the duodenum to the junction of the second and third portion of the duodenum. In addition, the *subpyloric dissection* is critical. As one follows the dissection of the greater curvature outside the right gastroepiploic artery from the spleen towards the pylorus, the greater omentum is divided along its entire length from the spleen to the second portion of the duodenum. By continuing the omental dissection all the way to the gallbladder (or gallbladder fossa if a cholecystectomy has been previously performed) the pylorus is 'unweighted' from the colon, and the gastroepiploic pedicle can usually be seen coursing behind the first portion of the duodenum. As the stomach is elevated anteriorly, posterior attachments between the antrum of the stomach and the

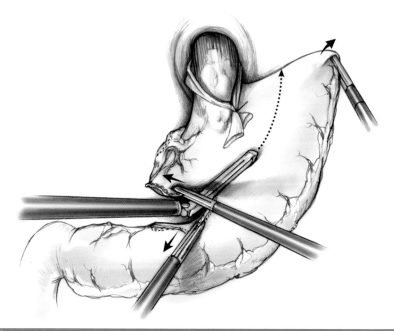

Figure 6.2. Laparoscopic creation of a gastric conduit. *Reprinted with permission from: Hunter J, Spight D, Sandone C, Fairman J, Eds. Atlas of Minimally Invasive Surgical Operations. McGraw Hill, in press.*

retroperitoneum are divided down to the level of the pylorus. When this dissection is complete the pylorus can be rotated cephalad such that it will nearly reach the hiatus! **If one cannot get the pylorus within a few centimeters of the hiatus, further mobilization should be performed**.

The next issue in obtaining an adequate length of gastric conduit to perform a tension-free anastomosis is the **creation of the conduit**. The narrower the conduit is, and the more the greater curvature is stretched by traction on the fundus as the conduit is created, the longer one can make an esophageal conduit. The limiting factors here are that very narrow conduits are more likely to become ischemic, while wide conduits empty poorly, so **we have settled on a conduit diameter of approximately 3-4cm**. As the stapler is applied to create the conduit, the fundus of the stomach is stretched towards the spleen and the antrum of the stomach is stretched towards the gallbladder. With this technique, we have almost always been able to get a very long conduit up to the neck without tension so that the anastomosis can be created along the greater curvature. While some surgeons have felt the need to make a small incision to create the conduit, this procedure is not difficult to perform laparoscopically (■ Figure 6.2).

The anastomosis

The next issue of significance in the prevention of leak is **construction of the anastomosis**. There will be ongoing debate as to whether a hand-sewn, single-layer, multi-layer, or stapled anastomosis provides the lowest rate of anastomotic leak. Amongst those who do a stapled anastomosis, the type of stapled anastomosis (EEA vs. GIA) will also have proponents and passionate debates. Because the primary risk factor for anastomotic dehiscence is poor tissue perfusion and not poor technique, it is difficult to determine, outside of a randomized controlled trial (RCT), the direct contribution of anastomotic technique to anastomotic leakage. But again: **sticking to first principles, the primary duty of the surgeon is to find a portion of the stomach where the blood flow is optimal**. Because the blood flow to the fundus of the stomach is often marginal, **the best place to perform the esophago-anastomosis is as low on the greater curvature as the conduit will allow without creating excessive tension**. Said another way, we always move our anastomosis several centimeters down from the fundus along the anterior wall of the stomach very close to the greater curvature in order to get the best blood flow possible. **This may allow resection of a congested or ischemic conduit tip, with a stapler**. While many surgeons feel it is necessary to invert any staple line by oversewing it, we have found this generally unnecessary. Nevertheless, the tip of the conduit is the most at risk for ischemia, so we will usually *invert* this staple line with a number of Lembert sutures when the anastomosis is done in the neck.

A global survey of anastomotic techniques turns up the following conclusion: **each expert has their own way of performing esophagogastrostomy, and in the experts' hands — all of them work.** The simplest of anastomotic techniques is a *single-layer* 'running' anastomosis of

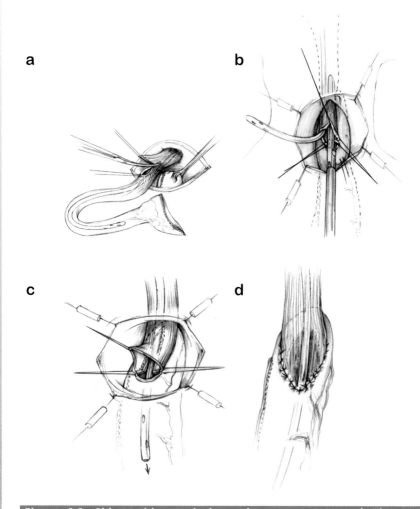

Figure 6.3. Side-to-side cervical esophagogastrostomy. a) The cervical esophagus is divided after the conduit has been 'dragged' up to the neck, attached to the resected portion of the stomach. **b)** An enterotomy on the greater curvature of the conduit is created, the esophagus is sutured to the stomach, and a GIA stapler is introduced to create a side-to-side anastomosis. **c)** The nasogastric tube is passed through the anastomosis. **d)** The esophagogastric enterotomy is closed with a running absorbable suture and interrupted silk sutures (two layers). *Reprinted with permission from: Hunter J, Spight D, Sandone C, Fairman J, Eds. Atlas of Minimally Invasive Surgical Operations. McGraw Hill, in press.*

Prolene® or monofilament absorbable suture (e.g. PDS® or Maxon™). This anastomosis has been best popularized by Drs. Law and Wong at the University of Hong Kong where their leak rates approach nil! At the other extreme are those, such as myself, who like the stapled anastomosis in the neck. Because of the lower morbidity of an anastomotic leak in the neck and the wonderful exposure that one achieves in this region we have always preferred this technique. In addition, the esophageal resection length obtained is maximal, so this technique can be applied to distal and mid-esophageal tumors. **Whether performing a transhiatal esophagectomy or a transthoracic esophagectomy the neck anastomosis provides an excellent functional outcome**. Like many, we initially sewed this anastomosis with standard techniques, resulting in leak rates around 20% (similar to the national average). Since making the transition to a side-to-side stapled technique with a GIA, as first described by Mark Orringer, our leak rate has fallen below 5% (■ Figure 6.3).

Postoperative considerations

Treatment of esophageal anastomotic dehiscence

Intrathoracic dehiscence

- **When a patient who has undergone an esophagectomy becomes acutely ill within the first ten days after surgery, the number one diagnosis is esophageal anastomotic leak**.
- The presentation can occasionally fool the unsuspecting house officer as **the first manifestations of leak are not fever and leukocytosis, but tachycardia and tachypnea, similar to a pulmonary embolus (PE)**.
- **PE or a myocardial event** are second and third on the differential list as causes for acute deterioration of a patient post-esophagectomy.

The patient who becomes ill in this fashion demands urgent care. If there is any doubt in the diagnosis (often there is), an EKG and a CT scan with a PE protocol can be performed quickly, minimally delaying re-exploration. If bile or *succus entericus* appears in the chest tube, clearly the CT is not necessary and an immediate trip to the operating room is warranted. While it is tempting to manage an esophageal anastomotic leak with a chest tube and an **internal esophageal stent**, the tube may not adequately drain the thoracic cavity, and the stent may not adequately cover the source of sepsis. **If the patient can stand it, a trip to the operating room is the best way to take care of this problem!**

In the operating room the right thorax should be entered through a posterior lateral thoracotomy and all fibrinous debris and fluid removed. The source of the leak can be found quite easily. **No attempts at suture repair should be made**; however, a small leak can be covered with a tissue flap such as an intercostal muscle. After repair, placement of multiple large drains near the site of the leak is mandatory.

Larger leaks may require the placement of a T-tube, which can be homemade out of two chest tubes, a right-angle tube and a smaller straight chest tube, which is nestled inside the larger right-angled chest tube with the tip brought out through a hole created at the right-angle bend. The T-tube is then placed so that one arm reaches above the site of dehiscence and one

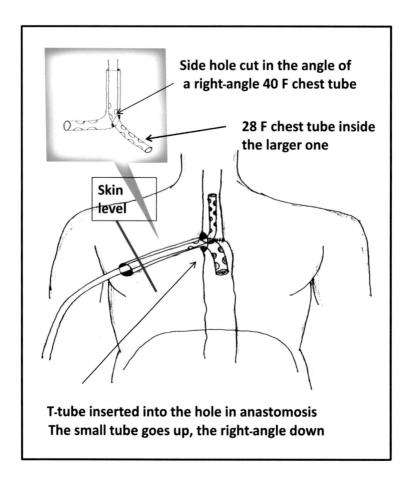

Figure 6.4. Our homemade T-tube for the management of intrathoracic esophageal leaks.

limb is directed distally. This 'combo' chest tube is then brought out through a stab wound between the ribs (■ Figure 6.4).

Occasionally, in a patient who is too ill to return to the OR for management of dehiscence, a coated endoscopic stent may be placed to provide 'source control'. This is usually used in combination with radiologic drainage, if a CT scan shows a fluid collection not being drained by the chest tubes currently in place. While stents may be lifesaving, they tend to migrate distally, and may not always completely control the anastomotic fistula.

If the gastric conduit is frankly dead, the esophagus and the gangrenous part of the stomach are separated. The necrotic portion of the stomach is removed with a stapler and the remnant viable stomach is *returned to the abdomen*. The remnant esophagus is freed to the thoracic inlet and an end *cervical esophagostomy* is performed. If a J-tube has previously been inserted, and the closure of the gastric stump is secure, it may not be necessary to reopen the abdomen at this juncture. However, enteral feeding access is crucial and a J-tube should be placed if it has not been done previously. The chest is then thoroughly irrigated and a large chest tube and closed suction draining catheters are placed in dependent portions of the chest.

Management of cervical anastomotic leakage

The cervical anastomotic leak presents as either a *wound infection*, *air in the soft tissues*, or a contrast esophagogram demonstrating extravasation. With the first two scenarios, we prefer to take the patient to the operating room for adequate cervical drainage: the wound is reopened, all pus is removed, and the space between the trachea and great vessels of the neck is re-explored with a finger. **No attempts are made to view the anastomosis as this would further disrupt it**. Instead, a soft, Penrose drain is placed inferiorly between the carotid artery and trachea and brought out through the neck incision. The neck incision may be packed open or loosely closed allowing room between the sutures for packing.

After drainage of a leak, we will wait until there is no further saliva coming through the Penrose drain, then test with a grape juice swallow (or any dye) followed by a contrast esophagogram to prove that the anastomosis is no longer leaking. Healing is usually complete within 1-2 weeks, unless the dehiscence is major.

Occasionally, the patient will develop a large amount of **subcutaneous emphysema in the neck**, usually as a result of a coughing spell that disrupts the anastomosis, especially if the gastric conduit is full of air. This complication can occasionally create sufficient neck swelling to cause airway compromise.

If the patient is stridorous, the incision should be opened at the bedside to allow evacuation of the air; then the patient should be returned quickly to the operating room for exploration and drainage.

If an esophagogram (usually performed seven days postop) demonstrates a **small contained anastomotic leak**, and the patient is completely *asymptomatic*, and the **wound is not infected**, we will manage that patient with first parenteral and then enteral antibiotics through the J-tube. The patient is kept NPO until the leak heals, as demonstrated with an esophagogram, performed weekly until healing is complete.

There is a frequent debate as to the **role of nasogastric tubes** in assisting the treatment of anastomotic leak. Some believe that an NG tube placed near the anastomosis will decrease the access of enteral secretions to the fistula, improving the rate of healing. However, there are inadequate data to support such a conclusion, and the patients are generally unhappy enough about the leak without having to suffer the replacement of an NG tube. In brief, in a patient who is ICU bound and horribly ill, we will place an NG tube in the conduit to decompress it. In patients who are not so ill, especially those with cervical leaks, we do not use an NG tube and allow the patient to live a reasonably normal life at home as the anastomosis is healing.

Management of abdominal esophageal leak after total gastrectomy and esophagojejunostomy

Total gastrectomy performed for gastric cancer is most frequently reconstructed with a Roux-en-Y esophagojejunostomy. Some surgeons prefer a straight limb, while others, including myself prefer the creation of a 'neo-stomach' by folding the jejunum back on itself and creating a *pouch* with several firing of the GIA stapler. With this approach the preferred anastomotic technique uses an EEA stapler sized to the caliber of the distal esophagus. Intra-operative quality control is attained by examining the anastomotic 'doughnuts' for completeness after staple firings, and performing a leak test with dilute methylene blue instilled through an NG tube at the completion of the operation. Nonetheless, anastomotic leakage may occur and is usually diagnosed after the warning signs of tachycardia and tachypnea are correctly interpreted as a leak. Confirmation of leakage with a CT scan or contrast esophagogram then follows.

Management may be non-operative (with antibiotics) for contained leaks in a well patient, but the **ill patient should be returned to the OR for exploration** (open or laparoscopic) and drainage of all fluid collections. Taking down the anastomosis is usually unnecessary, and **direct repair of a leak with sutures is futile, as the leak will quickly recur through the suture area!** —

as the primary reason for leak has not been corrected (usually poor blood flow). In addition, suture repair usually makes the fistula track larger by creating additional tension. If a feeding jejunostomy has not been previously placed *and* the patient is not terribly septic *and* the abdomen is not terribly contaminated, a jejunostomy tube may be placed. The healing of esophagojejunal fistulas is not always rapid. Persistent fistula drainage after exploration may warrant the placement of an **endoscopic covered stent**. For very persistent, chronic fistulas, fibrin glue, injected through an ERCP catheter endoscopically into the fistula tract, has been reported to facilitate fistula closure.

Long-term management of an anastomotic leak

There is always a question as what to do with a *non-healing fistula*, especially the intrathoracic fistula. These may be difficult problems. The first and foremost duty of the surgeon is to make sure all sepsis is controlled such that the nutritional condition of the patient in the hyper-inflammatory state created by the sepsis can improve. When a patient's albumin and pre-albumin remain below normal, it is often difficult to obtain healing, even in the face of adequate enteral nutrition. This generally indicates a hyper-inflammatory condition that suggests inadequate source control. Internal, endoscopic stenting may be helpful in restoring a catabolic state which will eventually lead to fistula closure. Rarely, injection of the fistulous tract with fibrin glue applied endoscopically with an ERCP catheter will facilitate fistula closure (see above).

Post-anastomotic fistula strictures

After an anastomotic leak, it is not unusual to have a stricture at the level of the anastomosis. Depending upon the amount of tissue loss, this might necessitate a number of esophageal *dilatations* with either endoscopic balloon dilatation, or Savary (wire-guided) rigid dilators. The more tissue loss, the more difficult it will be to maintain adequate patency. For tough strictures with tissue loss, I am a strong believer in *weekly* dilatations, occasionally using *injectable steroids* until an adequate lumen can be achieved. For recalcitrant strictures home dilatation by the patient has been effective at maintaining patency of difficult strictures, but is very rarely necessary. While **anastomotic revision** would be a common response to this problem in the abdomen, the options in the chest and neck are fewer, and the outcomes of anastomotic revisions in these regions are not generally acceptable. However, on occasion, especially if dilatation has led to an esophageal perforation, other means must be explored. Under these circumstances, the most common approach is to reconstruct the esophagus with a piece of **left colon**, brought above the area of stricture. A free **jejunal interposition graft** can also be used to bridge an area of conduit loss, using microvascular techniques.

In conclusion, the best way to treat an esophageal anastomotic fistula is to avoid it. While recurrent dilatations for stricture are not especially pleasant for the patient, a life-threatening leak is a whole lot worse. Generally, the cervical leak is much better tolerated both immediately and in the long term, and an anastomosis there is consequently our preferred method of esophageal reconstruction.

3 Stomach and duodenum [3]
Wen-hao Tang

The stomach enjoys a superb blood supply which however can be compromised in certain circumstances…

Pre-operative considerations

The Editors instructed me not to dwell on how we can improve the patient's condition before the operation so he is less likely to leak after it. I hope they have managed to cover this important topic in the previous sections of this book and chapter. But, please allow me to mention a pre-operative concern which is specific to gastric operations.

Preparation of the obstructed stomach

Longstanding **gastric outlet obstruction**, due to antral cancer or chronic duodenal ulcer is associated with **bacterial overgrowth** in the stomach — an organ which under normal circumstances should be virtually sterile. The *achlorhydria* typical of gastric cancer, or which follows prolonged management with acid-reducing agents, can also promote bacterial overgrowth. You do not want to operate on an atonic, distended 'bag', full of old food and foul-smelling liquids resembling feces. So, for the patients with chronic gastric outlet obstruction I recommend inserting a large-bore nasogastric tube and cleansing the stomach with warm saline until clean. Then place the tube on intermittent suction and continue irrigating once or twice a day, for 3-5 days.

---

[3] See Chapter 23 for leaks following bariatric operations.

Not only will this clean the stomach and thus reduce the risk of intra-operative contamination and septic complications but also alleviate distension of the stomach and improve its muscle tone. We hope that the anastomosis created in such a 'resuscitated' stomach will be safer and the gastric remnant less susceptible to delayed gastric emptying.

Do not forget prophylactic antibiotics! Remember that diseased stomachs are rarely sterile!

Intra-operative considerations

Preserving the gastric remnant blood supply and avoiding accidental injuries

It is true that the stomach which is fed by so many arteries has a superb blood supply, but there are situations in which the blood supply to the gastric remnant can be compromised endangering the safety of the anastomosis:

- In patients with a history of **previous splenectomy** or when **splenectomy** has to be added to the partial or subtotal gastrectomy (e.g. cancer invading the splenic hilum, accidental injury), be aware that the *short gastric arteries* (arising from the splenic artery) are no longer perfusing the gastric remnant. In this situation, if you ligate the *left gastric artery* at its origin, the remnant may become ischemic. Always ensure that the remnant is pink and bleeding generously — if not you have to resect it and fashion an esophagojejunostomy.

- When you dissect the first part of the duodenum, consider the gastroduodenal artery as the limit marker and do not dissect beyond the artery. Dr. J.E. Skandalakis remarked that the term "water under the bridge" applies not only to the relationship of the uterine artery to the ureter but also to the gastroduodenal artery and the accessory pancreatic duct. In one out of ten cases, the duct of *Santorini* is the only duct draining the pancreas, so ligation of the gastroduodenal artery with accidental injury of the duct could be catastrophic. In addition, the gastroduodenal artery should be carefully preserved to maintain an adequate blood supply to the duodenum.

- Some authors emphasize the need to be cautious when inserting sutures into the posterior wall of the duodenum during attempts to control the **gastroduodenal artery** (or one of its branches) at the base of a **bleeding duodenal ulcer**. They claim that sutures placed too deeply may catch the common bile duct. In my experience this is a somewhat theoretical danger, unless you are dealing with a *postbulbar ulcer* or your suture bites are deeper than a few centimeters ☺...

- Avoiding **injury to the pancreas** — especially to the pancreatic tail during mobilization of the fundus, or when a splenectomy has to be added — prevents *traumatic pancreatitis* or *pancreatic fistula*. Release of pancreatic enzymes could be deleterious to the nearby gastric suture line.

Reconstruction (repair and anastomotic techniques)

I do not need to remind you in detail of the well-established principles of bowel anastomosis (preserving adequate tissue vascularization, avoiding tension and keeping the suture lines watertight) for if I do the Editors will delete it. So let me go directly to the reconstruction of gastroduodenal continuity in specific situations.

Closure of perforated peptic ulcer

Simple closure of the perforated ulcer is best achieved with an omental **Graham's patch** — *omentopexy*. Insert a few 'through-all-layers' interrupted sutures through both edges of the perforation (placed vertically along the long axis of the duodenum so as not to narrow the duodenum) and leave them untied. Next, fashion a well-perfused pedicle of the greater omentum, flip it over the perforation, and tie the sutures gently — not too tight, not too loose — over the omental flap. Ask the anesthetist to inject a few hundred cc of 'blue-stained saline' through the nasogastric tube to ascertain that the patch is waterproof.

There are surgeons who tend to misunderstand what *omentopexy* should be: they first suture-close the perforation and only then cover the suture line with the omentum. But a suture repair of the edematous, friable edges of perforation is prone to leakage. Some surgeons omit omental patching altogether and simply suture the duodenal hole — this seems to be the emerging trend adopted by *laparoscopic* surgeons. Of course one can 'get away' with almost everything, and simple suturing is usually successful in small, fresh perforations. But I believe and there is some evidence, that in most duodenal leaks occurring after closure of perforated ulcers (not an uncommon complication — especially in series from the developing world), the lack of a properly performed omentopexy is the overriding factor. **So do not compromise — do it right the first time around, even if you choose to do it through the laparoscope. Plug — not only stitch!** And if you do not know how to do it laparoscopically then do it open. Duodenal leak is a devastating complication!

Repair of gastroduodenal injuries (traumatic or iatrogenic)

Fixing a hole in the stomach or duodenum can be considered an anastomosis — prone to leakage — and hence I mention this topic here.

The injured stomach, with its mobile and thick muscular wall and superb blood supply, is easy to fix. Just suture it, in one layer or two or use the linear stapler — whatever you do the gastric repair suture line is very unlikely to leak. Remember that in penetrating trauma you always have to follow-explore the course of the injuring agent, whether blade or projectile. Without opening the *lesser sac* and examining the posterior wall of the stomach you will miss through-and-through gastric injuries. I remember a patient undergoing laparotomy (not by me of course!) for a stabbed abdomen; a hole was found and repaired in the anterior wall of the stomach. The patient became critically ill over the next 24 hours and died: at autopsy a gaping hole was found in the posterior wall of the stomach. **Neglected holes in the UGI tract can kill within 24 hours!**

The duodenum with its thinner wall, fixed position, adjacent to the portal triad and pancreas, and constantly 'flushed' with activated erosive pancreatic enzymes, is a 'different fish' altogether — a shark rather than a carp! Duodenal suture lines are more leak-prone and when they leak the consequences are serious and difficult to manage. The spectrum of the severity of duodenal injuries is wide and over the years various techniques of duodenal repair have been introduced and forgotten — usually reported as 'case reports' or small case series, not amenable to proper assessment and comparison. But here are a few principles based on common sense and my own vast experience (as you know, experience improves your common sense and common sense makes your experience more positive…):

- Special care should be taken to assess the viability of the injured bowel wall and exclude injuries to adjacent structures (common bile duct, pancreas, portal vein, etc.).
- **'Simple', non-destructive laceration of the duodenum**, if diagnosed and operated upon 'early' (within ~12 hours) can be primarily repaired in a tension-free manner following minimal debridement of the bowel edges. The suture line has to be fashioned in transverse orientation in order not to narrow the duodenum.

- **Early diagnosed** injuries resulting in *tissue loss* that do not permit a simple repair are managed with **segmental duodenal resection**. If the length of the duodenal gap created permits the bowel ends to come together easily, it should be reconstructed with an end-to-end duodeno-duodenal anastomosis. However, if the bowel ends do not reach each other without tension (which is common for the second or third parts of the duodenum), then reconstruction with a Roux-en-Y duodenojejunostomy is necessary. The latter can be 'side-to-side' (if the duodenal defect is not circumferential) or 'end-to-end' — anastomosing the jejunum to the proximal end of the resected duodenum while the distal end is closed.

- **Late diagnosed** duodenal injuries (>~12 hours) are usually associated with peritonitis; furthermore, the tissues are already macerated by the corrosive admixture of leaking bile with pancreatic juice — predisposing to suture line dehiscence. Over the years multiple techniques have been proposed to 'support' such problematic duodenal suture lines — for example: *buttressing* the repair with *omentum* or a 'serosal patch' (the sero-muscular layer of an intact loop of jejunum is attached to the duodenum to cover its suture line). Even abdominal wall *muscle flaps* were used to cover the duodenal repair site. Another method used to treat **complex duodenal injuries** (often involving the pancreas) was the 'duodenal diverticulization', consisting of suture repair of the duodenal injury, antrectomy (plus truncal vagotomy to decrease the risk of anastomotic ulcer) and gastrojejunostomy (i.e. Billroth II) and tube duodenostomy (inserted through the duodenal stump). Some surgeons believe in the concept of **duodenal decompression** by inserting a T-tube into the second part of the duodenum whenever the duodenal repair is considered high risk (to some surgeons any duodenal repair seems 'high risk' ☺). Furthermore, a 'three-tubes-technique' has been advocated by a few 'tube-aficionados' — a T-tube in the duodenum, gastrostomy and feeding jejunostomy. **I am a 'tubophobe' however: I believe that the more tubes you insert into the bowel, the more holes you create, the more potential leaking points you create**. In my view, the best technique currently available to deal with 'problematic' duodenal repairs — if segmental duodenal resection is not required for destructive injuries — is **'pyloric exclusion' to be discussed** below as a treatment for postoperative leaks.

- In rare instances, destructive, **combined duodenopancreatic injuries** (when nothing is left to be repaired) would require a **pancreatoduodenectomy**. This of course has to be STAGED: first 'damage control', then optimize the patient and come back for the reconstructive phase.

- Needless to add that whatever you do, the periduodenal spaces should be **widely drained** so that any prospective leak will be well controlled and not require a reoperation. Of course, always think whether a **feeding tube, either nasojejunal or a jejunostomy** is indicated. And if you think about it then place one! (Read more about duodenal injuries in ⟳ Chapter 24.)

Avoiding leaks after partial gastrectomy

The Editors deleted half of what I tried to sell you in the first draft of this chapter, telling me that this is not "a manual of UGI surgery... but just a small book on complications". Nevertheless I wish to make a few brief points below.

Dealing with a 'difficult duodenal stump' after Billroth II gastrectomy
When the duodenum is normal this is rarely a problem: simply avoid transecting the duodenum too close to the pancreatic capsule — leave enough tissue to afford closure of the stump without tension, even if you choose to do it in two layers. However, when the first part of the duodenum is scarred by a **chronic duodenal ulcer** the closure of the stump may become difficult and prone to leakage. This, in the developed world at least, has become a rare situation but is still encountered in less privileged places where *proton pump inhibitors* are not being sold for a few dollars in Wall Mart. How should you deal with it? **The best management is prevention**: it is a very rare complicated duodenal ulcer that necessitates gastrectomy (e.g. perforated giant duodenal ulcer). **And even if gastrectomy is absolutely indicated why not choose a Billroth I gastrectomy, thus avoiding a duodenal stump altogether**. On how to do gastroduodenostomy in the presence of a large duodenal ulcer I would refer you elsewhere [4]. **In brief: if you do not create a stump then it won't leak!** There will always be a few surgeons who won't take my advice and will obstinately proceed with a Billroth II gastrectomy under adverse circumstances. For generations surgeons have designed 'fancy' closure techniques of the duodenal stump and gave each their own name (e.g. **Bancroft** — where the mucosectomized antrum wall is used to close the stump, or **Nissen** — where the anterior lip of the stump is sutured to the pancreatic capsule). Others even recommended avoiding the stump by anastomosing it with a Roux-en-Y loop of jejunum — turning a simple operation to a complex one. **But my advice is this**: if the probability of duodenal stump leakage is expected to be high, insert a **tube duodenostomy** — place a large and soft tube (a Foley will do) into the duodenal stump and close the stump around the tube (■ Figure 6.5) to establish a *controlled duodenal fistula*. Place

---

[4]   *Schein's Common Sense Emergency Abdominal Surgery*, 3rd Ed. Springer Verlag, © 2010: Chapter 17: 150.

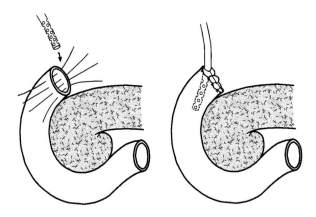

Figure 6.5. Tube duodenostomy.

a drain nearby to collect whatever initially leaks out around the tube. The tube can be clamped and removed when the fistula tract is matured. And then you may want to occlude the tract with fibrin glue (if you enjoy gimmicks).

Avoid kinking or angulation of the gastrojejunostomy

Avoid kinking or angulation of the *gastrojejunostomy* (I do so by suturing the jejunal loop to the stomach for 2cm beyond the actual anastomosis on both sides) as this may obstruct the afferent loop, thus raising its luminal pressure and compromising the duodenal stump's closure.

Insertion of a small-bore tube

Inserting a small-bore tube deep downstream into the *efferent* loop is often a good idea as this will allow you to start feeding the patient immediately after the operation. After having completed the posterior wall of the anastomosis ask the anesthetist to pass the tube and guide it under vision into the correct loop — not the *afferent* one. If you have a reason to suspect prolonged anastomotic 'troubles' (anastomotic failure, delayed gastric empting and so on) or your patient suffers from malnutrition, I would rather recommend placement of a *tube jejunostomy*.

Drains

For most **elective UGI operations, drains are normally not necessary**, except in patients at high risk of leakage (e.g. difficult duodenal stump, severe malnutrition, accidental pancreatic tail injury, esophagojejunostomy, etc.). I prefer using a (passive) soft and flat Penrose drain placed near the anastomosis and in Morrison's pouch. There are many hospitals in China where large sump suction drains are frequently encouraged, yet the incidence of bowel erosion is high because of pressure necrosis. I know that in the West, soft, small-diameter suction drains (e.g. JP) are commonly used. I am not aware of any randomized prospective trial comparing those drains ☺.

Postoperative considerations

In order to anticipate and diagnose complications, and take early action, it is crucial that the operating surgeon — yourself (the senior surgeon) — should review and touch-examine his patients at least twice a day, particularly in the early postoperative days. That optimal postoperative care facilitates anastomotic healing has been stressed in the preceding sections of this chapter. Remember that adequate nutrition is important — this is why you have inserted the feeding tubes during the operation! I have no doubts that enteral nutrition has great advantages over the parenteral one. To paraphrase Ambroise Paré, the great 16th century French surgeon: "I support him, God cures him."

Typically, upper gastrointestinal anastomotic leaks occur around the fifth postoperative day, but may occur sooner and also much later. The main clinical picture is unexplained systemic inflammatory response syndrome (don't tell me: "I never heard the term SIRS"), peritonitis and an abnormal amount and character of drainage. In some patients, especially the very obese (as you will read in ➲ Chapter 23), leaks may develop early without any abdominal manifestations — the only suggesting feature being a **sustained tachycardia**. This is also true for **accidental duodenal perforation during laparoscopic cholecystectomy or ERCP** — yes, these situations do not represent 'anastomotic leaks' but what we discuss in this chapter is relevant to the diagnosis and management of these conditions as well. Thus the key to saving the patient can be summarized in three words: SUSPECT, SUSPECT, SUSPECT! **If you do not suspect the leak today — tomorrow may be too late!**

You already know how to diagnose, confirm and delineate the leak using a water-soluble contrast study, with or without a CT scan. You also understand that occasionally early leaks may not be visualized but this doesn't mean that there is no leak: **sometimes you will have to reoperate based only on your suspicion!**

Your chief aim is to achieve SOURCE CONTROL — stopping the continuing contamination of the adjacent spaces. You may want to try to seal the leaking point — inserting a few sutures, patching with omentum — **but you** already know that such maneuvers are usually futile: it will leak again! Unlike the situation with small or large bowel anastomotic leaks, UGI structures are generally 'fixed' and usually not amenable to **exteriorization** or **proximal diversion**. So, in most instances your best and only lifesaving 'source control' option is adequate external drainage to obtain a controlled external fistula. **Remember this: your aim is to achieve a controlled fistula!** Of course, this task can occasionally be achieved (when the leak is 'contained') percutaneously without resorting to reoperation.

'End' vs. 'side' leak: this is an important concept in the management of UGI leaks. Look at ■ Figure 6.6. A **side leak** is a 'hole' in the wall of the stomach or duodenum 'irrigated' with the normal stream of gastroduodenal contents (saliva, gastric acidic juice, pancreatic alkaline output and bile). A leaking gastroduodenal anastomosis (Billroth I), a leaking gastric staple line after *sleeve gastrectomy* or an accidental duodenotomy are side leaks. An **end leak**, on the other hand, is relatively remote from the corrosive stream of biliary and pancreatic juices — for example: the duodenal stump after Billroth II gastrectomy, the leaking gastrojejunal anastomosis after Roux-en-Y gastric bypass for morbid obesity. **Remember**: adequately drained **end leaks** will form a controlled fistula which should close readily. Conversely, side leaks are much more difficult to control; they are less likely to close spontaneously. **So, when reoperating for a side leak you have to consider converting it to an end leak**, as I will specify below.

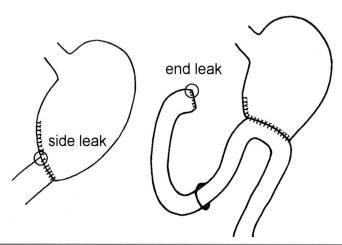

Figure 6.6. Side leak and end leak.

The management of leaks

Once the leak has been diagnosed, how are you going to manage it?

You know the principles already: a **contained** or **well-controlled** leak (through drains placed at the original operation) when the patient is 'well' (minimal SIRS, no peritonitis) can be managed conservatively, often assisted by CT-guided percutaneous drainage. If you are lucky, feeding tubes have been inserted already into the jejunum at the original operation — you can start using them immediately. If not start TPN; if the leak is unlikely to resolve within a week or so think about inserting a transanastomotic nasojejunal tube; this is not too difficult to accomplish with the aid of an endoscope.

On the other hand, when the **leak doesn't seem to be controlled (SIRS and peritonitis), do not hesitate much and reoperate! What to do? Three principles**:

- **Achieve better drainage** — establish a controlled fistula.
- **Insert feeding tubes**, if not already in place.
- **Convert side leaks to end leaks**.

Now let us be more specific.

Leaking duodenal stump
When reoperating for a **leaking duodenal stump**, your best bet is a tube duodenostomy (■ Figure 6.5). Oh yes — and wide local drainage. Also examine the gastrojejunostomy to make sure that the afferent loop is patent. The diagnosis of an afferent loop syndrome (kinked or angulated loop distal to the leak) can be excluded pre-operatively with endoscopy.

Leaking closure of perforated duodenal ulcer
When reoperating for a **leaking closure of perforated duodenal ulcer** you have more than one option. If the diagnosis has been made 'early' and the tissues still in relatively good shape you should do what should have been done originally: a proper omentopexy! Assure that it is watertight and place drains in the vicinity. **In neglected cases I would recommend adding a pyloric exclusion (see below).** I have to mention, however, that there are reports (from India) of successful management of a leaking omentopexy by inserting a T-tube into the perforation and local drainage. **No, there are no prospective, randomized studies to show which of the above approaches is the 'best' — you have to use your judgment and common sense!**

What to do with a leaking gastroduodenostomy?
The management of a **leaking gastroduodenostomy** (Billroth I) anastomosis is more complex. As you remember, this is a side leak, so if the patient and his tissues are 'stable' and his nutrition status not dreadful, I would opt for converting

it to a Billroth II reconstruction: dismantle the gastroduodenostomy, place a tube in the duodenal stump and add a nice gastrojejunostomy (hand-sewn — remember the tissues are edematous!); add drains and don't forget to pass a feeding tube down the efferent loop. In **desperate situations** I would recommend that you take down the anastomosis, fashion a tube duodenostomy, and bring the end of the stomach out as a gastrostomy. **This is a lifesaving procedure!** After a few months you can come back and join the stomach to the jejunum.

What to do with a leaking gastrojejunostomy?

This fortunately is a rather rare complication because both small bowel and the stomach have such an excellent blood supply, are mobile and so forth. I said "fortunately" rare because if it does occur it behaves like a 'side' gastric leak, combined with a proximal small bowel leak — and this makes its management highly problematic. If you reoperate for an 'early' leak (i.e. within a day or two after the index operation) and local circumstances are favorable you may be tempted to create a new gastrojejunostomy (preferably hand sutured). Otherwise, your best chance to save the patient is to **dismantle the anastomosis**, bring the gastric stump out as a gastrostomy and exteriorize the small bowel — with a feeding tube down the distal loop. This may sound a rather radical solution but if you are not radical now, there may not be a patient left for reoperation! If the leaking small bowel loop is proximal it may not reach the skin level: solutions for this problem are discussed below in the section on small bowel.

Leaking gastrostomies or PEG tubes (percutaneous endoscopic gastrostomy)

As a huge number of these tubes are being inserted around the world for feeding purposes in debilitated patients it is not a surprise that we encounter leaks from the insertion site. Most such leaks involve gastric contents leaking to the *outside* around the tube, a minor problem which is beyond the scope of this chapter; but what is to be done if you suspect that the leak is *inside*? Diagnosis is with a contrast study (+/- CT) via the tube. Contained leaks can be treated conservatively — the tube is left in place on gravity drainage waiting for the surrounding tissue to seal before repeating the contrast study and attempting feeding. As with any non-operative (and operative) treatment of GI leaks, **antibiotics are given**. Operative treatment is mandatory with free intraperitoneal leaks and signs of SIRS and peritonitis. In the absence of significant tissue edema, a purse-string suture can be reinserted around the G-tube and the stomach carefully attached to the abdominal wall all around the tube. Otherwise, the tube should be removed and the hole in the stomach carefully closed. Consider inserting a jejunostomy tube based on the condition of the patient and the degree of peritonitis.

Pyloric exclusion

I promised to describe 'pyloric exclusion'. Some surgeons recommend cross-stapling the pylorus, adding a gastrojejunostomy. I prefer this technique: place a small gastrotomy just proximal to the pylorus, grasp the actual *pyloric ring* with a tissue forceps and pull it out into the wound. With a running heavy non-absorbable suture close the pylorus, making sure to take bites of the actual muscle layer, not just the mucosa that is surprisingly thick; finally, anastomose a loop of proximal jejunum to the antral opening. Don't forget to guide a feeding tube into the efferent loop. Whatever suture material you have used to close the pylorus (some surgeons would use absorbable sutures) the closure will dehisce within a month or two (and the same applies to a stapled closure). The gastrojejunostomy will continue to be patent 'forever', prone to the risks of stomal ulcers, bile reflux and dumping — unless electively closed. For this reason some surgeons would omit the gastrojejunostomy — instead they would pass a fine-bore feeding tube (through the nose, or through a gastrostomy), through the pylorus and into the proximal jejunum and only then suture close the pylorus around the tube. Is this a better alternative? I don't know. Chapter 24 will tell you that some recent studies voiced doubts about the advantages of pyloric exclusion. Yet another controversy in a controversial field…

Another point: when reoperating for UGI leaks check <u>all</u> anastomoses. When one suture line leaks (e.g. duodenal stump) the others (e.g. gastrojejunostomy) are at risk of being 'chewed' by the surrounding infective/corrosive peritoneal environment.

Management of UGI fistulas

So now, thank God, when you have succeeded in controlling the leak you are left with an enterocutaneous fistula to treat. You are starting to see the end of the forest but it is — to paraphrase Winston Churchill — only the beginning of the end, if not the end of the beginning. The general principles of management are the same for all enterocutaneous fistulas, and these will be discussed below in the section dedicated to the small bowel. Here are a few points specific to the UGI.

The late Dr. Etienne Levy of Paris accumulated a large experience with gastroduodenal fistulas and his publications from the 1980s are worth looking at. He emphasized the corrosive nature of the effluent from duodenal fistulas and the method of controlling them. I successfully used his tactic a few times as follows: the duodenal hole is cannulated with a soft silastic tube. A few similar tubes are placed in the adjacent spaces; one tube serves to *continuously* irrigate the space with large amounts of saline, the other is connected to suction — this serves to dilute/neutralize the corrosive juices leaking around the duodenal tube. Eventually, over a few weeks, as the duodenum heals around the intraluminal tube, the suction tube drains only what is being infused into the irrigating tube. The irrigation is stopped, contrast is injected into the duodenal tube to confirm that nothing leaks around it and one by one the peri-duodenal tubes are removed. Over the next week or so the duodenal tube is gradually removed to lie outside the duodenal wall; it is completely removed when it dries up. **One**

has to ensure (with a sinogram) that the tip of the shortened tube is not abutting the duodenal hole as this impedes its closure!

> The technique we often use: one or usually two large, silicon drains with side holes are placed near the leak site at operation to achieve some sort of source control, carefully ensuring that the drains are not inside the hole preventing it from closing. Once the tract has formed, after about two weeks, one of the drains is shortened, about 2cm every three days, until the first side holes are visible and the drain is removed. Then the second drain is shortened in a similar way and finally removed. Often, the pressure of the external tissue overcomes the pressure of the lumen and the fistula closes. Even if not, it is a long fistula tract that can be later manipulated with glue, etc., if secretion is prolonged. **Ari**

There are many ways to win the battle. I offered you mine; I don't claim that mine is the best but I hope you will try it. We also say in China, "talk doesn't fight on the battlefield." So I will stop here.

4 Small intestine
Moshe Schein and Mark Cheetham [5]

Astonishingly, there is very little in the literature about postoperative leaks from the small bowel (SB). If you search "anastomotic leaks" — on Google, PUBMED or in the various books — you will find many articles and chapters on the incidence and management of leaks after colorectal, esophageal and bariatric surgery, but very little specific to leaking SB. Why is this so?:

- In comparison to anastomoses in the other locations — leakage from SB anastomoses is rare. The well-perfused, mobile, easily accessible SB is easier to anastomose and its suture line less likely to leak.
- Each of us has personal experience with only a few cases which we try to forget — one does not want to remember NIGHTMARES! And SB leaks are nightmares: you fire a few staplers, hop hop, so easy and fast. The patient should be farting and defecating in 3-5 days but instead his abdominal wound is soaked in bile. *Oy vey!* And if you do not manage him correctly and promptly he is likely to die.

In the absence of any series dedicated specifically to leaks from the SB we have to base our practice on:

- Lessons learned managing leaks in the colorectal and UGI situations.
- Our own experiences managing SB leaks produced (preferably) by others.

---

[5] Mark Cheetham authored the fistulas section — see "Management of the enterocutaneous fistula" on p132.

- The (larger) experience of others. Sitting in numerous M&M meetings and reviewing a large number of legal cases of anastomotic leaks, provided me with many examples on how NOT to treat SB leaks...

In the previous sections you have heard enough about "Pre-operative considerations". There is also no need to dwell again on how to create a safe small bowel anastomosis. So let us jump directly into "Postoperative considerations."

Postoperative considerations

The general principles of diagnosis and management laid down in the first section of this chapter are pertinent also to the SB and I do not want to repeat myself. What is true to UGI and colorectal leaks is true for the SB situation — the consequences of leak are varied: some leaks are localized, some are walled off, and some are 'free'. Some leaks find a way to the outside, through the drain or the incision, producing a controlled fistula, and some are uncontrolled. So, one has to tailor the treatment — non-operative management, PC drainage, or laparotomy — to the specific clinical scenario. In our other book on abdominal emergencies I wrote a chapter about the management of SB anastomotic leaks [6]. I don't want to be accused of self-plagiarism but for readers who don't have our previous book I will summarize here briefly the key points relevant to the topic.

Please note that the present discussion is relevant not only to leaking SB suture lines but also to SB leaks from **unrecognized incidental enterotomies** during the index operation. These can be caused by reckless use of diathermy or other energy sources (the plague of laparoscopy!), harsh retraction, traumatic separation of adhesions or blind insertion of lap trocars — real catastrophes! A postop leak is a leak — it doesn't matter whether it comes from an anastomosis or operative injury.

A few words about the diagnosis

As you already know, a 'visible' leak is a diagnostic no-brainer but the diagnosis of a 'concealed' leak is trickier in the SB compared to the UGI or the colon-rectum. **While a contrast study from *below*, or *above*, +/- a CT, usually confirms the diagnosis in the foregut or colorectal locations, it rarely does so in the SB**. In fact, the sensitivity and specificity of CT combined with oral contrast is very low in diagnosing SB anastomotic leaks!

---

[6] *Schein's Common Sense Emergency Abdominal Surgery*, 3rd Ed. Springer Verlag, © 2010: Chapter 50.

In most cases proved at relaparotomy (or autopsy) as having leaked from the SB, the pre-operative CT did not demonstrate extravasation of contrast outside the lumen of the bowel — the contrast may be flowing freely into the colon but this doesn't exclude a leak. Of course CT findings of free gas or liquid are common during the first postoperative days (and even beyond), but still — **the most frequent and thus suggestive CT feature in patients with a proven SB leak are air bubbles and fluid in the vicinity of the anastomosis**. Such allegedly *non-specific* CT findings, visualized in a patient with the 'soft' and *non-specific* clinical features hinting at a leak (as described in the first section of this chapter) are often the most specific indication that the patient is leaking from the SB. **In most cases, waiting for the 'dry drain' to show bile or feces, waiting for bowel contents to appear in the wound, waiting for contrast to pour into the peritoneal cavity, is like waiting for the *Messiah* — instead of the *Messiah* the *Malach HaMavet* (Devil of Death) will arrive...**

A few words about management

Again, if the SB leak is **well controlled** (through a drain or the wound), the patient is 'well', and you have excluded associated intra-abdominal collections (or managed them percutaneously) you can sit on your hands and manage the enterocutaneous fistula (see below). In all other cases **you have to reoperate in order to control the leak**.

As you will read in the following section about colorectal leaks, the message is clear: **never, never-ever consider a reanastomosis**. In the preceding chapters on esophageal and UGI leaks you learned that attempts at repairing leaks or doing a reanastomosis are doomed to fail. In the UGI situation it isn't easy to divert or dismantle the anastomosis. So, most surgeons would try to patch the leaking site and improve the drainage — knowing that 'patching' never works and that a few days later the leak will redevelop. The hope/aim is to achieve a controlled fistula which will, eventually, close. **What is true in all other anatomical situations is true for the SB: reanastomosis or repair will fail, and failure means disaster!**

I don't claim that 'repair' of a leaking anastomosis, or a reanastomosis, is never successful or has no place at all. I also understand the tremendous psychological urge experienced by the surgeon to try and restore bowel continuity at all costs! You resected a segment of small bowel — say for a Meckel's diverticulum — a relatively straightforward operation — and now, a few days later, you find yourself reoperating for a leaking anastomosis. Exteriorize the anastomosis? SB stoma? How are you going to face the patient and his family? So you think: hell, what a flop! Let me fix it ASAP... let me try it again, let's take the chance — anything to avoid a high-output SB stoma with its prolonged morbidity. Well, each of us can recall an isolated case where a repair/reanastomosis was successful, but the **overwhelming experience indicates a prohibitive rate of failure**. Attempts to close an intestinal leak, after a few days, in an infected peritoneal cavity are doomed to fail. By now, the patient is catabolic, his intestine swollen, the albumin level low, and in most cases the underlying factors which led to the leak in the first place are even more pronounced — he will leak again and a re-leak is almost equivalent to death. You may wonder why we nag you with this point *ad nauseum* in this chapter: it is because we see surgeons committing this sin again and again!

So what are the circumstances in which you can entertain the idea of reanastomosis (never-ever a simple repair!)?:

- When the leak presents within a day or two of the operation — usually caused by a technical mishap.
- When the bowel appears of 'good quality'.
- When the patient is stable and SIRS minimal.
- When the peritoneal milieu is friendly.
- When the albumin level is reasonable.

In such rather exceptional situations resect the leaking point or anastomosis and reanastomose carefully — I would do it by hand!

Otherwise you should resort to the logical and lifesaving option of exteriorization — at any level.

How to exteriorize?

The simplest way is to bring the leak to the skin level as a loop enterostomy. But this is not always easy. The now thickened intestine and mesentery may prevent the loop reaching to the surface of the skin. The fat-laden mesentery in our increasingly obese population doesn't make life easier. Commonly in such circumstances you have to leave the abdomen open (laparostomy) and the stoma must be sited away from the central abdominal defect — this further hampers exteriorization. Sometimes the solution is to divide the bowel, exteriorizing the ends separately, or even closing the distal end. If the leaking segment cannot be exteriorized you may have to drain it and divert by exteriorizing a more mobile proximal loop of SB.

Another viable solution when the bowel reaches the level of the peritoneum — but not the skin — is to create a tube enterostomy. Place a Foley catheter into the leaking hole, secure it in place with a purse-string suture, inflate the balloon (but not too much so as not to obstruct the lumen), and bring the catheter out of the skin. Suture the loop to the anterior abdominal wall around the tube; finally place suction drains in the vicinity to evacuate any bowel contents which may escape around the tube. In due time (usually weeks) when local and systemic sepsis is under control you will be able to remove the tube — but only after a contrast study shows no leak around it: *Voilà* — **you have created a controlled SB fistula!**

There are situations in which the leaking loop won't be able to reach the abdominal wall — for example, a leaking enterotomy just distal to the ligament of Treitz. Here you'll have to improvise: intubate the hole with a soft tube, place suction drains around to catch what's leaking around the tube and pray for a controlled fistula to develop.

Management of the enterocutaneous fistula

I wrote about this topic in our previous book[7] and elsewhere so I would prefer to let another expert offer his version — **Mark Cheetham** (the author of ➲ Chapter 14).

You did a difficult diverticular resection a week ago. This morning you are called to the ward by the nurse because there is small bowel content pouring from the wound. This is every surgeon's nightmare; what should you do? Firstly — resist the overwhelming urge to reoperate (we know you are a surgeon and that's what you do, but here there is a good chance you will make the situation worse). To steal a British Second World War slogan: "Keep calm and carry on."

SNAPP is a useful *aide memoire* in this situation although we did not invent this acronym:

- **Sepsis**. Aggressively treat sepsis. This involves resuscitation and giving appropriate antibiotics. **Have a low threshold for CT scanning** — sepsis in this situation may present with very subtle findings. If you find an intra-abdominal collection avoid operating; instead find the radiologist with the biggest *cojones* and get the collection drained percutaneously. Reserve surgery for situations when the patient has peritonitis or sepsis that cannot be controlled by percutaneous drainage. Reoperation carries a high chance of causing bleeding and further damage to the bowel — what has started with a 'simple leak' ends with multiple holes in the bowel and a laparostomy.

---

[7] *Schein's Common Sense Emergency Abdominal Surgery*, 3rd Ed. Springer Verlag, © 2010: Chapter 50.

- **Nutrition**. After sepsis, lack of nutrition is the most significant risk to your patient. Traditionally patients with enterocutaneous fistulas were always treated with intravenous nutrition (as an aside we dislike the term "TPN" — as, almost always, patients treated with i.v. nutrition are allowed to eat and drink as well). Consider this: a newly formed ileostomy often has an output of 1000ml/day — would you treat that with i.v. feeding? No, so why should a leaking distal small bowel anastomosis be different? Many patients with an enterocutaneous fistula may be maintained on a normal diet or with enteral feeding. With a proximal fistula, especially if the bowel has been exteriorized, consider instilling feeds into the distal limb; collect what is coming from above and infuse it distally. **There is no doubt that the outcome is better with enteral nutrition! So don't be lazy — be creative**.

- **Anatomy**. Define the anatomy: where does the fistula originate? Is there an associated collection? To define the anatomy accurately will require a combination of cross-sectional imaging and contrast studies (small bowel follow through and fistulograms). You may have difficulty in arranging some of these contrast studies; modern radiologists seem to have developed a distinct aversion to latex tubes, orifices and bodily fluids. You have to go with the patient to radiology and show them where to inject and what you want to see. Don't nominate your intern for this task: the patient may never 'forgive' you for inflicting the leak on him but your presence now could assuage the anger.

- **Protect** the skin. Small bowel contents contain proteolytic enzymes which will rapidly digest the skin around the fistula. You (and your enterostomal nurse — if you have one) need to protect the skin using stoma paste, suction tubes and stoma appliances. A certain degree of creativity is needed to construct something to protect the skin reliably for a good period of time. Rarely, inability to protect the skin will tip your hand and force you to operate early — in this situation do not try to be too clever and certainly do not perform an anastomosis. Raise a proximal stoma and get out (actually, just getting into the abdomen and making a stoma at this stage is a difficult and dangerous undertaking).

- **Plan definitive surgery**. Do not expect to operate soon. If you have made the patient 'safe' by doing the above then there is no hurry. We would wait until the albumin level is normal (in the acute phase albumin is a poor measure of nutrition but an excellent broad-spectrum indicator of poor outcome). This may take 6-9 months or so. Use this time to rehabilitate your patient and review the imaging studies. Many of these patients can be managed at home. Yes, we know that in some parts of the world facilities for i.v. nutrition or local care of fistulas are lacking; we know that the patient and family are pressurizing you to restore bowel continuity as soon as possible. But be resilient to the pressures — do not surrender! Of course, if your local facilities are not optimal and you can refer the patient to a larger institution then do it. Sometimes it is better to let others manage your disasters...

Of course, not all patients will need to undergo late definitive reconstruction. With proper supportive management, and in the absence of distal obstruction or loss of bowel continuity (i.e. when exteriorization was not needed), **about a third of postoperative small bowel fistulas will close spontaneously within six weeks**. Those that fail to close by this time will require elective reoperation. This, when performed on an anabolic, non-SIRS patient, in a less hostile peritoneal environment, will restore the integrity of the gastrointestinal tract with an acceptable risk of complications.

Remember: in unselected series of postoperative enterocutaneous fistulas, a third of patients die — the vast majority from neglected intra-abdominal infection.

Finally: when you are reoperating for an intestinal leak you are actually dealing with **postoperative peritonitis**. To do justice to this entity — including the management of abdominal compartment syndrome, and how to deal with the commonly occurring abdominal wall defects and complex 'exposed fistulas' within it — a few more chapters are needed. If you wish to see what we had to say about these matters please consult our previous book.

5 Large bowel and rectum [8]
Caitlin W. Hicks, Jonathan E. Efron

The actual incidence of anastomotic leaks following colonic or colorectal anastomoses is difficult to define, but ranges from 2-20%. This difficulty arises from defining who has a leak and whether the leaks are deemed clinically significant. Leaks are much more prevalent than we surgeons like to believe. Colorectal anastomoses are qualitatively different from colo-colic and small bowel anastomoses because of a multitude of anatomic and physiologic issues. When studied in all patients undergoing a low anterior resection, leak rates have been reported as high as 35%! Although a surgeon never likes to admit to the possibility of a leak, it is important to maintain a low threshold of suspicion for leaks since the associated mortality may be as high as 35%. By working effectively to prevent, identify, and manage leaks early in the course of their development, we hope to minimize the morbidity and mortality that can devastate affected patients.

---

[8] See also Chapter 14.

Pre-operative considerations

Prior to surgery, patients should be screened for any comorbidites that may place them at increased risk for an anastomotic leak. The general factors found to be associated with anastomotic leaks were discussed in the first section of this chapter. When identified, consideration should be given to correcting the potential risk factor prior to elective surgery, if possible. Here are a few considerations which, we believe, are of special importance in colorectal surgery.

Immunocompromised patients

Immunocompromised patients are generally at the highest risk for anastomotic breakdown because of impaired wound healing. **Patients who have been on chemotherapy within one month of surgery or have been using steroids and/or other immunomodulator therapy deserve special consideration during operative planning to ensure that they are fit for surgery — physically and psychologically**. If possible, patients using high-dose steroids (>40mg prednisone) and other biologic immmunomodulators (e.g. infliximab) should be weaned from therapy at least one week before surgery. If not possible, **proximal diversion is highly recommended**.

Obese patients

Obese patients (body mass index, BMI >30kg/m^2) also deserve special consideration, since their common comorbidities (hypertension, diabetes, sleep apnea, etc.) put them at a higher risk for postoperative complications in general, and anastomotic leaks in particular. Obese patients undergoing elective surgery may be encouraged to pursue a weight loss regimen prior to their procedure, but this is not always feasible within an appropriate time frame and is often not achieved anyway. The increased weight from extra mesenteric fat or appendices epiploicae can put tension on the anastomosis despite adequate bowel mobilization, and maneuvers such as a high ligation of the inferior mesenteric artery should be considered in obese patients to relieve this tension. **Maintain a low threshold for proximal diversion in those patients who are morbidly obese** (BMI >40) — not forgetting the added morbidity of stomas exteriorized through an obese abdominal wall (isn't the practice of surgery a little similar to a Russian roulette?).

Malnourished patients

Patients who are malnourished, with significant weight loss (>10% of bodyweight) and albumin <3.0g/dL, should be considered for pre- and/or peri-operative nutritional supplementation. Although not directly associated with reduced leak rates, nutritional support has been shown to improve overall postoperative outcomes in malnourished patients with gastrointestinal cancer. All surgical patients should start early enteral nutrition postoperatively, and total parenteral nutrition (TPN) may be necessary for those in whom enteral feeding is not possible, particularly in the malnourished. Correcting significant malnourishment with 4-6 weeks of TPN prior to elective surgery should be considered if enteral feeding is not possible, especially in patients with chronic conditions such as inflammatory bowel disease.

Mechanical bowel preparation

Mechanical bowel preparation in patients undergoing elective colorectal surgery was traditionally thought to protect against anastomotic leaks and other infectious complications, but there is little or no evidence to support this notion. Recent evidence indicates that preparation with oral antibiotics may reduce the rate of wound infection. The routine use of mechanical bowel preparation as a means to reduce anastomotic leak rates is not indicated, especially in open colonic surgery; however, it may help reduce the rate of abdominal wall complications. The use of bowel preparation for low rectal resections and laparoscopic procedures is currently less clear due to a paucity of data on the subject; however, cleansing the colon of stool makes it easier to manipulate laparoscopically because it is lighter. Having the rectum and sigmoid colon clear of solid stool facilitates stapled anastomosis when performing low anterior resections. Multiple randomized prospective trials have demonstrated that there is no difference in anastomotic leak rate between patients who have undergone mechanical bowel preparation and those who have not; however, recent data indicate those patients who perform a bowel preparation with oral antibiotics prior to colorectal resection will have lower surgical site infections. We currently perform mechanical bowel preparations with the addition of oral antibiotics. Since initiating this practice we have seen a reduction in our surgical site infection rate. (For the British take on this issue read ➲ Chapter 14.)

History

History of Crohn's disease and history of radiation to the resected area increase the leaking risk. Be ready to divert.

Intra-operative considerations

The main intra-operative factors increasing the risk of anastomotic leak include a high volume of **blood loss** (i.e. >500ml) and a **low anastomosis**. An anastomosis within 5cm of the dentate line almost doubles the risk and some experts suggest that any extraperitoneal anastomosis should be included in this high-risk group. In general, **the risk of leak following extraperitoneal resection of the rectum is inversely related to the distance of the anastomosis from the anal verge**.

Anastomotic technique

Multiple studies comparing stapled and hand-sewn anastomoses have demonstrated equivalent results for the two techniques. Most low colorectal anastomoses are performed by stapling, given the difficulty of suturing in the pelvis. The invention of EEA staplers (yes, we have to acknowledge that the Russians were the pioneers...) was undoubtedly a significant advance in the surgical management of rectal cancer.

Divert or not to divert?

There is significant debate surrounding the use of proximal diversion during the initial surgery in order to reduce complications occurring from a leak. Although diversion has not been shown to reduce the incidence of anastomotic leak, there is evidence suggesting that **the morbidity and mortality resulting from a leak is decreased in patients who are diverted**. Notably, a low rectal anastomotic leak that is not diverted will often lead to pelvic inflammation causing scarring in the deep pelvis, particularly near the anorectal ring. This scarring may significantly affect the overall function of the colo-anal or ileo-anal anastomosis, worsening urgency and frequency seen with 'low anterior resection syndrome'. Of course, stomas are not without their own risks (e.g. peristomal skin irritation, dehydration, obstruction), and the **complications of stoma reversal** can be significant (e.g. anastomotic leak, wound infection, fistula formation, bleeding, and hernia). **There is no right answer as to whether a patient should or should not be diverted at their initial operation.** However, from the information available it seems sensible that those at high risk of an anastomotic leak should be diverted. When an anastomosis is felt *not* to be intact because of a positive air test or obvious defects are visualized in the anastomosis, the best solution is to **redo the anastomosis**. However, when a colorectal anastomosis is low in the pelvis, this may not be feasible and suture repair of the anastomotic defect with proximal diversion is mandatory. Disease states requiring **hand-sewn colo-**

anal anastomoses such as ultra-low rectal cancers or rectal dysplasia in patients with colitis also require proximal diversion. Stapled anastomoses that are performed near the dentate line that have evidence of a defect can often be repaired with greater ease through the anus than via an abdominal approach; proximal diversion is recommended if this is required.

The pre-operative considerations discussed above, surgeon experience, and specific procedure performed should all play a role in the decision about diversion. **In general, if you think that a patient may need a proximal diversion — they probably do**.

Ileal pouch-anal anastomosis (IPAA) procedures are associated with a 5-10% leak rate. The risk may be even higher among patients using high-dose steroids (>40mg prednisone) or biologic immunomodulators (e.g. infliximab), although this is a topic of some debate. It is a rare patient who does not have some tension on their ileal pouch-anal anastomosis, therefore patients undergoing IPAA procedures are generally diverted because of this high-risk status. In general, the same principle regarding diversion that we recommend for other colorectal procedures should be applied to IPAAs: **if the notion that a patient might need proximal diversion crosses your mind, do it**. In general we divert all immunosuppressed patients undergoing IPAA.

The role of drains and intraluminal devices

Other intra-operative considerations to reduce anastomotic leak include the use of mechanical intraluminal devices and pelvic drains:

- The role of **pelvic drains** in preventing leaks is controversial but we routinely place pelvic drains after proctectomy with a low anastomosis. There are no data to support or refute their use but our routine practice is to place them for any anastomosis below the peritoneal reflection. They are removed on postoperative day two or three if the drainage is serous. Yes, we know, many surgeons would omit pelvic drainage all together.
- **Intraluminal devices**, including transanal decompression, intraluminal, and biodegradable protective devices, have been employed in a number of animal and non-randomized human studies with low leakage rates. However, data from randomized clinical trials evaluating these devices are lacking, and their use is often time consuming and costly. There has also been some worrying evidence of worsening overall leakage rates with the transanal stent. Thus we do not currently endorse the use of any mechanical intraluminal device to prevent anastomotic leaks, and recommend that surgeons take caution when

utilizing innovative devices that have not been proven to be of benefit in well-constructed randomized, prospective trials.

Postoperative considerations

The key postoperative considerations in managing a colorectal anastomotic leak are early detection and intervention.

Timing

Anastomotic leaks following colonic or colorectal anastomoses usually occur between postoperative days five and ten, most commonly on postoperative day seven. However, a leak may occur anywhere between 24 hours and three weeks following surgery, so it is imperative that surgeons maintain a heightened awareness for potential leak symptoms throughout this time period.

Signs and symptoms

Signs and symptoms of an anastomotic leak can be highly varied, making the clinical diagnosis a difficult one. Patients may present with low-grade fever, tachycardia, hypotension, or respiratory difficulty. Occasionally, the only sign that something is amiss may be chest pain or a cardiac arrhythmia. Abdominal pain and tenderness may be diffuse or localized, **but is often difficult to distinguish from normal postoperative incisional pain**. As a result, sometimes the best method of assessment is how the patient's pain on examination compares to his/her pain from an earlier time point; worsening tenderness or pain that changes from localized to diffuse should be considered worrisome for leak until proven otherwise. Similarly, patients with pain out of proportion to their procedure — for example, a patient who underwent a laparoscopic right hemicolectomy that reports pain so severe that he/she cannot get out of bed — should be approached with a high suspicion for leak.

Some patients with leaks will have nausea, vomiting, and bloating that is consistent with **ileus**, but others will continue to pass flatus and have bowel movements. **Remember: the return of bowel function does not rule out the presence of an anastomotic leak** [9]. In fact, if a patient with a possible leak is

---

[9]   I recall a patient with a totally disrupted colorectal anastomosis who experienced massive diarrhea-infected intraperitoneal fluids decompressing through the open rectum [Moshe].

having bowel movements, the surgeon should use this to his/her advantage and check for blood in the stool: **the presence of hematochezia, low-grade fever, and tachycardia is almost certainly indicative of leak** — calling for immediate diagnostic steps and intervention.

Diagnosis

Patients with signs of sepsis and diffuse peritonitis belong in the operating room undergoing re-exploration. Those patients who have some indicators of sepsis but are clinically stable and without diffuse peritonitis can be observed while undergoing further work-up with radiological studies. A gentle rectal exam may confirm the presence of, or rule out, anastomotic leak in patients who have had a colo-anal or ileo-anal anastomosis. While the exam may be uncomfortable, severe pain and discomfort are highly suspicious for anastomotic disruption. Drainage of pus after digital exam is also concerning and if disruption of a low anastomosis is suspected, examination under anesthesia with transanal drainage is appropriate if there is no evidence of diffuse peritonitis.

It should be noted that diagnosing a leak in both immunocompromised and obese patients can be difficult, the latter because of difficulties performing an adequate abdominal exam and the former because they may not be able to mount an effective systemic inflammatory response. Thus the threshold for suspicion of leak must be low in both of these groups to prevent any delay in diagnosis. These patients often need radiological exams to help the surgeon confirm the diagnosis, and if there is doubt early return to the operating room.

Diagnostic work-up

The gold standard for diagnosing a colorectal anastomotic leak is a *Gastrografin®* *enem*a. However, a CT scan of the abdomen and pelvis with i.v. and rectal contrast is becoming increasingly more common, especially since the sensitivity of this modality is higher than that of the enema alone. CT also allows for better delineation of surrounding anatomy, including identification of abscess cavities, and definitive treatment via CT-guided percutaneous drainage if appropriate. Either a Gastrografin® enema or a CT scan with i.v. and rectal contrast is appropriate for working up a patient with suspected anastomotic leak, and the choice of one modality over the other should be based on availability, local expertise, and surgeon preference. **It is important to note that barium should not be used in the diagnosis of bowel leak because of its**

significant inflammatory effects in the peritoneal cavity. When performing either of these tests in a patient with a low anastomosis, the surgeon must ensure that the balloon on the catheter used to infuse the contrast is not inflated. Inflating the catheter balloon in patients with a low anastomosis may obscure the anastomosis and prevent visualization of the leak. **It is also helpful if the surgeon is present during the study both to assist with the catheter insertion and to view the exam**. Gastrografin® enemas are dynamic tests and need to be visualized in real time to obtain maximum benefit from the test. In many academic institutions they are delegated to junior radiology residents who may not have the experience and knowledge needed to perform or interpret the tests. Indeed the art of the contrast enema is being lost as a greater emphasis is placed on CT scans and MRIs.

Management

All patients with anastomotic leaks require a course of broad-spectrum i.v. antibiotics, regardless of the size or extent of the defect. An **anti-fungal drug** should be included in this regimen if the patient has been in hospital and/or on proton pump inhibitors. **Beyond this, management of a colorectal leak depends on whether it is free vs. contained, major vs. minor, and symptomatic vs. asymptomatic**.

Free leaks
Free leaks are associated with generalized peritonitis and sepsis, and require urgent laparotomy following a short period of hemodynamic resuscitation. In the operating room, the leak should be located and identified as a **major defect** (>1/3 of the anastomotic circumference) or **minor defect** (<1/3 of the anastomotic circumference). Minor defects can be managed through **primary repair, proximal diversion** (with either a loop ileostomy or loop colostomy), and peritoneal toilet. This option also requires that the proximal and distal bowel appears viable and healthy. Often all that can be done to achieve closure are large full-thickness simple sutures. **Drainage of the anastomotic repair** and evacuated abscess cavity is strongly recommended. Major defects should be managed more aggressively, including **complete take-down of the anastomosis** with creation of an end colostomy, wide drainage, and peritoneal toilet. If a large amount of stool is found in the distal colon or rectum, then **rectal irrigation** is also recommended, along with leaving a transanal rectal tube for decompression. At times the rectal stump after take-down of the anastomosis may be so inflamed that closure is not possible by either staples or sutures. In these cases wide drainage with a transanal rectal drain such as a large *Malecot* catheter is recommended in addition to multiple transabdominal pelvic drains.

The use of large (number one) chromic sutures will often allow the surgeon to suture very inflamed tissue thereby approximating the bowel wall.

Contained leaks

Contained leaks can be managed by CT-guided drainage (in the case of an intraperitoneal leak) or examination under anesthesia with transanal drainage (in the case of extraperitoneal leaks) and i.v. antibiotics. In these cases, if there is worsening pain or signs of sepsis following initial treatment, laparotomy should be considered and management should proceed as outlined above. If the patient's condition improves with drainage and antibiotics, observation alone is sufficient. **Contained leaks managed via percutaneous drainage** will either heal spontaneously or form a **controlled fistula**. Patients should be assessed for the presence of a fistula via a fistulogram, either through fluoroscopy or a CT scan, following resolution of sepsis. Long-term drainage with gradual drain removal may allow for spontaneous healing when the abscess cavity collapses (usually after 2-3 weeks of drainage). If a repeat fistulogram shows no further connection between the anastomosis and the cavity after 6-8 weeks of drainage, the drain can be removed. If a connection remains, continued drainage is recommended until the patient can undergo reoperation to address the defect. **Reoperation should be deferred for six months**, if possible, to allow for resolution of intra-abdominal inflammation. **Frequently, an anastomotic stricture will develop following a contained leak**. These strictures may require interventions such as endoscopic balloon dilatation or (for low anastomoses) transanal dilatation. Repeated dilatation may be required and should be pursued prior to reoperation; however, if reoperation is required, repeat colo-anal anastomosis is possible with adequate postoperative function.

Asymptomatic leaks

Asymptomatic leaks occur in as many as 10% of colorectal anastomoses, and are most commonly diagnosed following a routine Gastrografin® enema prior to stoma reversal. Observation alone is usually sufficient in these patients, as most such leaks will heal spontaneously.

In summary, we can try and prevent anastomotic leaks following colorectal surgery by considering all potential risk factors pre- and intra-operatively that may contribute to their development and attempting to correct those that can be corrected prior to operating. However, not all risk factors are modifiable, and leaks are an indisputable complication of some procedures. Low anastomoses and patients at high risk for leak should be proximally diverted to reduce morbidity following any potential leak, and surgeons should maintain a high suspicion in the first two weeks postoperatively. Any patient with a suspected leak should be worked up via a Gastrografin® enema and/or CT of the abdomen and pelvis with i.v. and rectal contrast. Management should be based on whether the leak is free or contained, major or minor, symptomatic or asymptomatic. Mortality rates from colorectal anastomotic leaks range from a few percent to as high as 35%. Some short-term morbidities for these patients include wound complication, prolonged ileus, hernias, and delaying adjuvant therapy for stage 3 and 4 cancer. Longer-term issues are usually related to intestinal function with worsening 'low anterior resection syndrome' seen in patients that leak. The fibrosis that develops after pelvic sepsis worsens urgency, frequency, and incontinence secondary to stenosis and lack of rectal pliability. **Approximately 20% of these patients eventually end up with a permanent stoma secondary to poor function**. Notably, leaks after cancer surgery result in decreased long-term survival.

With an appropriate preventive and management strategy, we can minimize the complications associated with anastomotic leak, and improve outcomes of patients undergoing colonic or rectal resections. **Finally, when in doubt — reoperate! In the end this decreases the morbidity and mortality associated with anastomotic leaks. Early reoperation saves lives!**

"Anastomosis is like your baby: you may have fun creating it, but then it affects your life immensely; it makes you anxious for its safety and integrity, and quite often wakes you up at night. But if it matures as a healthy and functioning creation... your pride and satisfaction are endless."

Danny

Chapter 7

Abdominal wall dehiscence

Moshe Schein, Paul N. Rogers, Ari Leppäniemi and Danny Rosin

There are few things more embarrassing to a surgeon than the sight of his recently operated patient, his abdomen gaping, and the gut spilling out all around...

Such a catastrophe occurs either because you did not close the tummy properly or it should not have been closed at all. And because we are all such good surgeons, and possess superb judgment, our incidence of *complete* postoperative abdominal wound dehiscence should be negligible. Over the last 20 years we do not recall having to take a patient back to the operating room to reclose a burst abdomen. But from time to time we have had to do it for other surgeons (e.g. gynecologists) and this experience provided us with the opportunity to learn what they did wrong, and to savour the sweet-sour taste of *Schadenfreude* ☺.

From colleagues working in the developing world (e.g. India), and from the literature, we learn that in some deprived environments dehiscence of the abdominal wound is still quite common, with some centers lucky to gather up to 60 cases over four years. This obviously reflects the fact that they have to operate on neglected, undernourished patients under adverse conditions — often lacking proper suture material or even training.

Let us start with some **basic definitions**: like everything in surgery (and life) so too dehiscence has a spectrum:

- **Complete dehiscence**: is full partition of the fascia and skin. Loops of small bowel — if not glued in place by adhesions — eviscerate or are completely exposed at the base of the gaping wound.

- **Partial dehiscence**: is a separation of the fascial edges of the wound without evisceration but often with exposure of the underlying viscera. The fascial gap varies in width and length — in some cases you may glimpse a loop of bowel at the bottom of the defect; in others the only sign of dehiscence would be some serosanguineous peritoneal fluid seeping through the wound.

In some series, cases of *complete* dehiscence outnumber the *partial* ones. But this is an artifact: while the true incidence of the former is known, that of the latter is not. In an unknown number of patients, partial dehiscence remains *covert* or latent with the skin intact (some surgeons preferring not to be aware of it...), only to present later as incisional hernias. So partial dehiscence is 'good news', in the short term — you do not need to reoperate; in the long term it heralds the development of an incisional hernia. And this gives us an opportunity to discuss the prevention of this late complication of surgery — so common that many surgeons do not even consider it a 'complication'; they shrug — "s**t happens".

Dehiscence, be it complete or partial, is associated with significant morbidity and mortality. Obviously, local and systemic factors contribute to such outcomes, but proper management is crucial in lessening the impact of this complication.

Pre-operative considerations

To prevent this complication you have to understand its etiology. Abdominal closure fails for one, or more, of three main reasons:

- **Patient faults** — this seems to be the main problem.
- **The suture breaks** — rare!
- **Poor surgical judgment or technique** — not so rare...

Patient faults include multiple systemic and local factors (see ■ Table 7.1), presenting before the operation or developing after it, which render the tensile strength of the fascial closure inadequate. These factors cause either *poor tissue healing* or increased *intra-abdominal pressure* (IAP) — allowing the sutures to cut through the fascia. You'll find a few of these factors in most patients who suffer dehiscence.

Naturally, some of the patient-related predisposing factors can, and should, be modulated before any elective operation (including cessation of smoking) as described in ➲ Chapter 2. This can't happen with emergency procedures

Table 7.1. Factors predisposing to abdominal wall dehiscence.

PATIENT-RELATED		SURGEON-RELATED
Poor wound healing	Increased intra-abdominal pressure	Judgment
Hypoalbuminemia — poor nutrition	Ileus or early postop small bowel obstruction	To close fascia or leave open? Close the skin only?
Systemic or local infection (deep wound infection)	Obesity	Choice of **incision**: *midline incision* responsible for most cases!
	Ascites	
Shock (reduced perfusion of abdominal wall)	Chronic cough	Choice of **suture material**
Anemia	Vomiting	Inadequate **closure technique**
Hypoxia		
		Placing **stomas** or **drains** through the main wound
Uremia		
Malignancy		
Corticosteroids		
Uncontrolled diabetes		

which, therefore, are typically more susceptible to dehiscence. Other than this, dehiscence is prevented in the operating room...

Intra-operative considerations

You can prevent dehiscence by the following.

Choosing a 'correct' incision

Vertical incisions — especially midline — are much more prone to dehiscence than transverse ones. Not only are midline incisions subjected to greater disrupting mechanical forces but in general they are chosen for 'bigger' operations, and favored in emergency situations — in sicker patients. Of course, the length of the incision does matter; and so minimal access surgery is relatively immune to this complication.

Thus, choose the abdominal access carefully in each case: Can we do it laparoscopically? Do we really need a midline incision here? Can't we remove the right colon through a transverse incision? Even when converting from a laparoscopic procedure to an open one do not rush to a midline incision. Yes, when converting from a laparoscopic appendectomy it is so tempting or allegedly convenient to 'connect' the subumbilical trocar site with the suprapubic one. But the risk of dehiscence and other complications is lower for the muscle splitting RLQ incision (⮌ Chapter 17). **In general, apply the concepts of 'minimal access' also in open surgery!**

Correctly closing the abdomen

Abdominal closure: if it looks all right, it's too tight — if it looks too loose, it's all right.

Matt Oliver

Any fisherman can teach you this: you lose the big fish either because the line breaks (not strong enough for the weight of the fish, damaged or poorly handled), the knots slip (at the junction with the hook or lure) or the fish manages to break away from the hook or lure. Commonly the fish slips away during a botched *landing*. Any avid fisherman who is also a surgeon (like Ari or Moshe; Danny runs marathons, Paul prefers golf!) knows that the two professions share numerous principles (e.g. patience and attention to detail). And this applies to abdominal closure as well.

If you choose an optimal suture material and avoid damaging it with your instruments; if you know how to throw 'safe' knots and a sufficient number of them, then the **chief cause of dehiscence will be the tissues' failure to hold the sutures** — the patient's fault. A more detailed discussion of the 'correct' abdominal closure you can find in our previous chapter [1]. The following is a brief summary:

- **Ensure optimal abdominal wall relaxation**. Ask the anesthetist to help you land the fish! Not by handling the net but by seeing to it that during closure the patient is fully asleep and relaxed. Some anesthetists wake up from their slumber (or drop yesterday's *Wall*

---

[1] *Schein's Common Sense Emergency Abdominal Surgery,* 3rd Ed. Springer Verlag, © 2010: Chapter 43.

Street Journal), when they sense that you have completed the anastomosis, or closed the perforation, and decide to wake the patient too. *(Indeed, why should they have to wait at the end of the operation for the anesthetics and muscle-relaxants to metabolize rather than drink coffee or get the next patient ready?).* But struggling with fascial closure in a non-relaxed abdomen — the patient thrashing up and down like a hooked fish — the viscera bulging out... is a recipe for poor closure and injury to the underlying bowel. When this happens, stop what you are doing, remove your hands from the operating field, and say calmly to the anesthetist: "I am not going to proceed until the patient is fully relaxed...". (Or in the UK: "I say old chap, are you completely sure this patient is fully relaxed?"). Meanwhile you can continue discussing fishing with your assistants.

- **Choose the optimal suture material.** For abdominal closure avoid rapidly absorbable suture material such as *chromic* or *dexon*. Also shun braided non-absorbable materials like silk which are associated with chronic, infected sinus formation. For single-layer closure of midline incisions use either heavy non-absorbable monofilament (e.g. nylon or *Prolene®*) or heavy 'delayed' absorbable monofilament such as *PDS®* or *Maxon ™*. For layered closure of transverse incisions you can use any of the above (we prefer an absorbable suture material) — even a heavy *Vicryl®* will do.
- **Use 'mass closure' for midline incisions.** On how to do it see the footnote [1].
- **Transverse incisions** are closed by most surgeons in two layers of continuous sutures. The first includes the peritoneum and posterior fascia (if present), the second approximates the anterior fascia.
- **Careful, layered closure of the subcutaneous layer and skin guards against *complete* dehiscence if the fascial suture line gives away.**

Moshe describes a recent case: A gynecologist performed an abdominal hysterectomy (in an obese patient) through a midline incision. He closed the abdomen using continuous Prolene® for the fascia and staples for the skin. The patient was sent home the next day with no abdominal binder. Five days later, over the weekend, she presented to the emergency room (ER) with what the ER doc suspected to be 'wound infection'. He removed a few skin staples to be greeted by prolapsing loops of intestine. I was called to reclose the abdomen.

Closure of the subcutaneous layer (interrupted absorbable sutures through the subcutaneous fascia) and suture closure of skin with interrupted sutures (we use interrupted nylon 3-0 or 4-0, in 'mattress' fashion) provide additional support and strength for the abdominal wall closure. So even if the underlying fascial closure fails, the intact superficial layers prevent complete dehiscence and often hide the partial one — producing 'closed dehiscence' — until the hernia develops.

- **Support the abdomen with binder**. We advise most patients to wear a Velcro abdominal binder after any laparotomy — whenever ambulating, for six weeks. We apply the binder over the dressing while still in the operating room. Obviously, the tightness of the binder has to be adjusted to the abdominal girth; it should not be so tight as to produce intra-abdominal hypertension. Not only does the binder support the healing fascia but most patients swear that it alleviates incisional pain.

'Retention sutures' in the high-risk abdominal closure

Classically, in patients with multiple systemic (e.g. advanced cancer) or local (e.g. peritonitis, obesity) factors predisposing to wound dehiscence, 'retention sutures' (some call them 'tension sutures') were and still are used today by many surgeons. These heavy 'through-and-through', interrupted sutures take bites of at least 2cm through all abdominal-wall layers, including the skin, preventing evisceration but probably *not* the occurrence of late hernia formation. There is no doubt that such sutures can effectively close the most horrendous looking abdominal incisions — **but at what cost?**

Such sutures cut through the skin and produce parietal damage and ugly skin wounds and scars. Fascial and skin ischemia may contribute to superficial and deep wound infections. But the main problem to consider is that **forcibly closing a distended-bulging abdomen with retention sutures commonly produces intra-abdominal hypertension** and its offspring — the **abdominal compartment syndrome** with its well-known deleterious physiological consequences. For example: if you approximate the abdominal wall under excessive tension in a hugely distended abdomen do not be surprised when your patient is not able to come off the ventilator, or that he becomes oliguric.

The first author never uses retention sutures (the others would use them extremely rarely), believing that those patients who do well after closure with those ugly sutures would do equally well without them; and those who do poorly should have had the fascia left unsutured. Clearly, the traditional obsession of surgeons with closing the abdomen at all costs has diminished over recent years with the improved understanding of the adverse consequences of closing abdomens which should be left open. **In situations**

Table 7.2. Abdomens which cannot or should not be closed.

The abdomen cannot be closed:

- After major loss of abdominal wall tissue following trauma or debridement for necrotizing fasciitis.
- Extreme visceral or retroperitoneal swelling after major trauma, resuscitation or major surgery (e.g. ruptured abdominal aortic aneurysm).
- Poor condition of fascia after multiple laparotomies.

The abdomen should not be closed:

- A reoperation planned within a day or two.
- Closure possible only under excessive tension creating intra-abdominal hypertension (IAH).

when the abdomen cannot be closed or should not be closed (■ Table 7.2), **laparostomy is advisable**. For details about laparostomy read our previous chapter [2].

Closing the skin only (a 'planned' hernia)

You have just completed a laparotomy for small bowel obstruction within a giant incisional hernia. You resected the strangulated loops of intestine, completed the anastomosis. Next you replace the bulging viscera within the peritoneal cavity and try to close the abdomen. You cannot use mesh because of the significant contamination. But when you start approximating together the edges of the fascia the anesthetist (a smart one!) warns you that the *peak inspiratory airway pressure* is above 35mmHg — suggesting significant elevation of the intra-abdominal pressure (IAP). This is the classical indication for closing the skin only — avoiding intra-abdominal hypertension as well as the morbidity associated with laparostomy. **How to do it**: always spread the omentum, if available, over the viscera; approximate the subcutaneous layer with interrupted (strong) *Vicryl®* and the skin with 2-0 nylon interrupted mattress sutures, taking bites of at least 1cm. Although non-absorbable mesh is contraindicated in this situation, considerable assistance may be obtained from the use of absorbable mesh placed under the skin; it won't prevent a hernia but it will make complete dehiscence much less likely. Apply an

---

[2] *Schein's Common Sense Emergency Abdominal Surgery*, 3rd Ed. Springer Verlag, © 2010: Chapter 52.

abdominal binder. **And for God's sake: do not let anyone but you touch or remove the skin sutures**. Keep them at least for three weeks. What to do with the ensuing hernia is another story but a **planned hernia is much better tolerated than fascial dehiscence or laparostomy!**

Postoperative considerations

After the operation, anything which exerts excessive tension on the fascial suture line — anything elevating intra-abdominal pressure — contributes to the risk of dehiscence. Thus, severe coughing, retching, vomiting, abdominal distension and constipation should all be avoided. But we hope your closure was solid enough to endure the elevated pressures.

Some claim that wound infections predispose to fascial dehiscence. We are not sure whether this is really true for superficial wound infections — a more plausible explanation for such an association would be that both such complications share similar risk factors (e.g. malnutrition, emergency surgery, etc.).

However, there is no doubt that **deep SSIs** can chew up the fascial repair leading to dehiscence. It is unclear in such cases what came first, the chicken or the egg, as in some cases (those that "should not have been closed" — see above) it is possible that the extra-tight fascial sutures 'strangulate' the fascia, predisposing it to infection. **Any deep SSI may be associated with intra-abdominal infection; often neglected forms of the latter initially reveal themselves through dehiscence.**

Recognize the warning signs

Educate your residents and staff (and yourself) to recognize the signs heralding fascial dehiscence: **moderate to large amounts of serosanguineous fluid draining from the wound during the first postoperative week**. That this is not pus but intraperitoneal fluid is lost on non-experienced doctors who then rush to remove "a few sutures" believing that they are treating a wound infection. An hour later the nurse calls them back: "Hey Doc, I think his belly is open!" — "What the f…!" (■ Figure 7.1).

As a **general rule** (and this applies not only to sutures but also to staples, tubes, drains, lines): **do not allow anybody to remove anything from *your* patient's body that has been placed by you**. It is not easy nowadays to implement such rules within our modern, pseudo-democratic environment of health care, but try you must.

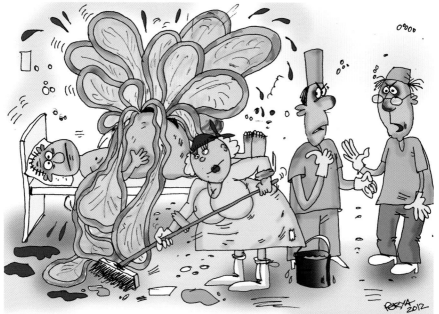

Figure 7.1. Surgeon to his buddy: "I don't understand what happened — I used PDS 2..."

Management of dehiscence

This quotation is from one of many online texts of surgery:

> *The seepage of serosanguineous fluid through a closed abdominal wound is an early sign of abdominal wound dehiscence with possible evisceration. When this occurs, the surgeon should remove one or two sutures in the skin and explore the wound manually, using a sterile glove. If there is separation of the rectus fascia, the patient should be taken to the operating room for primary closure. Wound dehiscence may or may not be associated with intestinal evisceration. When the latter complication is present, the mortality rate is dramatically increased and may reach 30%.*

We believe that the advice it provides is totally wrong! But unfortunately it reflects the recommendations given in other modern texts as well. Treated according to the above recommendations the patient's abdomen is resutured with retention sutures (see above). But why is the mortality so high? **The dehiscence itself is not responsible for the high morbidity and mortality — it is the conditions predisposing to dehiscence and the emergency reoperation to correct it that contribute to poor outcomes.** Forcing the distended intestines back into a cavity of limited size may kill the patient by producing intra-abdominal hypertension with all its deleterious physiological effects.

We believe that by and large, partial dehiscence can (and should) be managed conservatively and only complete dehiscence must be operated upon.

Partial dehiscence

Partial dehiscence is best managed conservatively. The viscera are not falling out so why rush to reoperate? In our experience the natural course of a partially dehisced wound is to heal by granulation and scarring with or (rarely) without the formation of an incisional hernia. On the other hand, reoperating through such a friable wound, in an ill patient, involves the additive risks of anesthesia and abdominal re-entry while not precluding an eventual hernia. If the bowel is partially exposed we approximate the skin to cover it. Otherwise, the wound is managed as any open wound (⊃ Chapter 5) until healed.

Complete dehiscence

Complete dehiscence necessitates an operation to reduce the eviscerated abdominal contents. What to do at laparotomy after the viscera have been reduced depends on the perceived cause of the dehiscence. **Closing the abdomen without attending to the 'deeper', underlying pathology (e.g. draining pus, exteriorizing an anastomotic leak) is equivalent to closing the coffin on top of a living patient!** You can resuture the fascia when a broken suture or faulty closure technique is the assumed cause. But only if local circumstances permit — the fascial edges can be approximated without excessive tension and the fascia is viable and not grossly infected. If this is not the case you should leave the abdomen temporarily open, using one of the temporary abdominal closure (TAC) methods described (see footnote [2] above). As mentioned above, skin closure only is another option. In brief, avoid abdominal reclosure if the cause of the evisceration is still present, or if you predict the need to re-explore the abdomen within the next few days.

We hope that after reading this chapter you will agree with the following:

- Abdominal dehiscence is a *symptom* rather than a *disease*.
- Sometimes, dehiscence of the abdomen represents a spontaneous decompression of intra-abdominal hypertension, and thus could be considered a 'beneficial' complication.
- You have to operate for complete dehiscence with evisceration; resuture it or treat it as a laparostomy.
- Partial dehiscence is best treated conservatively.

Happy fishing!

Chapter 8

Ileus and early postoperative small bowel obstruction (EPSBO)

Moshe Schein

> *The truth is that most patients [with early postoperative intestinal obstruction] will improve without you ever knowing whether it was a mechanical obstruction or 'just' an ileus.*

If you discover an effective method to prevent intraperitoneal adhesions or a remedy to prevent or treat postoperative ileus you'll deserve a Nobel Prize! Until then we are all left to face these two often exasperating conditions which blight our surgical lives. You did a wonderful, bloodless laparoscopic hemicolectomy; you've strictly followed "fast track surgery" and "rapid discharge" protocols. Alas, on the fifth postoperative day, your patient — whom you'd promised would be at home, munching his favorite macaroni & cheese, within two days — is still lying in his hospital bed, with an abdomen like a balloon, nasogastric tube in his nose, looking at you depressingly. What a nuisance!

Is this early postoperative small bowel obstruction (EPSBO) or 'just' an ileus? It could be either and in many cases, as stated in the above aphorism, we will never know the answer, which will become irrelevant when the patient, eventually, starts farting. In this chapter we will not deal with the general topics of small bowel obstruction or colonic obstruction (which are addressed in our previous book [1]) but focus on **ileus and EPSBO developing immediately after abdominal operations**.

---

[1]   *Schein's Common Sense Emergency Abdominal Surgery,* 3rd Ed. Springer Verlag, © 2010: Chapters 21 and 25.

In some countries the terms "**ileus**" and "**obstruction**" are used to describe the same condition; however, the prevailing wisdom distinguishes between these entities:

- **The term "ileus" describes a "paralytic ileus"** which develops after abdominal surgery. It affects, to some degree, the whole length of the gastrointestinal tract from the stomach to the rectum. **Notably, ileus can develop also after non-abdominal surgery or trauma** (e.g. severe burns, spine fracture, massive resuscitation, severe sepsis…).
- **EPSBO** refers to mechanical obstruction of the small bowel (that of the colon is extremely rare) due to two main mechanisms: **adhesions** or incarceration within an **internal hernia** (e.g. unsutured mesenteric defect) or an **external** one (e.g. trocar site). By 'early' we mean the first 30 postoperative days.

Whereas postoperative ileus is deemed a *physiologic* phenomenon — some laziness of the intestine is 'normal' — EPSBO is considered a 'complication'. But when ileus is **prolonged** beyond what is expected proportional to the specific operation then it begins to look like a complication.

Pre-operative considerations

There is not much *before* the operation you can do to prevent ileus or EPSBO except careful selection of the operation and optimal preparation of the patient as outlined in previous chapters.

The **expected duration of the postoperative ileus** correlates broadly with the magnitude of the operation performed and the underlying indication. Major dissections, prolonged intestinal displacement and exposure, denuded and inflamed peritoneum, residual intra- or retroperitoneal pus or clots, are all associated with a prolonged ileus. **We always list the possibility of postoperative ileus in the informed consent and mention it during the pre-op discussion**: "you know, most patients like you would drink and eat and go home a day after an uneventful appendectomy. But occasionally, the intestine may become lazy after being manipulated, or if the appendix is perforated… and we find pus. In that case your tummy may be bloated and you could even need a tube in your nose for a few days." When the patient and family are aware that the intestine could become 'lazy' after the abdominal operation — and if it does, it is not your fault, but a 'shit happens' phenomenon — they will accept the prolonged ileus more gracefully.

While a certain degree of ileus is expected after the operation, **the development of EPSBO is unpredictable**. You have to invest effort *during* the operation to prevent it (see below), but there is nothing you can do before the operation except warn patients undergoing specific procedures which are susceptible to it. **EPSBO is more likely to occur following small bowel operations, especially when performed to treat small bowel obstruction (SBO), both adhesive and malignant**.

It appears that in general, laparoscopic procedures, as distinct from open surgery, **lower the long-term risk of adhesive SBO**. It seems likely that this applies also to EPSBO although this is unproven. (But see below regarding EPSBO after bariatric lap procedures.)

Intra-operative considerations

Striving to do a perfect operation is your best strategy to prevent both ileus and EPSBO.

Prevention of ileus

The less you do, the less you manipulate the bowel, the better. **The key** is: gentle dissection and handling of tissues, not denuding the peritoneum unnecessarily, careful hemostasis to avoid hematomas, evacuation of all contaminants, not using the cautery like a flamethrower. Prolonged exposure of the intestine should be avoided — wet it periodically with warm saline, and protect it from retractor injury inflicted by well-meaning but slumbering assistants. In addition: avoid letting the small bowel hang out outside the belly on one side for a prolonged period and don't let it get blue while being busy with other things. **Of course, the longer the operation, the higher is the risk of ileus**. The anesthetist can contribute his share to the genesis of ileus by flooding the patient with i.v. fluids — **edematous bowel tends to be sluggish!**

Prevention of EPSBO

At the end of what you have done take care to close any mesenteric or peritoneal defects which could become a site for internal hernia, incarcerating the small bowel. Of course, doing this can be more demanding during laparoscopic procedures and this explains the increased incidence of strangulating SBO after laparoscopic bariatric operations (⟳ Chapter 23). Rough surgery, producing injury to the peritoneal surface, not only contributes to ileus but also fosters the early fibrinous adhesions that cause EPSBO. **Remember: the more adhesions you lyse, the more new ones will form.**

Therefore, limit adhesiolysis to the minimum necessary to obtain the exposure needed for relief of the obstructing adhesions — that is, if you are operating for SBO. **Lysis of chronic non-obstructing adhesions should be avoided because they 'lock' the small bowel in the open position — dividing them is counter-productive.** Do not leave behind 'foreign bodies' to which loops of bowel can adhere and subsequently obstruct: for example, 'lost' gallstones, long knots of non-absorbable sutures, or misfired staples or clips. At the end of laparoscopic procedures **carefully close trocar sites** (>5mm), including the underlying peritoneum — these are not an uncommon site for bowel incarceration in the postoperative period. **Drain sites**, if you still use passive rubber drains (I wonder why?), should not be so wide as to allow the intestine to be caught within the fascial defect after removal of the drain. The same applies to **stoma sites**. At the end of the operation, replace the small bowel in position, let the loops fall in and lie comfortably — you can fold the small bowel into nice, lazy curves like placing a hosepipe into a bucket; remember that jejunum belongs to the upper abdomen and ileum to the lower ☺. Avoid leaving omental defects through which the bowel may prolapse; if necessary detach the omentum, or what is left of it, from the abdominal wall and let it cover the viscera, protecting it from the fascial suture line. When closing the fascia take care not to catch intestine in the suture line — insert your finger again and again to check that the intestine has not been included. We are not impressed with any currently fashionable but costly products (e.g. X-film adhesion barrier) offered by the pharmaceutical industry to prevent postoperative adhesions. Are you?

Should you leave a nasogastric (NG) tube at the end of the operation?

Some 30 plus years ago, when I was a lowly resident, the answer to this question was straightforward: "of course!" You did not see a post-laparotomy patient leaving the OR without a tube in his nose. And if you dared to omit the NG tube you would be crucified by your chief. But, luckily there has been some progress over the years and surgeons realized that not all patients need an NG tube after abdominal operations; instead, we have to use them selectively (see also ➲ Chapter 2).

This is an opportunity to remind ourselves about **the actual function of the NG tube — what can it accomplish after the operation?:**

- It prevents *aerophagia* — the continuous swallowing of air which tends to accumulate in the stomach and intestine paralyzed by postoperative ileus, contributing to abdominal distension.

- It decompresses the 'backwash' into the stomach of intestinal fluids which accumulate in the paralyzed small intestine — or above a site of mechanical obstruction — thus alleviating intestinal distension, which otherwise contributes to the ileus.
- By decompressing the distended stomach it prevents pulmonary **aspiration** of gastric contents: a devastating complication which could develop in susceptible postoperative patients unable to protect their airways (e.g. obtunded patients with depressed gag reflex, sedated patients on mechanical ventilation).
- We said it before and we'll say it again: the NG tube does *not* protect distally-placed bowel anastomoses as liters of juices are secreted each day distal to the decompressed stomach.

So if the NG tube can accomplish all the above why not use it routinely? Because:

- Many studies have shown that **most patients do not benefit** from it: their physiologic ileus is limited and not shortened by the NG tube.
- **NG tubes produce complications**: they interfere with breathing, contributing to pulmonary complications, cause gastric erosion, reflux esophagitis and contribute to fluid/electrolyte imbalance.
- **Patients hate them!!!** Every surgeon should experience a tube down his nose at least once — what about you?

What then are our indications to leave an NG tube at the end of the operation?

- **After an emergency operation** when intra-operative findings predict that a significant ileus is expected. For example: diffuse peritonitis, ruptured abdominal aortic aneurysm.
- **After an emergency operation** to treat intestinal obstruction (small bowel or colonic) or intestinal ischemia where ileus or EPSBO are highly predicted.
- **After laparotomies for trauma** where visceral edema and abdominal compartment syndrome are predicted.
- **After major elective abdominal surgery** involving extensive dissection, bowel manipulation and tissue trauma — for example, pancreatectomy.
- **To prevent gastric distension and aspiration after any operation** when the patient is unlikely to be able to protect his airway (e.g. patients with head trauma).
- **In any patient who goes to the ICU for mechanical ventilation.**

- **In selected UGI operations**:
  - a transanastomotic tube for feeding purposes;
  - to prevent distension in the presence of a high-risk suture line (e.g. duodenal).

As you see, this is not a major intellectual exercise but a simple strategy based on clinical judgment and any such list would be controversial even before completely read. Essentially after any significant emergency laparotomy the patient in the recovery room or ICU will have an NG tube; the opposite is true after elective procedures, here tubes can be omitted in many cases. **If in doubt then leave a tube — you can always remove it the next morning!**

Postoperative considerations

Let us now return to the case scenario mentioned at the beginning of this chapter. So we are now four days after the hemicolectomy and the patient — to whom you'd made the promise about being at home, munching his favorite food, within two days — is lying in his hospital bed, with an abdomen like a balloon, nasogastric tube in his nose, looking at you depressingly. His family is jittery. **What now?**

Well, most probably you are dealing with a *physiological* **postoperative ileus** which should resolve gradually — the small bowel should resume activity almost immediately, followed, a day or so later, by the stomach; the colon, being the most sluggish, is the last to start moving. The magnitude of such ileus is unpredictable — in some patients it is negligible, in others more significant; some would just bloat a little, others would vomit and require insertion (or reinsertion) of the NG tube, which has been omitted or removed earlier.

However, failure of your patient to eat, pass flatus or evacuate his bowel beyond five days after a laparotomy (or laparoscopy) signifies a persistent-prolonged ileus and this should start worrying you. Now you have to make sure that this is 'only' an ileus and there are no underlying conditions which prolong it. You have also to exclude the possibility of EPSBO. You have to take further diagnostic steps:

- **The clinical differentiation between ileus and EPSBO is extremely difficult**. In both conditions the abdomen is distended and can be tender (distended loops of bowel are tender!). Dogma and textbooks teach you that in ileus the abdomen is *silent on auscultation* while it should be *noisy* when mechanical obstruction is present. Unfortunately, the recently operated abdomen doesn't always behave according to rituals or textbooks — abdominal auscultation for peristalsis is as accurate as the horoscope. Not that one cannot tell whether the abdomen is *silent* or *noisy* but that it doesn't accurately distinguish between ileus and EPSBO. **If the patient has been already passing gas or feces and then stops, the likelihood that you are dealing with EPSBO is much higher**. But overall the clinical picture tends to be non-specific.

- **Any evidence of ongoing SIRS should make you think about the possibility of complications smoldering within the abdomen**. For example, the soft signs of developing anastomotic leak include ileus (⮌ Chapter 6). A persisting ileus is a warning sign that things are not *kosher* — inside the abdomen or possibly even outside it (e.g. pneumonia).

- **Radiology. Plain abdominal X-ray** in ileus would typically disclose significant gaseous distension of both the small bowel and the colon. However, EPSBO is often 'partial', featuring distended loops of small bowel as well as variable quantities of air in the colon. Very rarely will a plain X-ray provide you with a specific diagnosis. Therefore, in this day and age a **CT of the abdomen and pelvis with water-soluble contrast (through the NG tube) is the way to go**. It will diagnose, or rule out, potential causes of ileus and it will help you differentiate between ileus (contrast reaches the colon) and EPSBO (contrast fails to reach the colon). If you do not have a CT at your disposal a '**Gastrografin® challenge**' through the NG tube is a reasonable alternative (see below).

How to manage this patient?

With abdominal distension, expect vomit at any time.
Ivor Lewis

- **Pass an NG tube** — if not already in — to relieve distension, nausea and vomiting, and measure gastric residue. Of course, patients hate the tube and by inserting or reinserting it you 'admit failure' — that the postoperative course is not as uneventful as you wished it to be. But having 'pity' on the patient and delaying insertion is counter-productive. The NG tube will promptly improve the patient's symptoms and is the mainstay in the management of prolonged ileus and EPSBO — hastening its resolution.

- As already mentioned: **search for and correct, if present, potential causes of prolonged ileus**. A hematoma, an abscess, an anastomotic phlegmon or leak, postoperative pancreatitis, postoperative acalculous cholecystitis — all can produce ileus or mimic EPSBO.

- Measure and correct **electrolyte and fluid imbalances** (e.g. *hypokalemia* contributes to ileus. Remember: *hypomagnesemia* has to be corrected to allow amendment of potassium levels!).
- Consider starting **parenteral nutrition** if ileus/EPSBO continues beyond a week. Remember: hypoalbuminemia causes edema of the bowel and thus adds to the ileus (*hypoalbuminemic enteropathy*).
- **Opiate agents** used for postoperative analgesia suppress bowel motility and thus promote ileus. Use them prudently. Obviously, the less pain, the less the demand for opiates. Therefore, laparoscopic surgery is advantageous and so is postoperative epidural anesthesia.
- There are studies suggesting that **manual abdominal massage** and munching **chewing gum** can alleviate ileus. There is nothing wrong in trying these harmless modalities. We encourage patients to chew gum. Let the wives or partners massage their tummies…
- **Drugs**. Although erythromycin and metoclopramide are effective in resolving postoperative **gastroparesis**, neither has been shown to be effective for small bowel ileus or colonic ileus.
- **You should encourage the patient to ambulate as much as possible and frequently change position when lying in bed** (from side to side). It shifts the loops of bowel, stimulating motility and, in the case of EPSBO may lyse the early, soft adhesions responsible for it. We cannot offer any high-level evidence for this but it seems to make sense. At least it might prevent atelectasis and DVT.
- As already mentioned, on **postoperative day five we would obtain a CT with contrast**. If the prolonged ileus is totally unexpected following the index procedure (e.g. a repair of a small umbilical hernia), we would image the abdomen even earlier, looking for a correctable mishap. The water-soluble oral contrast agent (*Gastrografin®*) we use with the CT reduces intestinal edema and hurries intestinal transit — **we believe in its therapeutic benefits, speeding the resolution of ileus as well as EPSBO**.
- Occasionally, when features of SIRS are absent (no worry about infective or inflammatory underlying causes of ileus), rather than order a CT we would start with a **Gastrografin® challenge**: instill 100cc Gastrografin® through the NG tube, clamp the tube and get a plain abdominal X-ray after 4-6 hours. Seeing the contrast rush to the rectum means that whatever the problem was, be it ileus or EPSBO, it has now resolved. Often, when you arrive at the patient's room, to announce the good news and remove the torturing pipe from his nose, you find him happily busy moving his bowel.
- In the absence of intra- or extra-abdominal causes for ileus, and when the 'ileus' does not respond to the Gastrografin® challenge, your working diagnosis is EPSBO, which in most cases (exceptions

discussed below) is caused by early, soft, flimsy, inflammatory adhesions and, in the majority of cases, resolves spontaneously within two weeks. **The risk of strangulation in adhesive EPSBO is negligible**; therefore, **do not rush to reoperate; treat conservatively, with an NG tube and nutritional support, for 10-14 days — in fact, sometimes you have to wait longer — even a month!** Failure of resolution forces you back to the OR, for an operation which may prove difficult and hazardous because of the typical early and vascular adhesions cementing the bowel at many points. **Remember: the key is patience!** You are under constant pressure from the patient and his family to "do something". But do not surrender! Typically, on postoperative day nine, just before you decide that enough is enough — let's go to the OR — the patient will have an explosive BM. Hurrah!

Think outside the box

What we have discussed so far are general considerations, but of course each patient is different and has to be considered individually.

Do not forget that postoperative patients can develop ileus-producing abdominal complications which are not directly related to the index operation. For example:

- **Mesenteric ischemia** due to mesenteric *venous* thrombosis has been described after major open abdominal surgery and laparoscopic procedures. Mesenteric *arterial* thrombosis, attributed to prolonged pneumoperitoneum in susceptible patients, has also been described even after an uneventful laparoscopic cholecystectomy. Mesenteric ischemia due to a *low-flow state* can develop in any critically ill patient. Again: the presentation in the postoperative patient is non-specific: **ileus! Think about it and... use the CT!**
- **Incarcerated external hernia**. An elderly woman develops marked abdominal distension two days after ambulatory repair of a ventral hernia. She is readmitted with the diagnosis of 'ileus', which persists. A few days later a **strangulated femoral hernia** is diagnosed on the CT — how embarrassing! **Remember**: increased intra-abdominal pressure and bowel distension which follows the operation may predispose to incarceration of abdominal wall hernias which were until then asymptomatic. Careful and complete physical examination of the patient would have revealed the femoral bulge on readmission. Only superheroes can see through clothes, for the rest of us it helps to look at the femoral area after taking down the jeans and the underpants ☺. **Always fully examine the patient — avoid tunnel vision!**

Table 8.1. Early postoperative small bowel obstruction (EPSBO) after specific operations. Modified from: Schein's Common Sense Emergency Abdominal Surgery, 3rd Ed. Springer Verlag, © 2010: Chapter 48.

Index operation	Question	Consideration
Laparoscopy	Is the bowel incarcerated within a trocar site?	Early CT If yes — reoperate now!
Colostomy, ileostomy	Is bowel incarcerated behind the emerging stoma?	Early CT If yes — reoperate
Major pelvic resections	Is bowel prolapsing/ incarcerated into the new pelvic space?	Early CT Consider reoperation
Laparotomy for SBO	Did you relieve the actual source of obstruction?	CT Usually wait and see
Appendectomy	Is there a collection or abscess, phlegmon of stump?	Early CT Usually responds to antibiotics +/- percutaneous drainage
Carcinomatosis	How extensive? Resectable?	Consider avoiding operation, palliative measures such as gastrostomy
Intestinal anastomosis	Consider anastomotic obstruction	See text above

Always take into consideration the specific index operation which preceded the ileus or EPSBO (■ Table 8.1). A few main points are outlined below.

EPSBO after laparoscopic procedures

Adhesions are responsible in half of the patients and small bowel incarceration at the port site in the other half (■ Figure 8.1). In most of these latter cases the bowel is caught at the site of insertion of 10 or 12mm trocars

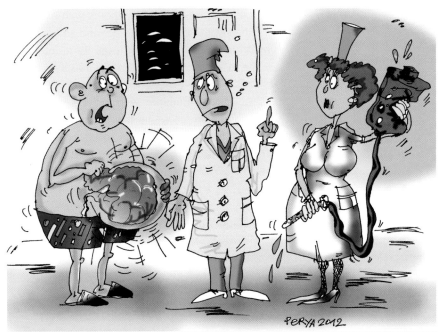

Figure 8.1. A patient after laparoscopic cholecystectomy. Surgeon: "Let us try a large enema!"

and the umbilical port site is the commonest. Adequate closure of the fascial defect does not preclude the possibility of trocar site incarceration of bowel; a strangulated Richter's hernia (an incarcerated 'knuckle' of small bowel) may develop, with the bowel caught in the preperitoneal space behind a well-repaired fascial defect. **Physical examination is rarely diagnostic but CT is — use it early and liberally in the post-laparoscopy patient who develops features of ileus/EPSBO!** Incarcerated or strangulated hernia at the trocar site mandates an immediate operation to relieve the obstruction; you can carry it out through the (extended) actual trocar site obviating the need for a formal laparotomy. **Remember also that laparoscopic procedures are prone to 'bizarre complications'**: gallstones can be 'spilled' or 'lost' during cholecystectomy producing inflammatory masses to which intestine can adhere; residual segments of inflamed appendix can be left *in situ* after lap appendectomy producing local ileus or EPSBO; and the incidence of accidental injury to adjacent viscera (responsible for ileus) is not negligible. Always suspect!

The 'hostile' abdomen

This describes a small subgroup of patients in whom the findings at the index operation suggest that any further surgery to relieve the obstructive process would be perilous and pointless; for example, patients with extensive **radiation enteritis** in whom persisting obstruction can be defined as "intestinal failure" and who are best managed with long-term parenteral nutrition. Indiscriminate reoperations in these patients may lead to massive bowel resection, multiple fistulas and death — any experienced surgeon has a few personal horror stories of this condition. Patients with diffuse **peritoneal carcinomatosis** at the index operation also fall within this group. **In general, only one-third of patients with 'malignant' bowel obstruction from peritoneal carcinomatosis will have prolonged postoperative palliation.** Persistent EPSBO in such patients is a gloomy warning that reoperation should be avoided and future palliative treatment planned — a gastrostomy tube for example. Finally, some patients (fortunately rare) develop a 'frozen abdomen' — intractable SBO caused by dense, vascular and indivisible adhesions which glue the bowel at multiple points. The wise surgeon knows when to abandon a precarious dissection before multiple enterotomies are created; and understands that reoperation should be avoided. Prolonged parenteral nutrition over a period of months, with complete gastrointestinal rest, may allow the adhesions to mature — with resolution of the SBO, or at least allowing a safer reoperation.

Anastomotic obstruction (⮑ Chapter 6)

Intestinal anastomoses at any level may narrow early after the operation and cause UGI, small bowel or colonic obstruction. Most such early postoperative anastomotic obstructions are 'inflammatory' in nature due to local edema. They should resolve spontaneously within a week or two. Avoid hurrying to reoperation; often a gentle passage of an endoscope — if the anastomosis is within reach — confirms the diagnosis and 'dilates' the lumen. Remember also that 'mini' or 'contained' anastomotic leaks can present with obstruction — not only at the anastomotic site. The adjacent small bowel can adhere to the inflamed anastomotic phlegmon, causing EPSBO or local ileus (for example, duodenal ileus producing delayed gastric emptying due to the adjacent leaking ileocolic anastomosis). Contrast study (preferably with CT) is diagnostic. You know already how to treat the leak after reading ⮑ Chapter 6.

Colonic ileus

In some postoperative patients, colonic ileus dominates the picture — the patient **being extremely distended and abdominal images showing massive dilatation of the colon**. This typically develops in debilitated patients not only after abdominal surgery but after any major procedure (e.g. hip replacement). Other terms commonly used to describe this condition are **Ogilvie's syndrome** or **colonic pseudo-obstruction**. If the usual steps (NG tube, avoiding opiates, correcting electrolytes — potassium!) are not helpful, then pass a well-lubricated rectal tube (the soft rubber one which is unlikely to perforate the rectum). If this fails the literature supports treatment with **neostigmine** to 'stimulate' the colon, either as a single bolus of 2-2.5mg or infusion of 0.4mg/h over up to 24 hours. It has to be given in a monitored setting, as both bradycardia (have *atropine* ready!) and bronchospasm can occur. Oral or NG administration of polyethylene glycol (17g in 250cc) up to three times a day has been recommended as well. **Obviously, before considering such therapies you have to be sure that this is not a mechanical colonic obstruction!** Inserting a colonoscope to suck out the colon and rule out mechanical obstruction is another option — which becomes the method of choice when the cecum (on abdominal X-rays or CT) is very large (>10cm), denoting danger of impending rupture. Finally, a **Gastrografin® enema** can be both diagnostic and therapeutic.

When to remove the nasogastric tube?

We have left this question to the end because the answer is so nebulous: the **NG tube should be removed when no longer needed**. This means when clinically the ileus or EPSBO has resolved. In our minds there are no practical formulas or guidelines which can be universally applied as each patient is different. Using a cut-off volume of NG tube aspirate as an indicator that the NG tube can come out is inaccurate as well: the problem may have resolved while the NG tube continues to syphon out significant volumes of foregut juices. **Hence, look at the whole clinical picture**. If in doubt cap or clamp the tube for 12 hours before removing it and observe how this is tolerated by the patient. Always warn patients, especially those who each morning beseech you to remove that insufferable tube, that occasionally it will have to be reinserted. By the way, **inserting the NG tube can be made atraumatic and more tolerable**; there is an art to it with which you have to become familiar, doing it better than the nurses. Soften the tube in hot-hot water just before insertion (or use a silicon NG tube), spray the nostril and the oropharynx with *xylocaine* and lubricate the tube. Have the patient sit up with his head semi-flexed; when the tip of the tube reaches the oropharynx let him take small sips of water through a straw — the ensuing swallowing will guide the tube into the stomach. Confirm the correct position by auscultation of the stomach while injecting air or get a plain X-ray. An incorrect position is extremely common but easily preventable if you do it yourself or check that it has been done properly.

In most cases you won't ever know what has caused the problem because it will resolve spontaneously. Was it an ileus or an EPSBO? But who really cares if the patient is doing well?

Chapter 9

Minimal access surgery

Danny Rosin

> *Laparoscopic surgery is the one case where a resident can destroy the remainder of a patient's life, and your mental health and well-being, with one squeeze of the clip applier or one cut of the shears.*

> **Jeffrey Young**

The aim of laparoscopic surgery is to achieve the same goals as open surgery, using a technique that reduces surgical trauma, and therefore hastens recovery. However, the road to such a glorious target may be bumpy and may even lead to fatal accidents. The numerous complications associated with minimal access surgery — gleefully cited by non-believers and antagonists ("I told you so…"), and commonly hushed or understated by champions of laparoscopy ("I never have any complications…") — can be divided into three main groups:

- Complications **specific to the technique** — like access injuries, or pneumoperitoneum-related morbidity.
- Complications that, although **seen in open surgery, may be made more likely ('augmented') by use of the technique** — like bile duct or bowel injury.
- Complications **associated with the procedure performed**. These complications may happen regardless of the approach (like anastomotic leaks); in some cases the laparoscopic approach is 'blamed', justifiably or not, but in others the procedure may be done exclusively or mainly by laparoscopy (e.g. sleeve gastrectomy) so direct comparison with the open procedure is difficult.

In this chapter I deal mainly with the first group, and refer a little to the second one. Procedure-specific complications, even if performed laparoscopically, will be described in the appropriate chapters.

Pre-operative considerations

Even in operations for which laparoscopy is the default approach, like cholecystectomy, choosing laparoscopy should always be weighed in comparison to the equivalent open procedure. "What would I, and the patient, gain from laparoscopy, and what can we lose?" is a mandatory question that should never be answered flippantly. The gain is usually in the patient's recovery, but can also be in the surgeon's comfort in performance. The loss may be in operating time or in expense, and sometimes in technical difficulty, **but the main loss is the hazard of complications that may have been avoided by choosing an open approach (■ Figure 9.1).**

Selecting the correct procedure is always important, but even more so when considering an approach that may subtly influence the choice of the procedure. **Preferring laparoscopy in all circumstances may compromise the surgeon's**

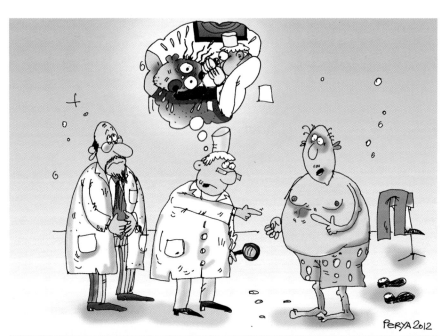

Figure 9.1. "Hey Chief, what about removing this lipoma transgastrically, you know, NOTES... didn't you see the YouTube clip?"

choice, for example, by restricting options to a simpler procedure that may not solve the patient's problem, or may lead to a missed pathology.

Intra-operative considerations

After selecting laparoscopy as the preferred approach, **planning the procedure** then begins. How do I gain access to the abdomen? Is a blind entry appropriate? How many trocars? In which positions? The limitations of minimal access should be well understood. Compromises should be avoided and the surgeon should be working in optimal conditions (exposure, visibility, including even the surgeon's comfort and ergonomics). For example, the addition of just a single trocar may reduce the risk of inadvertent injury by allowing better exposure of the operative field and by providing the surgeon with a better dissection angle.

Reasons for difficult laparoscopy

Laparoscopic surgery is highly technical. Safety is very dependent on ease of performance and any technical difficulties may increase the risk of unwanted outcomes. **Remember: some of the more horrid complications happen in simple, easy and quick laparoscopic operations, due to lack of attention to detail or incorrect technique**. Even so, it is generally true that the more difficult the surgery, the higher the chance of complications and a bad outcome.

Access
It seems that the debate between proponents and opponents of the 'closed' approach, using a blindly inserted Veress needle, will never be settled. As in most debates, the truth may lie somewhere in the middle, and *selectivity* is the key. A previously scarred abdomen may be made safer to enter by using an open approach, although some surgeons will swear by their mother about the safety of *Palmer's point* in the left subcostal area. I wouldn't bet on my mother's life for such a cause. On the other hand, in **obese patients**, insistence on the open approach may result in diving through the fat, via wide and deep wounds, increasing the chance of **wound infection** and **incisional hernia**; so a smaller, closed entry may be less prone to complications.

View
The optimal view is mandatory to achieve accurate dissection and avoid injuries, and is a prerequisite for safe laparoscopy. The reasons for a

suboptimal image are numerous, and familiarity with the technical equipment, its weaknesses and how to troubleshoot each one are mandatory, and can only be learned with practice and experience. Even the most expensive system with HD, 3CCD, 3D (or any other letter combination that adds to the $$) may suffer from a broken lens, burnt light cable, incorrect white balance or just smoke, vapor or condensation on the tip of the scope — turning the laparoscopic experience into the annoying and dangerous guesswork of a half-blind surgeon.

Correct surgical planning may also significantly affect the view. Plan the location of the trocars to optimize the direction of the scope and the working ports. This is particularly important when operating on pathology that is not fixed, for example, bowel obstruction. **Make sure you choose the appropriately angled scope that will enhance your field of view and allow 'peeking' behind obstacles**. Try to achieve the best retraction you can, moving bowel and omentum away — using all kinds of table positions and angles. You need a cooperative anesthetist[1], and good fixation of the patient to the table, with straps and supporters; this should be routine in every laparoscopy! Adding one or two 5mm ports to assist in retraction may improve your well-being as a laparoscopic surgeon for a negligible price and no added morbidity.

Equipment

Optimal laparoscopy is dependent on availability and functionality of multiple pieces of hardware, starting with the electronic equipment on the 'laparoscopy cart', the CO_2 system, the laparoscopic instruments and other accessories like various energy sources and laparoscopic ultrasound. Each of these elements can go wrong and hamper the smoothness of the laparoscopic procedure. But even when everything functions flawlessly, it is still in your hands to choose the correct tool for the action, and use it wisely. Making compromises by using inadequate or malfunctioning equipment is a recipe for increased difficulty and greater risk of complications: the wrong grasper may tear the bowel, the peeled insulation may cause inadvertent electro-thermal injury, and the blunt scissors will tear the tissue or just drive you crazy.

Lighting

Although modern laparoscopic systems make use of high-definition images, intense light sources and dense fiber-optic light cables, and thus minimize the likelihood of blundering in the gloom, still no system is immune from the

---

[1] *I know lots of anesthetists who regard laparoscopic surgery as a means by which straightforward operations that used to be done quickly now take hours and inevitably involve vast quantities of disposable kit.* [John MacFie].

difficulties of darkness, especially if maintenance of the equipment is not optimal. Several common factors should be kept in mind:

- **Small-diameter scopes transmit less light**: if the view is too dark — zoom out, and if the light is still not enough replace the scope with a thicker one.
- **Blood in the surgical field absorbs light**. Keep your field clean and dry. Use common tricks, like inserting a piece of gauze to clean the blood, absorb it and cancel its optical effects.
- **'Chain of components'**. Since multiple factors can lead to inadequate lighting and image quality, familiarity with all potential (and common) problems will allow you to perform a systematic check, and isolate the culprit: an old and weak light bulb, a burnt or broken fiber-optic cable, a broken lens in the scope, or just insufficient gain or inadequate settings of the camera.

Local conditions

The findings inside the abdomen have a major effect on the ease with which any laparoscopic procedure will be carried out. Inflammation makes anatomy less clear, and dissection more difficult and bloody. Whether the procedure can and should be continued laparoscopically depends greatly on the surgeon and his/her expertise, but a **low threshold for conversion should guide the safe surgeon when dealing with hostile abdominal conditions**. Other conditions that will make your life tough are discussed below.

Adhesions

Once a contraindication for laparoscopy, adhesions resulting from previous surgery no longer deter dedicated and determined laparoscopic surgeons from completing their task... but nevertheless, higher rates of complications, especially those related to bleeding and intestinal injury, are expected in the presence of adhesions. Access should preferably be away from old scars, and despite optimistic reports by brave and dexterous surgeons **we highly recommend that you stick with the open-access technique** in these cases; that is, if you wish to continue to be considered a safe surgeon. Even if a bowel injury does happen when you carefully dissect the abdominal wall — it is less likely to be missed with catastrophic consequences. After entry has been achieved, assess the amount and severity of adhesions, make sure you have enough working space, and consider whether you feel you can safely deal with them. **Calling for assistance and converting are two excellent choices you can make at this point**. When lysing adhesions during the procedure your best strategy is to stay in the correct surgical plane — that of loose adhesions.

This is the plane that can be separated by cold, sharp dissection, with minimal bleeding, and no need for thermal energy that may endanger the bowel.

Distension

Bowel distension decreases the available space and makes laparoscopy riskier, more difficult and sometimes impossible. Bowel obstruction is the classic example of a condition in which laparoscopy may provide an excellent solution, but severe distension may prevent it from being practical or safe. Apart from lack of working space, the distended bowel is more difficult to manipulate, and may be thin and friable, easily prone to perforation. Injury to an obstructed bowel may lead to a major spillage and consequent severe and even lethal sepsis. **Remember: converting because you are "forced to" is ALWAYS worse than converting because you have "decided" to do so**.

Fat

Like the factors mentioned above, obesity is no longer a contraindication for laparoscopy, and actually it may be the most common indication for laparoscopic surgery nowadays... but still, operating on a fat person is always more difficult. In most cases, the advantages of laparoscopy, if successful, are more prominent in obese patients. Different types of obesity may also make a difference, and may be gender-specific: a patient with huge thighs or buttocks may have surprisingly little omental fat.

Volume, pressure and muscle relaxation

Abdominal wall compliance is a major determinant of the working space available for the laparoscopic surgeon. A thick, fat wall, or a highly muscular one, may limit the abdomen's distensibility, and result in a small volume and 'crowded' abdomen, and often requires the use of a higher insufflation pressure. A thin, post-partum lady may be considered the optimal patient from this aspect. **The key to a 'convenient' laparoscopy is good muscle relaxation. A compliant anesthetist equals a compliant abdominal wall**, so keep a good relationship with him/her, and never let him wake the patient up before you're really done. Loss of muscle relaxation in the last few minutes of the operation not only will annoy you but may spoil your perfect laparoscopy by an unnecessary complication: failing to control a bleeder, inadvertently injuring a loop of bowel that was pushed away from the surgical field, or failing to close the fascia adequately and having an incarcerated hernia a few days later.

Laparoscopy-specific complications

Access complications

Gaining access to the abdominal cavity, at the beginning of every laparoscopy, has been implicated as a major risk factor for laparoscopic complications. Penetrating the abdominal wall may result in injury to superficial and deep blood vessels and to abdominal organs and viscera. Minimizing these risks has been the subject of numerous discussions, focusing mainly, as I mentioned above, on the 'closed' vs. 'open' access. Dedicated preachers exist on both sides, but it seems that most laparoscopic surgeons will settle on either side of the fence, almost equally divided, based on their education, habits and personal experience, with no clear advantage to either technique. In the 'real world', away from the so-called 'centers of excellence', access complications still occur with annoying persistence and frequency. From time to time you may hear about such a case — always produced by somebody else (a gynecologist? ☺), somebody who managed to insert a trocar directly into the aorta.

Familiarity with the various access techniques and devices (like optical trocars), and wise selectivity, is the key to minimizing your risk of injury while inserting the first laparoscopic port (and remember — injuries have happened with the second and third port as well, despite 'under-vision' insertion). Blind creation of a pneumoperitoneum using a Veress needle is widely practiced with minimal morbidity, but even 'Veress enthusiasts' should recognize high-risk situations in which the open alternative is safer, like the scarred abdomen or the presence of distended bowel. Despite some avid supporters and even 'positive' publications, we recommend avoidance of blind trocar insertion without a pneumoperitoneum. Going through the umbilical stalk, using a 'semi-open' technique, is another good and safe option.

Abdominal wall bleeding

Injuring a major vessel in the abdominal wall should be rare with umbilical or periumbilical penetration, but typically may occur with a secondary, laterally placed trocar. The most commonly injured vessel is the **inferior epigastric artery**, which may result in a significant abdominal wall hematoma. Transilluminating the abdominal wall helps to identify the vessel and avoid it, but this may be ineffective in obese patients. Blunt, blade-less trocars are safer in this aspect. **Portal hypertension** may result in multiple abdominal wall venous collaterals, and bleeding from these high-pressure veins may ruin your beautiful laparoscopy before it even started.

Remember to check all trocar sites for bleeding before the end of the procedure: extract under vision trocar after trocar — the trocar may have provided tamponade for the bleeding which will become manifest after its removal.

There are many ways to control bleeding from the abdominal wall, ranging from local pressure (a Foley catheter may help, with the balloon inflated and pulled back), to the use of coagulation, clips and sutures. A **suture passer** may be especially helpful in this situation, and a nice figure-of-eight suture placed around the fascial incision will quickly achieve what minutes of repeated tissue charring failed to do.

Injury to deep vessels

Nightmare stories about this float around the surgical community; they are seldom published in medical journals but feature in the legal (malpractice) literature — at least in countries where legal recourse is available to harmed patients or those relatives who survive them. **Blind and forceful insertion of the Veress needle or the first trocar, especially in thin patients, may result in injury to the great vessels in the retroperitoneum**. In non-obese patients the distance between the skin of the abdomen and the anterior border of the spine is surprisingly short, so injuries to the aorta, vena cava or iliac vessels are relatively easy to create — if you don't follow careful insertion procedures as outlined above. **Investing a few extra minutes in gaining safe access can prevent a horrendous disaster!**

Blood in the needle or the trocar (even if not hitting the ceiling), free peritoneal blood or hemodynamic deterioration should alert you to the possibility of inadvertent injury. A quick laparoscopic exploration, with a good suction in hand, may reveal an easily controlled bleeding source like a small mesenteric branch. **But an immediate conversion**, control of the bleeding point by pressure, letting anesthesia catch up with the situation and summoning help (another surgeon with vascular expertise) is the way to go. **Remember: a delay of a few minutes, while you scratch your head about what to do next, may mean death. Seeing only RED through the camera is a GREEN light to a macrolaparotomy!**

Bowel injury

Adhesions to the abdominal wall are a major risk factor for injury while gaining access to the abdominal cavity. Using an open approach for the first laparoscopic port is highly recommended, but does not completely eliminate the risk, as bowel can be injured even during a slow and careful open approach. For example, during mini-laparotomy to insert a Hasson trocar, a loop of small bowel could be 'pinched' together with the peritoneum by the clamp and inadvertently opened. **However, the risk of MISSED bowel injury is greatly reduced by the open technique**. Remember that a blind trocar may go through and through a stuck bowel loop, and therefore may go unnoticed!

If a bowel injury occurs and is immediately diagnosed, repair should be completed carefully, without compromising safety for the sake of continuing laparoscopically. **Mini- or even formal laparotomy, full identification of the injury, lysis of adhesions and a meticulous repair should be your goal.** Plans for the laparoscopic procedure should be re-evaluated: in most cases the procedure can proceed as planned, but some operations may require modifications, like the use of mesh to repair an abdominal wall hernia. Consider aborting the procedure and reschedule, or modify the procedure to reduce the infection risk (e.g. open, non-mesh repair, accepting the higher risk of recurrence, instead of laparoscopic repair using an intra-abdominal mesh).

Missing a bowel injury (a typical example is duodenal injury during laparoscopic cholecystectomy) results in severe sepsis and extremely high mortality rates. Defending it in court is impossible. So, carefulness during the procedure, and awareness after it, is your best strategy to avoid this mess. Read also ⮌ Chapter 6.

Pneumoperitoneum

Pneumoperitoneum is the established method of obtaining a convenient working space for laparoscopy. Alternatives, such as abdominal wall lifting, never gained acceptance, mainly due to being cumbersome and less practical. **The price for using a pneumoperitoneum is two-fold: the gas being used and the intra-abdominal pressure.**

CO_2

Despite attempts to use various other gases, like helium, xenon, nitrous oxide and simple air, CO_2 is established as the standard insufflation gas, solubility being its great advantage. The risk of catastrophe due to **gas embolism** is decreased with CO_2, as even if it enters the venous system (the risk is higher in hepatic surgery) it quickly dissolves in the blood, and is evacuated through the respiratory system. **The main adverse effect of a CO_2 pneumoperitoneum is postoperative pain**, due to the acidity created by the formation of carbonic acid. Use of low pressure (12mmHg or even less, depending on the abdominal compliance), and complete CO_2 evacuation at the termination of the procedure, should reduce the severity of this pain. **Hypercapnia** may result from prolonged procedures in patients with compromised respiratory function. Increasing minute-ventilation helps the anesthetist get rid of CO_2 and correct the resultant acidosis, but occasionally the procedure should be stopped temporarily, or even converted to open surgery.

Intra-abdominal pressure

Increasing the intra-abdominal pressure (IAP) is non-physiologic, and therefore results in pressure-related pulmonary and hemodynamic changes. Despite multiple experimental studies demonstrating various effects on pulmonary pressure, increased cardiac after-load and decreased pre-load, and reduced renal and splanchnic circulation, actual ill-effects of a pneumoperitoneum in clinical practice are rare. **Nevertheless, extra care is needed in compromised situations or susceptible patients**, as even minor elevations of IAP may be significant in failing kidneys; and reduced mesenteric flow may be the trigger for ischemia in an already compromised bowel in a patient with septic shock treated with inotropic drugs. **Make it a habit to use lower abdominal pressure if possible (try 2mm Hg below what you intended...), enough to create sufficient working space**. Again, adequate muscle relaxation is important to achieve adequate abdominal wall compliance — make sure you get what you need from the anesthesia team. Lastly, in **some situations you may want to avoid a pneumoperitoneum altogether**: consider the frail 'old duck' with a cardiac ejection fraction of 15%, presenting with acute cholecystitis. Do you want to pump her abdomen with gas? Wouldn't percutaneous cholecystostomy be safer?

Laparoscopy-'augmented' complications

Visceral injuries

The unfamiliar approach, the different viewing angle, the limited field of view, the indirect handling of tissues — all these factors may increase the risk of specific complications which are less frequently encountered in open procedures. Passing instruments in and out, sometimes through 'blind' areas outside the surgical field, can result in injuries to adjacent organs and viscera. This is more common with an instrument passing through a remote port — by a less experienced assistant — but nevertheless it's your responsibility to avoid it!

Missing a visceral injury is, unfortunately, more likely to happen in laparoscopy. While a bleeding injury is evident in most cases, bowel injury is more difficult to detect, if it happens outside the surgical field, or if it is small and not easily seen. Laparoscopic adhesiolysis not infrequently results in a miniature perforation that may go unnoticed as spillage is prevented due to the positive intra-abdominal pressure. **Partial thickness damage to the bowel wall**, as in thermal injury, manifests usually only *after* the operation. Defective insulation may cause injury along the instrument shaft away from the surgical field, and energy sources can cause heat dissipation and thermal injury adjacent to the operative field. Commonly, clinical manifestations develop a few days after surgery, with late perforation and resultant peritonitis.

Before you terminate the laparoscopy move the camera around and look beyond the operative field: did you cause any trauma? And remember the old dictum: the source of any postoperative problem resides at the operative site unless proven otherwise!

Apart from missing an iatrogenic injury, **laparoscopy carries the risk of missing the actual pathology, or a coexistent one**. Although visual exploration may sometimes be easier and more complete by laparoscopy (compared to a limited incision like McBurney), the lack of manual palpation contributes to the risk of missing pathology like a colonic or gastric mass, or a retroperitoneal (pancreatic) lesion. With extensive pre-operative imaging so frequently used nowadays the chance of missed pathology is diminished, but if a patient does not improve after your negative exploration consider the possibility that your laparoscope has missed something important. For example, the upper abdominal symptoms which prompted laparoscopic cholecystectomy for 'symptomatic cholelithiasis' are caused by an undiagnosed carcinoma of the pancreas. **Use your little grey box to think outside the box** ☹.

Bleeding

Bleeding during laparoscopy may happen while entering the abdomen or during the procedure itself; it could range from a minor (but nagging) ooze to a major, life-threatening venous or arterial bleed. While in general laparoscopic procedures result in less blood loss than the open alternative, if bleeding does occur it disrupts the course of the operation, is more demanding to control, and may lead to complications associated with the blood loss itself and the attempts to control it (➲ Chapter 3).

There are numerous devices, maneuvers, techniques and tricks to control bleeding during laparoscopy, and the more experienced the surgeon, the more likely it is for the bleeding to be safely controlled laparoscopically. Local pressure, hemostatic agents, electrocoagulation, clips and ligatures can all serve the purpose of hemostasis, and are safe when the bleeding source is well identified. **However, blind attempts at clipping in a pool of blood, or excessive electrocoagulation, are a recipe for complications, some of them catastrophic**. For example, blind clipping to control a bleeding cystic artery may result in common bile duct (CBD) injury or stricture, and excessive coagulation may result in thermal injury leading to a CBD stricture, a right hepatic artery pseudo-aneurysm, or a duodenal injury and late perforation.

Confronted with significant bleeding, it's your task to make some quick decisions: Can the bleeding be controlled laparoscopically? Can you do it

or do you need assistance? Can you temporarily control it and wait for assistance? Do you need to convert now?

For the laparoscopic novices among you: don't forget that the laparoscopic view is magnified — a small fish looks like a shark. So what at first glance seems a major arterial pumping could be a bleeding arteriole. **Do not panic! Wash, suck and look again**.

Conversion

Conversion from laparoscopy to open surgery is considered by some to be a failure, but it is better conceived as a calculated decision to complete a safe and successful operation — the access being just the means and not the goal. While it's difficult to draw the exact line at which a change of surgical strategy is mandatory, and conversion is inevitable, it is better to err on the safe side. The thought of your colleagues' reaction, and the 'shame' associated with conversion, should not deter you, the safe surgeon, from reaching the correct decision and acting upon it. **Always consider what you lose and what you gain by conversion**. You should consider calling for help, as fresh eyes and hands may push the operation forward or solve a problem you are struggling with, but remember: **conversion can always be explained, and considered a safe option, while failure to convert in time is hardly respected or defendable. And the one who really loses from a wrong decision is the patient, not you**. (Nay, at the end of the day you'll lose as well...).

Reasons for conversion may vary, from a non-progressing operation due to difficult dissection, through a complication that needs repair like bowel injury, to an emergent situation like uncontrolled bleeding. **The ideal conversion will be the result of a thoughtful calculation — made relatively early during surgery, before any complication intervenes — that the operation cannot be completed laparoscopically**. Opening the abdomen after an hour of futile dissection is a sign of surgical stubbornness and lack of sound surgical judgment. As you know, the duration of operation does matter: converting a difficult appendectomy after an hour of manipulation — with the appendix now in pieces — is how septic complications are produced. And when you audit your laparoscopic experience, you should analyze the converted cases within the laparoscopic group ('intention to treat') — not the open — to avoid bias.

You should also remember that conversion is not a panacea, and a difficult operation may continue to be difficult as an open procedure as well. Some of the complications may happen at the conversion (cutting through bowel stuck to the scar), or after it. Not a few CBDs were transected after converting a difficult cholecystectomy. **However, converting after the injury has been created won't let you off the hook**.

Postoperative considerations

As is true for any operation, laparoscopy does not end at the suturing of the skin. Complications may manifest themselves hours or days after surgery (and even months or years, if hernias in scars are included). Overall, convalescence after laparoscopy is expected to be smooth with relatively little pain and quick recuperation. Small scars and early feeding and mobilization should minimize 'regular' complications like wound infection, pneumonia or DVT. Other 'non-laparoscopic' complications, like anastomotic leak, are expected to occur at a similar rate as after open surgery.

Therefore, any alteration from the expected postoperative course should alert you, the surgeon, to a possible complication that should be actively investigated or ruled out. Excessive pain, tachycardia, fever, abdominal distension or prolonged ileus may be signs of a complication that may be still hidden and warrants further studies, imaging or even re-exploration.

The decision to proceed with further investigation and possibly return to the operating room is never easy, and surgeons tend to downplay the situation and ignore hints that something may go wrong after what seemed like a successful operation. Consulting with other surgeons is often productive and eye-opening, but is a privilege not always available for solo surgeons.

After laparoscopy, even the slight suspicion of a complication should prompt you to exclude it! The fat lady three days after an 'uneventful lap chole' is still not well. Measure the liver function tests, order a CT. **It is better to prove that everything is *KOSHER* rather than miss a bile leak**. In the case when re-exploration is needed, the option of **repeat laparoscopy** is possible, first as a diagnostic tool but also as a therapeutic procedure, if appropriate. The exact nature of the complication, coupled with your ability to solve it, should direct the choice of the procedure, with the patient's safety guiding this decision.

With laparoscopic surgery, coupled with modern "fast-track surgery", short hospital stay is the rule. **As a consequence, complications may manifest themselves after the patient is already home**. A detailed explanation about possible warning symptoms and signs, with the relevant directions if and when the patient should contact you or return to the ER, is extremely important. This allows early detection and treatment of complications, that otherwise may be neglected and treated too late.

I want to conclude with a comment which may sound like a **cliché** but is an important one. In this day and age of super-specialization, with many laparoscopic surgeons focused on a narrow spectrum of laparoscopic procedures, it is crucial that they preserve their general surgical judgment and skills. Laparoscopic surgeons must be able to know the operative field not only through the video camera — this is indispensable for the effective management of complications. **A good lap-surgeon has to be a solid general surgeon. Period.**

In this chapter I have tried to open your mind... to make laparoscopic surgery as safe as open!

> "Human mind, like parachute; works best when open."
> A Chinese proverb

Chapter 10

Dealing with patients, families, lawyers and yourself

Avi Rubinstein and Moshe Schein

Surgery is the most dangerous activity of legal society.
P.O. Nyström

The title of this chapter may appear weird but it makes sense: **if the patient and his family are satisfied then you won't have to see a lawyer. Wouldn't this improve the quality of your life?!**

The business of surgery shares much with any other service business. What is true for the hotelier, the sommelier and the butcher should apply to you — your job is to satisfy the customer and if, for some reason, right or wrong, he is displeased or peeved (e.g. the $250 Bordeaux was vinegary, the hotel room stank or the anastomosis leaked), you have to know how to manage the situation, placate the customer — keeping the lawyers at bay.

This is not intended to be a treatise on 'malpractice', nor is it a manual of 'risk management'. It is just some informal advice on how to please your patients before and after the operation, to protect yourself against the hassle of complaints and the plague of lawsuits. **Consider this**: if you are an American general surgeon, the probability that you are currently involved in a lawsuit is around 15% — by the age of 65 it's very unlikely that you will not have been sued at least once. Nothing can completely protect you from a frivolous lawsuit but the counsel offered below could help you defend yourself and perhaps win in court.

We won't dwell on the legal process involving cases of assumed or proven surgical negligence in the various countries. Legal systems differ greatly from place to place — in the US it is the jury that decides, in Israel it is the judge, in Scandinavia each case is arbitrated by a special tribunal and in India the offending surgeon is occasionally lynched by the mob. **But wherever you practice, the fundamentals of human interaction are the same: if you damage the patient, if you make him resentful, he may seek revenge by whatever measures are available to him. For this reason, the following discussion is universal!**

Careful **analysis of litigated cases**, irrespective of whether negligence is proven or not, serves as a superb teaching tool on how to avoid and treat complications and dodge entanglement in a legal muddle — any surgeon who acts as an expert witness (for the plaintiff or the defense) will tell you this. With this in mind, and to enrich this chapter, we invited a veteran malpractice lawyer (A.R.), who before dedicating his life to the glorious practice of suing surgeons was a (neuro)surgeon. His pearls of wisdom are scattered throughout this document.

Whatever we write, we don't preach 'defensive medicine'. We don't subscribe to the notion that "a CT scan a day keeps the lawyer away" — wasting resources, torturing patients with unnecessary tests or procedures ("for the lawyers or the jury") is the hallmark of an insecure surgeon. Instead, practicing 'correct' surgery, using your common sense and careful documentation are your best tools. **Furthermore, smiling and being non-arrogant should be part of your personality; that you are a surgeon doesn't mean that you can't be a 'nice guy'.**

> *Patients sue not when the patient gets angry with the doctor,*
> *but when the doctor gets angry at the patient.*
>
> **Thomas J. Krizek**

Each chapter in this book outlines optimal ways to avoid complications in particular situations and to deal with them once they develop. Below we'll highlight additional general measures to practice safe surgery, satisfy the patients, please the ever watching 'big brother' and famish the plaintiff lawyers.

General considerations

> *Surgeons must be self-confident. The problem is when that*
> *self-confidence becomes arrogance.*
>
> **Alden H. Harken**

Communication

Proper communication is the key! Good rapport with the patient and his family before and after the operation — especially if complications arise — is critical. Empathy, warmth, compassion, sympathy, patience, sincerity are your allies. Arrogance, detachment, condescension, rashness, evasion are your enemies — potentially deadly sins. **Remember**: the factor determining whether the deceased patient's wife would say "Dr. Kumar's such a compassionate surgeon... he did whatever he could to save my husband..." or "That arrogant bastard Kumar has killed my husband!" is your attitude and the way you communicate. **Body language** matters a lot: even if rushed, force yourself to listen, mask your inherent 'surgical touchiness' — any minute invested in the relationship with the patient and his family will pay off! **Watch what you are saying** — everything leaving your mouth has potential repercussions. If you say that the child needs an emergency appendectomy because the appendix has probably perforated then you must see to it that the operation is done NOW. No delays are acceptable to the family — anxiety, anger, resentment are increasing minute by minute. Gather all the facts before you say something! **Proper communication with everybody** involved in the care of the patient is equally important — consultants, residents, partners, nurses, OR team. **Convoluted lines of communication result in havoc and system failure — a leading cause of complications**. But it is not the 'system' that will suffer anguish and sleepless nights; it will be you! So communicate precisely with all the above to ensure that your patient receives the care you want him to receive. **As you know, hospital systems are as dangerous as war zones; your job is to protect the patient from the system**, by doing so you protect your own butt. And this brings us to the next item.

Documentation

A key principle in *real* 'defensive medicine' is *not* to order unnecessary tests but to document everything you're doing and **why** — including why you are not going to order the test. Some surgeons believe that 'excessive' documentation could be used against them by the lawyers but this is an absolute nonsense. Our vast experience with malpractice cases shows exactly the opposite— that **detailed documentation is your best defense line**. If sued, all that you (and your lawyer) have to do is to convince the judge and/or jury that the patient has received optimal expert attention: **that serious intellectual activity was invested in decision-making, which in turn was based on a proper assessment of the clinical picture and the test results obtained; that everything was explained and the patient's**

concerns noted and addressed. There is no need to write or dictate prolonged monologues — just mention the essentials: what a good clinician believes it is important to know. Include your assessment, what you contemplate and your dilemmas: "I decided to take the patient back to the OR because..." or "I decided to postpone the reoperation because...". Always indicate with whom you consulted and the advice you received: "I called the Infection Disease consultant. He advised me to stop the antibiotics and take cultures..." Investing five minutes in proper documentation at the end of the encounter (always enter date and time!) is not only useful to PYA (protect your ass) but it also improves your management — forcing you to sit down, ponder and reflect: "What should I do? Perhaps I'm wrong?" Think about it this way: whatever you write in the chart (it's a permanent record!) reflects on your practice more than your actions in the OR (only a few see this and... forget...). Be aware that lawyers and expert witnesses scrutinize the whole chart, not only what you've written but also what the nurses, residents and others had to say. **Often, in successfully litigated surgical cases we see extreme discrepancies in the chart**. This is a typical example: the surgeon enters in the chart each morning, "...patient doing well, abdomen soft, passing gas" and leaves for the day; a different nurse enters each shift (three times a day), "patient not well, complains about pain, received morphine, vomited once..." Now, how can any lawyer successfully defend such a surgeon? Clearly, to survive you have to be as facile (and honest!) with the pen as you are with the scalpel! **Remember: what has not been documented did not take place!**

Timing

The clock is ticking! As with anything in life also in surgery *time* and *timing* are vital in their impact on complications, outcomes and litigation. One of the most common terms used in lawsuits is DELAY. Delay to diagnose, delay to review the tests, delay to obtain consults, delay to treat, and delay to diagnose/treat failures. **So, do not postpone, do not temporize, suppress or deny — do it now!** And if it can wait then document why... "Frequent dilemma: take your wife for dinner or the patient back to the OR?"

Behavioral practice

The behavioral practice of surgeons is a more significant source of poor outcomes (and litigation) than technical misadventures alone. Commonly, it's not what you do in the OR (assuming that you are a qualified surgeon) but outside it that harms your patient and your reputation (see ■ Table 10.1).

Table 10.1. Flawed behavioral patterns associated with litigation.

(Percentages sum to >100% because there was more than one flaw per case.) *Based on analysis of 460 'closed' malpractice claims against general surgeons in the USA (Griffen FD, et al. Violations of behavioral practices revealed in closed claims reviews. Ann Surg 2008; 248: 468-74).*

Nature of flawed pattern	%
Poor communication with patient and/or family	34
Failure to pursue abnormal symptom or test result	25
Failure to pursue a postoperative problem	25
Failure to assess a surgical problem before surgery	19
Failure to enlist support of a proper consultant	14
Failure to see patient in a timely basis	13
Failure of cross coverage or continuity of care	12
Failure to communicate with consultants	10
Failure to stay within proper scope of practice	10
Failure to assess comorbidities before surgery	6
Failure to follow the patient long enough after surgery	5
Failure to check test results	5
Failure to maintain other practice patterns	14

Denial and wishful thinking

Denial and wishful thinking are powerful human defense mechanisms with which you have to engage in perpetual combat. Oh yes, "the anastomosis looks a little dusky, but it should be OK" or "it is only ileus, he can't be leaking" — how easy it is to look away! Don't behave like a 'surgical ostrich', burying your head in the sand. **As a surgeon you have to be a cheerful optimist and a dour pessimist at the same time!** Without a healthy measure of optimism you could not engage in such risky endeavors; without a measure of 'background pessimism' you won't be able to correct what went wrong. **The secret is: be optimistic before the operation and pessimistic after it — until the patient has fully recovered.**

Manage the patient as your own family

Finally, and this is a cliché — but a cliché that will live forever: **manage each patient as if he or she were a member of your own family.** Close your eyes and imagine that this is your father, your daughter or your wife lying on that stretcher in the ER… or even it is yourself: how would you want to be managed in such a situation? **Well, why should patients be treated differently from your loved ones?** Remember your own experience as a patient, or when your parents were hospitalized — it wasn't always rosy, eh? Try to be better!

Pre-operative considerations

> The degree of negligence is the inverse of the lack of diligence.
>
> **Tom Horan**

Whether it is an elective case, when you act at leisure, or an emergency one, when each minute counts, you have to prepare for war like a responsible commander-in-chief. That your forces have to be well trained, fed, and briefed is obvious, but you also have to think about diplomatic repercussions and prepare the ground for any contingency that might develop after the battle — especially if things go wrong, as they often do.

Specialty

Do not operate/practice out of specialty — every lawyer will tell you that it is a potentially lethal transgression! If the 'Whipple' you performed (the first in five years!) did wonderfully well, the patient will send flowers (and hopefully a bottle of 21-year-old single malt), you will walk on water, and your rivals will raise an eyebrow and await their chances to nail you 'the next time'. But if the Whipple complicates — as it often does — hell will break loose. Of course, when the situation is **life-threatening**, and there is no *alternative*, you may be forced to act outside your field of expertise. So it would be reasonable to operate on an actively bleeding hepatic adenoma even if the last hepatectomy you saw (as an assistant) was during your residency 15 years ago. There is a caveat, however, the *other* option: was the patient stable enough to be treated with angiographic embolization, which is readily available in your hospital? Isn't the other surgeon in your hospital (your declared enemy!) a superb hepatic surgeon? If so, the plaintiff's expert witness will scoop enough dirt to nail you! Even a *solo* practice in a remote (rural) location doesn't give you an absolute license to perform outside your usual scope. In elective cases, you have always to consider the option of **referring out** and even **emergencies** can be problematic. For example: in the middle of the night you repaired a complex hand injury; infection developed and the patient lost a few fingers. One can foretell what the lawyer will ask you during the deposition: "Dr. McDonald, are you a hand surgeon? Are you board certified in orthopedics? Couldn't you have dressed the hand and shipped the patient to the hand surgeon in the University Hospital of Dundee?" Again, **always document**: "patient was offered transfer to another center but elected to undergo the operation locally" — that is if you are confident that you know what you're doing…

'New' or 'experimental' treatments

Beware new or experimental treatments. <u>Remember</u>: "Be not the first by whom the new is tried, nor yet the last to lay the old aside." And: "When technology is the Master, the result is Disaster."

Indication

"The lesser the indication, the greater the complication." The importance of a 'correct' indication for any operation is stressed *ad nauseam* in each of the chapters of this book. You can *get away with* almost anything, even removing almost normal organs for flimsy indications — that is, if things evolve smoothly. So, nobody will raise an eyebrow if you do an *internal sphincterotomy* for acute anal fissure in a patient you saw first a few days ago. But if you render the patient incontinent be ready to reply to the question: "Dr. Rasputin, why didn't you attempt to heal the fissure with conservative treatment? Did you ever hear about diltiazem ointment, stool softeners?" **Of course, the indication for operation, and alternative treatments, has to be clearly documented by you in the chart!**

Delay

Avoid postponement, avoid delay, avoid procrastination. Yes, we have mentioned the time factor just above but delays of all sorts are your mortal foes!

Consent

Consent is not just a piece of paper! The standard, pre-printed form available in your hospital, which the patient is made to sign — agreeing to whatever operation and whichever additional steps are deemed necessary during it — is not the *real* consent. The real process of informed consent is not a somewhat confused, hurried and embarrassed first-year resident addressing a pre-medicated and anxious patient — the patient lying down, the doctor hovering above him — an hour before the operation. The real informed consent should be taken always by the **operating surgeon himself**, discussing, at leisure, with the patient and family **indications, alternatives, benefits, expected postoperative course and potential complications**. Everything has to be explained and repeated as many times as necessary, using language and terms comprehensible to the party involved. Teaching aids like booklets, pictures, even YouTube operative clips are useful — we find a pen, a piece of paper and a few simple drawings less intimidating.

The key is honest disclosure: never underestimate the risks involved, prepare the patient and family that bad outcomes are possible. Be specific. Honesty means also that 'new' or 'experimental' procedures are presented as such: "I would like to perform a new 'single-port' laparoscopic thyroidectomy, the guys in Mayo have been doing it successfully, I watched them doing it and I'm confident that I can do it as well... the alternative would be..." [Please do not take this example seriously!]. **Disclose even your 'learning curve'**. Yes, it is not easy to admit that you completed only five sleeve gastrectomies — while the guy on the other side of the corridor has done 1000! The consent process can be hastened during **emergencies** but never bypassed. A personal note signed by you, on the electronic chart, on paper — even a few words scribbled on the actual consent form — attesting that a factual informed consent has been taken may prove invaluable one day.

Diplomacy!

Wars are usually preceded by intense background diplomatic activities. The same applies to your own battle — the planned surgery. From the first encounter with the patient, in your office, the ER, wherever, you have to establish adequate rapport with the patient's family. You have to spot your potential allies, the ones with whom you'll deal with after the surgery, when the setting could become unpleasant. Acknowledge each member of the family — look into his or her eye. The fat ugly one, sulking at the end of the room, not appreciating your famous sense of humor [1], is exactly the one who may initiate the lawsuit against you (■ Figure 10.1).

> *Risk management begins just when you first meet the patient and family.*

---

[1] *Use humor with patients and families judiciously — you must stop all attempts at humor after the first blank look.* [Leo A. Gordon].

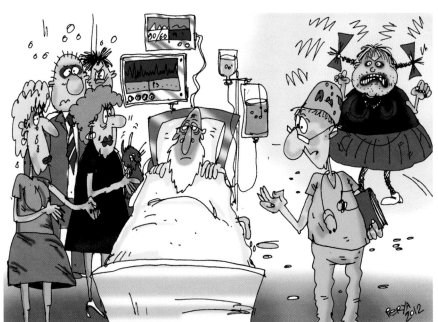

Figure 10.1. Do not ignore the ugly daughter hiding in the corner of the room — she may be the one who becomes your enemy!

Intra-operative considerations

Surprisingly (for some it won't be a surprise), in most litigated cases, **intra-operative events — including technical misadventures — are not the main reason behind lawsuits**. Instead, it is what came to pass before the operation (e.g. delay in diagnosis) or after the operation (e.g. failure to recognize the consequence of the technical misadventure) which fuels the lawsuits (look at this reference [2]). This reflects what J.L. Yates wrote in 1905: "There is a tendency always to attribute fatalities… to sins of omissions, whereas the many evil results of the sins of commission are given much less consideration." In other words (see ➲ Chapter 1), **people do accept that 'shit happens' but when it happens they want you to diagnose and treat it effectively**.

Yet another surprise: **most technical errors in a study of surgical malpractice claims in the USA occurred in routine operations performed by experienced surgeons** (look also at this reference [3]). Atul Gawande, who

---

2   Griffen FD, *et al*. The ACS's closed claim case study: new insights for improving care. *Journal of the American College of Surgeons* 2007; 204: 561-9.

3   Regenbogen SE, *et al*. Pattern of technical error among surgical malpractice claims. *Ann Surg* 2007; 246: 705-11.

co-authored that study said: "The real problem isn't how to stop bad doctors from harming, even killing, patients. It's how to prevent good doctors from doing so." Of course, experienced surgeons tend to operate more and do more complex procedures, making them prone to technical mishaps. **But let us not forget that the vast majority (>95%!) of surgical errors are never subjected to litigation**, and so we don't know who is *overall* more prone to technical error — experienced or inexperienced surgeons? The frequency of error could also depend on the type and location of practice; teaching hospitals and academic surgeons were over-represented in the cited study.

Be that as it may, an uneventful and perfectly performed operation reduces the probability of postoperative complications, creating fewer opportunities for you to blunder, mismanage and be sued for. Avoidance of specific perioperative complications is emphasized all over this book but here are a few points we wish to reiterate:

- **The few minutes just before the operation provide you with another opportunity to engage in 'diplomacy' and improve safety**. Whatever you do, make the effort, nay, make it a routine, to visit the patient's bedside before he's wheeled to the OR. "So, today we are repairing your recurrent hernia, right? You wanted to have spinal anesthesia. Do you remember that we've discussed that removing the testicle could be a good idea? Are you still OK with it? Show me the hernia again… it's on the right side, correct?" Acknowledge again all members of the family present — probably you'll see a few new faces: the son who just flew in from Alaska or the daughter who drove from her University in Helsinki. Shake their hands and *schmooze* a little. "Is there anything that you wish me to clarify?" The whole *spiel* will take five minutes. Dedicate this time and look like a *mensch* — not a frickin' robot!
- **Always read your own notes before the operation** (that is, if you didn't do it early in the morning), to remind yourself about the nitty-gritty of the case. Yes, the nurses and OR staff will go over the check list *de jour*, mark the operative site and 'time out' will be conducted (⊃ Chapter 2), but all such precautions are prone to human error so conduct you own QA process.
- If you work in a system allowing trainees to operate unsupervised (this is common in many countries but prohibited in the US) **be in the operating room or nearby (readily available) from the start of the operation**… until its end. **Remember**: it is you who is responsible when your resident resects the common bile duct while you give a superb lecture to a class of medical students about bile duct injuries.
- Now do yourself a great favor and read Dr. Richard Karl's excellent piece on "**Staying Safe: simple tools for safe surgery**" — available online as a PDF [4].

---

[4] http://www.facs.org/fellows_info/bulletin/2007/karl0407.pdf.

- **OR culture matters. The atmosphere in the OR should be serious and relaxed at the same time.** *Serious* to avoid distractions, *relaxed* to allow open dialogue with each member of the team — welcoming questions and comments. The intern holding the retractor may have a valuable thing to say and also the scrub nurse. Listen to them! The airline industry endorses a policy of a 'sterile cockpit': below 10,000 feet no discussion is allowed unless it concerns matters to do with the conduct of the flight. Often the operation is more complex than landing an airliner so make everybody shut up (including the anesthetist who suddenly has the urge to boast about his recent trophy fish), switch off the radio, and focus on the operation. There is time to unwind and time to tense up — you decide when and dictate the pattern! Let us not even start ranting about cell phones… (the use of cell phones is forbidden in my OR [Moshe]).
- **See to it that members of the patient's family receive regular dispatches *during* the operation.** This is paramount if the procedure proves to be longer than the family has been led to expect. So if the 'lap chole' has to be converted let the husband in the waiting room know why he's still waiting. In certain situations it is best to pause the operation, unscrub and go to talk with the family: "I found an inoperable cancer, our only option is to do a colostomy…" — let them take part in the decision-making: this is the 'real' defensive surgery!
- **Never leave the operating room without thanking each member of the team — then go and talk to the family.** But don't go out and tell the family that "everything went smoothly and as expected" while the resident is still busy closing the abdomen — unpleasant surprises could be embarrassing.
- **Never leave the hospital before you are confident that the patient is awake, well and in the recovery room and that you have left somebody informed and responsible for any eventuality; even then be readily available to come back.** It is not uncommon for city surgeons to rush to another hospital (usually the private one…) before the case is finished — doesn't time = money? But starting a fresh case 25 miles away, while your previous case is crashing, is not too healthy to your career; nor is it beneficial to your coronaries. A renowned chairman in an American metropolis completed resection of a GI cancer, let his team 'mop up behind and close', went out to the family to report a successful operation and then took a cab to the airport. The patient died in the recovery room. The chairman lost his job. **The moral of the story: don't plan any elective operation if you are not able to provide, in person, the postoperative care.** This is true even if you work with partners who provide excellent cross cover for you. Another legal case we were involved with: a surgeon did a 'lap chole'

and immediately left for the Alpine ski slopes. Patients and families never forgive **abandonment**! (see below).

- **Dictate or write down the operative report at the end of the operation, even before you start the next case**. Do it while the operative details are fresh in your mind. You do not need to produce a mega document *à la* Tolstoy or Dickens but it has to be proportionate to the complexity of the procedure that it has to reflect — what exactly has been done and why. Be honest about mishaps and how they were managed. **When complications develop after the operation a detailed 'op report' may turn out to be your best ally**. When a severe CBD injury is diagnosed after lap chole which has been described in a three-line op report as "uneventful" or "routine", the legal battle has been lost. But if the op report describes a careful lysis of dense adhesions, attempts to achieve the "critical view" and so forth… your case may be defensible. In other words: don't be lazy, narrate the conduct of the operation but there is no need to be a *nudnik*! **Remember**: an experienced reviewer can gauge your surgical personality by reading your op notes.

Never refer to an operation as "just a…". It reflects lack of appreciation for surgical pathology. For any procedure in surgery can result in horrible complications. The vagaries of human biology assure this.

Leo A. Gordon

Postoperative considerations

As long as the abdomen is open you control it. Once closed it controls you. This is relevant, but to a lesser extent, for other cavities.

Always assume that the source of complications is at the site of the operation — unless proven otherwise.

These two adages, sometimes paraphrased, are repeatedly stressed in this book and for a just cause. They should become your postoperative *mantra*, obliging you to be constantly on the alert and suspicious!

So what would be your response once you have realized that your postop patient suffers a serious complication? We are all different but like *mourning* or *grief* one can describe a common pattern.

The Kübler-Ross model, commonly known as "The Five Stages of Grief" could be applied to our situation:

- **Denial** — this, hopefully, is not what we surgeons engage in when facing a complication. We do not look away, pretending that it doesn't exist. Instead, we face it head on!
- **Anger** — "Hell, why did it happen to me? I did such a good operation…"
- **Bargaining** — "After all, it is not my fault. Why did he wait so long? And he was so bloody obese! And anyway, why didn't the frickin' internist stop the frickin' anticoagulation?"
- **Depression** — "I'm fed up. What's wrong with me? Shouldn't I start thinking about quitting? Perhaps I should stop doing major surgery. Am I aging?"
- **Acceptance** — "Oh well, shit happens; only those who don't operate do not have complications!"

Others [5] describe four phases characteristic to surgeons' reactions to adverse events:

- **The Kick**. The surgeon experiences symptoms of stress and anxiety, the magnitude of such a response correlating with factors such as the age of the patient, the nature of the operation, the severity of the complication and the pre-existing rapport with the patient and his family.
- **The Fall**. The surgeon constantly ruminates about the case (we tend to replay the past events over and over again in our mind, like in a broken video), often asking "Was it my fault?" — sometimes looking for somebody to blame.
- **Recovery**. Gradually the surgeon calms down, realizing that one has to move on, but continues to be reflective. Coping mechanisms include discussion with the patient and family, analyzing with colleagues what went wrong and learning lessons for the future. For some, standing up at the morbidity and mortality conference to declare *mea culpa* can provide *catharsis*.
- **Long-term impact**. It all depends on the number and frequency of accumulated complications and the surrounding environment. Some learn to live with it, developing a 'thick skin'. In the more sensitive types it can lead to *burnout*. As surgeons age, their response to complications tends to become more drastic: most take it deeper into their hearts but the *psychopaths* erase it immediately as if it has never occurred — the "Professor Ferdinand Sauerbruch Syndrome" (read about his life and old age).

---

[5] Luu S, *et al*. When bad things happen to good surgeons: reactions to adverse events. *Surg Clin N Am* 2012; 92: 153-61.

Some additional advice on how not to piss off patients with complications and their families follows below.

Disclosure

Timely and honest disclosure of what happened and why, followed by the plan and the prognosis is indispensable. Lying, hiding, suppressing information... "not looking directly at their eyes", promotes alienation, suspicion, distrust, and later on, lawsuits. **Openness and sincerity, while not totally eliminating legal risks, are the key to maintaining a proper relationship with the 'patient-family complex',** facilitating the continuation of care — allowing you to 'fix the problem' and thus redeem yourself. And yet, there is nothing more difficult than to stand before the patient's wife, sons and daughters, gazing at their accusing eyes, absorbing their disbelief, anger and frustration and confessing that you, together with the system have screwed up. Of course, it is not always your fault. Shit happens and you should try explaining it.

What about disclosure of 'near misses'? It depends... we do not think that you have to divulge near misses which have no implications whatsoever for the patient's prognosis. For example, your resident has almost divided the ureter but you stopped him at the last moment — true, your own heart rate increased momentarily but otherwise one can forget about it. On the other hand, **we believe that any near miss that could affect the patient's recovery has to be openly discussed.** For instance — unexpected blood loss: "when we tried to clamp the aorta just above the aneurysm the renal vein was torn and we struggled to stop the bleeding... we managed eventually but lost lots of blood... now everything seems to be under control... yes, we completed the procedure as planned. I just want you to know that Hans received ten units of blood and this obviously puts him at higher risk for infections and his kidneys may have suffered as well. Why did it happen? Well, it was a huge aneurysm and it sat directly on top of the vein... and there were multiple adhesions from his previous colectomy which made exposure very, very difficult."

Whether you disclose or not and how much depends also on the 'local culture'.

A surgeon from Russia wrote on SURGINET:

"In my country if you find a retained instrument or tampon at relaparotomy you should remove it in such a way that nobody sees. And then call personally the surgeon who did the first operation and tell him about his fault. We try to hide it from the patient and nurses..."

For most of us such behavior is unthinkable. If you are brave and clever, and we hope that you are, you could try and change such a dismal culture! Anyway, try not to forget that the walls in the OR may have eyes and ears…

Interestingly, it is not fear from litigation which inhibits candid disclosure. Canadian surgeons are much less likely to be sued than their US counterparts but just as likely to hide the truth. We are told that "to err is human", perhaps we should add that "to lie is human" as well?

Abandonment

Abandoning your complicated patient to his or her fate is a huge mistake. It breeds bitterness, hate and desire for revenge. **The bigger the complication, the more significant its consequences, the more intensive should be your personal commitment to the management of the patient**. Oh, sure, we know how unpleasant and stressful it is to watch, day in and day out, the patient pouring enteric juices from his gaping abdomen (following your perfect gastric bypass). You many think, "the residents can look after him, they don't need my daily involvement…" But the family will think otherwise: "that frickin' Professor, he fucked up so badly and now he has lost interest. And he took the money, the SOB!…" Well, if this is the case they are right in thinking so and to seek revenge. **Advice: see the complicated patient as often as you can, stop by when you walk by his room, touch him, chat with the family**. Even if his condition is desperate and he is busy dying, even if he has been transferred to a different ward or another hospital — keep in touch and show interest! **People want to be respected until the end.**

Documentation

We apologize for the repetition but careful and detailed documentation of your ongoing involvement in the **postoperative** care is imperative. Always mention the exact date and hour. Again: **avoid or explicitly justify factual conflicts with what has been entered in the chart by others. Discrepancies** provide ample ammunition to lawyers — they cherish it! Unfortunately, it is our experience that such inconsistencies are extremely common. **So spend a few minutes to browse what the night nurse has written**. Never ever 'doctor' the chart, trying to modify what you have already written, and signed, or to 'insert' a new entry into an earlier date (this has become more difficult with **electronic charts**). Lawyers are expert in detecting such attempts which help them to tighten the rope around your neck.

Second opinion/transfer

Do not *shed* responsibility but *share* it. Accept responsibility for your complications but share the responsibility for its treatment. Get advice from wise older colleagues, even if you know how to proceed. A **second opinion** boosts your temporarily wobbly confidence. To the family an opinion from another expert is tremendously reassuring — get one before they ask for it. And if they do, never decline their wish with an (arrogant) excuse that you know what you're doing. **The same applies for shipping out to another hospital**: if you believe that the patient's chances could be improved by transfer to a higher level hospital then just organize it promptly. Yes, your ego may suffer as well as your reputation (you obviously do not want the guys in the Ivory Tower to see your disaster...) but what really counts is the final outcome. This is not a politically correct statement but a true one: it is better for your reputation that the patient doesn't die from complications in your small or rural hospital. The common perception is that mortalities after operations in a rural hospital are *because* "of the inexperienced surgeon or poor care" while in the Ivory Tower they die *despite* "the best efforts of the excellent doctors in the great hospital".

Post-discharge issues

Once you have operated on a patient he is yours — hanging around your neck like an albatross. Operating is fun — postop care is a heavy burden. The endorphin-fed euphoria you feel at the end of the procedure can be rapidly replaced with worry or even gloom... lasting until the final recovery; and this often doesn't end when the patient walks out of the hospital. Actually in this era when patients are dispatched home ASAP — ejected from the hospital after a lap colectomy even before they have farted — your direct involvement with the patient's care has to continue beyond the hospital's wall:

- At discharge provide patients with accurate instructions, preferably written, about *everything* (e.g. wound care, medications, signs to watch for and report, contact numbers). **Remember: in some patients the risk of DVT, and the need for prophylaxis, does not end at the parking lot of the hospital**.
- Do not wait for the patient to call you, or turn-up, too late, in the ER, with problems. Instead, call them (or let your staff do so) every day to ensure that their progress is uneventful.
- Should your patient need readmission, be there for him, even if he's admitted to the medical ward for treatment of his pneumonia. After all — **you are his surgeon!** And this may not be just pneumonia...

Money matters

*And thou shalt speak unto him, saying, Thus saith the LORD,
Hast thou killed, and also taken possession?*

In the Hebrew version of the Bible:

Haratsachta vegam yarashta, correctly translated as:

Have you murdered and also inherited?

1 Kings 21:19

Patients who suffer significant complications resent having to pay (out of their own pockets!) for a botched operation and the cost of treating such complications. **Thus, do whatever you can within your system to diminish the financial burden incurred by the harmed patient.** If you practice in a 'private system', be it 'official' or 'under the table' (oh yes, in many parts of the world surgeons do accept, or even demand, thick envelopes stuffed with cash!), hand the money back! This is called 'damage control'. However, again, there may be differences around the world. Some claim that to return money is tantamount to admitting liability. Waiving charges for follow-up procedures may be prudent.

*There are only four forms of incentive that I now, in my 27th
year as a surgical chair, recognize: cash, money, cash money,
and everything that can be converted into cash money.*

Josef Fischer

Legal considerations

*Doctors are just the same as lawyers; the only difference is
that lawyers merely rob you, whereas doctors rob you and kill
you, too.*

Anton Chekhov

*The only thing jurors hate more than cocky surgeons are
cocky lawyers.*

Whether harmed patients can protest, sue or hope to be compensated — and for how much — for the damage inflicted on them by their surgeons depends on the local legal system and culture. Many of you, living in, for example, Russia or Sweden, have never been exposed to a lawsuit; in the former the patients mostly remain uncompensated, in the latter the welfare state looks after them. On the other hand, in the US (it has been said that two-thirds of the world's lawyers live in the USA) and in certain countries (like Israel), the dangers of being sued are ever present like a constantly gathering hurricane.

Surgeons do not like lawyers, to say it mildly. To anyone who has been sued this is not surprising. But don't you agree that harmed patients should be able to express their grievances and be compensated? In the absence of a better and fairer system lawyers (well, some of them) are only doing their job. After reading this book we hope that you will know how to behave so that even when you are pursued (frivolously or not) you may prevail. Now here is some additional perspective that may help you to this end:

- You know by now why you're being sued: you had bad luck, did something stupid or managed to irritate the patient. Occasionally, the accusations against you are frivolous. **But what motivates the plaintiffs — patients or the families they left behind?** Often it is feelings of bitterness, anger and even hatred towards the surgeon and/or the system. When they present at the lawyer's office they may seek vengeance — they want a payback for the suffering, slight, or lost life! *If this is not possible, let us at least get some money!*
- **The vast majority (95%) of adverse surgical events due to error never lead to legal claims.** Once the case goes to court the plaintiff's chance of prevailing is no more than 20-30%. Most frivolous claims are dismissed, but although this doesn't compensate you for the wasted time and the emotional torment during the prolonged legal battle, you see that overall the legal system handicaps the patients! This is good news for you but bad for patients who are being harmed and not compensated. These figures refer to the USA; sorry, but we cannot provide you with data specific to your own country.
- **A reminder on what is the standard of care (SOC)**: the watchfulness, attention, caution and prudence that a *reasonable* surgeon under similar circumstances would exercise. **Failure to meet the SOC is negligence.** The 'problem' is that the 'standard' is often subjective, disputable and variable from place to place and from judge to judge. All this uncertainty feeds armies of lawyers and escalates the cost of care.
- We recommend that you read this excellent monograph debunking many perceived myths: "The truth about medical malpractice litigation" [6].

---

6 http://files.cttriallawyers.org/em/2012/0120-2054/MedMalFactSheet2012F.pdf.

The good thing about the standard of care is that there are so many to choose from.

In conclusion: not all medical negligence leads to complications and not all complications are caused by negligence. One can look at negligence from multiple angles and point out various etiologies such as ignorance, stupidity, over-confidence, carelessness, arrogance, greed — all part of the human condition.

To all the above we have to add a GLUE, binding it all together — the SYSTEM's dysfunction or failure, resulting from disorganization, apathy and miscommunication between humans who make up the system. We see the system failing all the time, every day we see near misses... we see numerous examples of negligence. It is so common that often we don't even stop to raise our brows or shrug our shoulders.

So at the end of the day each of us has to fend for himself... to actively or proactively and constantly maintain an anti-negligent awareness and attitude. We have to study how human nature works and play the system... but even then... even with all the check lists, QA bodies raining on us... we cannot completely win. **We have to rely on ourselves!**

> "Medical practice has also evolved so that now a defensive element tempers the physician's diagnostic and therapeutic approach... defensive medicine, with its economic and emotional consequences, is a pollutant byproduct of society that should be eradicated."
>
> **Seymour I. Schwartz**
>
> "On the sick bed we see man, as he is as well as who he is. He in turn, if we give wholly of ourselves, sees something of the secret in us. Here rather than in our societies, our laboratories, our hospitals, or our universities, is our future. We'll keep it or lose it on the same field."
>
> **J. Engelbert Dunphy**

And finally — Danny's list of the ten commandments:

- Be nice.
- Keep routines.
- Avoid shortcuts.
- Think again.
- Don't overdo.
- Know your limits.
- Respond — appropriately and in time.
- Disclose.
- Consult and refer.
- Be nice.

Chapter 11

The developing ('Third') World

B. Ramana

Privatization is presented as being the only alternative to an inefficient, corrupt state. In fact, it is not a choice at all... it is a mutually profitable business contract between the private company (preferably foreign) and the ruling elite of the Third World.

Arundhati Roy

The Third World

Many of you will have only heard of the Third World without even having smelled it once. No doubt, some of you will be living there all your unhappy lives, but Westerners need to know more, much more. The very nature of how schizophrenic (read crazy) such societies can be results in bizarre and troublesome situations that are hard for the *sahibs* to stomach.

Consider the contradiction of a patient dying of peptic perforation in a dilapidated Government Hospital because a bed was not available (or that he was operated upon too late), and another who perhaps had a ureteric injury during a robotic lap hysterectomy in a fancy private clinic at the same city (■ Figure 11.1). You can experience such wild variations in the nature of surgical complications when you are a third-world surgeon or surgical student. It is comforting to hear (yes, I admit *Schadenfreude!*) from some of my American friends that one can find third-world conditions and contradictions even in the USA — take certain hospitals in New York for example. And third-world medicine is not limited to the Indian sub-continent or to Africa. One need only look at

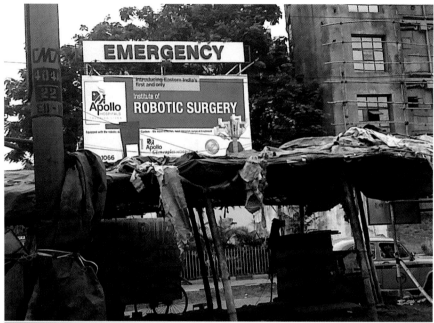

Figure 11.1. The 'Third World'— Institute of Robotic Surgery.

Russia with its huge gaps in the quality of surgical care between the public and private sectors to see that the 'Third World' can be found in many places.

General considerations

The third-world medical system suffers from numerous maladies that together contribute to the incidence and character of surgical complications:

- **Poor training** amongst surgeons, assistants, OR technicians and nurses: many surgeons have done their first hemicolectomy or Whipple operation while in practice, having never trained for these procedures.
- **Poor or no regulation** of medical practice: anyone can get away with anything!
- **Quacks operate**. Or "the janitor flew the plane because he thought he could, while the pilot took to the toilet seat."
- **Industry-driven procedures**: no FDA to impede the progress of science ☺!
- **Lack of hygiene and sterility**: cockroaches and rats are known to roam in many hospitals. I have found maggots in drain tubes while a

medical student/resident! (They could have been beneficial however — unclogging the tubes).

- Patients often present with **advanced/neglected disease**: you need to do a rotation here to know what I am talking about!
- **High workloads**: would you believe I used to do 20-25 procedures (mostly laparoscopic) in a day? And many others do insanely high volumes. As an historic legacy surgeons feel obliged to add a few zeroes religiously against the number of operations they have done. I joke that we Indians discovered the zero, and we take this fact too seriously!
- **Support system flaws**: the surgeon does a great job, but the ICU support is pathetic, and the patient is lost at dawn. Not a rare event.
- **Economic considerations**: procedures may be unnecessarily done for profit (correct me if I am wrong but isn't this also relevant in developed countries like the US?). On the flip side, lifesaving procedures may not be done in time because of the patient's financial limitations (the patient cannot pay!). Insurance coverage is poor and inconsistent.
- **Autopsies are not popular**, so you don't learn from your patient deaths.

Any one of you poor souls who have to survive, or thrive, in such an environment, and who is as outspoken and brave as I (☺), would be able to add a few examples to the above politically incorrect list. How much I would have loved to conclude the chapter at this point with a declaration: "the prevention and management of complications in the Third World should be exactly the same as in the developed world. Please consult the other chapters in this book…" Unfortunately, however, the situation is hopeless and unlikely to improve (like the chances for long-lasting peace in the Middle East). Therefore, I will continue to scribble some specific advice on **how to prevent and treat complications under our chaotic conditions — how to survive in the jungle!**

Pre-operative considerations

- **View any old man or woman brought in a stretcher/trolley with caring skepticism**. By this, I mean that you are empathetic to the patient's suffering, but watchful as to the harm you may inflict on him/her by poorly tolerated surgery. Often, these are malnourished, neglected end-stage cases with low albumin, a bad chest, and the works. Work up these cases medically and counsel the family exhaustively as to the risks involved.
- **Any cancer is locally advanced or metastatic unless proven otherwise**. This is not a blanket irresponsible statement, but merely a

rhetorical exhortation to you: are you sure that the 'Whipple' or esophagectomy you are planning is really beneficial to the patient? What if there are already metastases in the celiac axis nodes, for example? It is common for surgeons in the Third World to skip a CT scan to save the costs of treatment. The question arises if an unnecessary laparotomy is a more expensive and risky investigation, or not. The verdict in favor of imaging seems pretty strong.

- **Treat obese patients with the respect the condition demands**. Do not omit DVT prophylaxis when indicated. I have had to help surgeons whose uneventfully done operations ended in sudden death in the ward. One feature in common in all these was the absence of awareness about DVT/PE and the need for prophylaxis.

- **Do not jump on a peritonitis case and operate immediately**. Assess his hemodynamic status and whether he needs vigorous pre-op fluid resuscitation: usually he does! Antibiotics are invariably started on admission, but they may need to be changed for better results. Old timers have this confident and dismissive notion that once you open the abdomen and let out all the toxins, the kidneys will pick up and the patient will get well. I have seen surgeons sign death certificates soon after this statement. Learn from others' blunders. Or make your own. Your choice.

- **Do not do non-indicated or unnecessary surgery!** I am not aware of any Level I evidence for this, but bad things do happen in such operations. You don't need to remove those lily-white appendices. No, I insist, please let them be.

- **Operate within your core competence!** A gynecologist lost his license when he lost a patient after an appendectomy. No big deal, even a gynecologist can remove an appendix, you say? Well, not when the patient is a *male*. This makes it medically indefensible.

- **What minimum tests are to be considered mandatory?** Do not waste resources investigating the young patient due for a routine operation. Save them for the elderly patient, the obscure diagnosis, the GI cancer patient, the unwell postop patient, and so on. That said: some younger patients may have had valve surgery for rheumatic heart disease. Don't miss out on this bit of history: get the echo and cover for endocarditis. **Before all major surgery, serum albumin should be mandatory**. The point that needs to be noted is that you may need to defer your operation (like a Whipple or colectomy) until you nutritionally rehabilitate the patient, as reflected by a better sense of well-being and a higher level of albumin. "But this is not practical!" you may say? Well, be prepared for bad outcomes then.

- **What can one leave out?** When the fancy radionuclide assay and PET/SHMET scan are not available, you do not have a choice. Play with what you have, using maximal common sense and supra-maximal ethical standards.

- **Adequately brief people!** Teach in simple terms the nature of the operation, and what could go wrong: do it! If patients 'run away' that is their right. Forget it. **Never regret lost cases**.

- **What is a safe way to start doing a new procedure?** Keep a proctor, and be confident of handling a complication. For example, if your procedure is laparoscopic, then handling a complication by opening up should be within your reach. Anything less is unwise in your own interests, let alone the patient's.

- **When to say "no" to a patient?** When you feel that the operation is likely to be a surgical execution, you should say "no". At the peripheral level of the community, this may mean referring out to a bigger hospital. The signs are usually writ large on the wall: moribund patient, low albumin, anemia, end-stage disease and overall features flashing the 'neglected patient' sign in red.

- Let's say you get an admission of a patient in shock and a history of a 'lap chole' five days back, all signs screaming "my bile duct has been injured"! **Refer out or call for help**, unless you have the training and experience to handle complex biliary reconstruction. When you find the patient's relatives to be untrustworthy, refer out! This is more common sense than anything else here.

- **Trust is a two-way relationship**. Refuse to enter into a tight financial contract with the patient ("pay me x for doing y, all expenses covered"). While it is common practice in many third-world hospitals and communities, it is potentially harmful and actually a **conflict of interest**. Out of such conflicts arises mortality. **Your longevity as a surgeon depends likewise on the longevity of your patients**.

Intra-operative considerations

Much of the bad news that comes out after operations in the Third World does so for diverse reasons related, once again, to the surgical team, the patient and the health care system. Please excuse any repetition, for there is bound to be some overlap.

The surgical team

In many of the *chalta hai* ('anything goes') societies, best exemplified in the Indian subcontinent, a horrendous complication is often the result of an operation being done by someone who should not have been there. Some examples include: janitors suturing wounds and giving injections, gynecs doing appendectomies in male patients, GPs doing piles, hernias and breast lumps, and so on. Many examples we see in the field will be met with disdain and disbelief from readers, so more of these will not be mentioned here. What we need to understand here is that the treating team is at fault in a large number of cases.

Many anesthetists are not really qualified professionals. They may be administering age-old (and unsafe) drugs when newer, short-acting versions are preferred. Examples of archaic drugs that are still used include gallamine (a long-acting paralyzing agent) and ether. Even in a city like Mumbai, some surgeons themselves act as anesthetists! Yes, they give spinal anesthesia or ketamine and then scrub up for an appendectomy or hernia repair, while a nurse holds a mask over the patient. Disaster feels tempted to visit such quarters.

A qualified surgeon may have a complication because he is tempted to handle a case that he has little experience with. He may also be in the learning curve of a new technique and mess up a case in the absence of a proctor (an

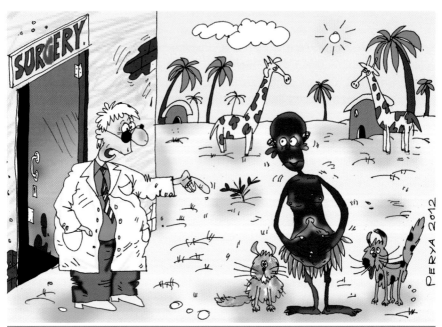

Figure 11.2. Surgeon: "I am going to fix it through a single-incision laparoscopy. To reduce costs, I'll use a mosquito net rather than a costly mesh." Patient: "Yes Sir, Doctor, but could you use the robot?"

all-too common phenomenon). An example: multiple intestinal perforations occurring during a ventral hernia repair and remaining undetected until late in the postoperative period. Another: ureteric injury during a lap anterior resection. You may say this would be valid for surgical incompetence anywhere in the world. I would agree. However, in the Western world, one would expect greater checks on a surgeon's freedom to do procedures and more severe punishments for major transgressions (arguably). **In the Third World, regulation is often a joke** (■ Figure 11.2).

The patient

The third-world patient probably deserves a special genus for himself. It seems disease has to be forced to throw its last cards on the table to be noticed by its host. Some examples: a 25lb abdominal tumor, a mesenteric cyst extending from pelvis to diaphragm, a massive, fungating breast cancer riddled with maggots, a 'watering-can' perineum with 12 external openings of an anal fistula and a 7cm-long bile duct stone, to mention just a few.

Almost invariably, patients with advanced disease come with economic weaknesses and impaired immune and nutritional status. They are high-risk cases even for a haircut, as we say in typical third-world black humor. Being poorly read, these patients may be wrongly guided towards quackery and homeopathy. After months of this, they seek proper medical help, now worse off in terms of health and financial strength.

Often, old patients are abandoned by their children to escape financial drain and the daily trudge to the hospital to hear continuing bad news. Without family support, medical care also suffers, as stressed-out nurses and ward staff focus on more demanding patients whose families would complain in the case of deficiencies in service.

The system

In many countries across the globe, disasters occur in spite of great surgical services. Infrastructural deficiencies themselves set the stage for unique complications, the kind not thought of by the originators of the operations, perhaps! Let me give you a personal example: I was visiting another state and was doing a lap chole on a patient who had previously undergone an operation for a hydatid cyst of the right lobe of the liver. While I had the harmonic scalpel for dividing the extensive adhesions, the hospital experienced intermittent **power outage**! The power was going and coming back every few minutes. Surgeons across the Third World have since shared similar nightmarish episodes. Many hospitals have their own generators to escape this problem. In spite of this, compromises inevitably occur. Often a long procedure may be done without air conditioning, with wall-mounted or floor fans maintaining the circulation of air — and spores...

Other infrastructure problems may be:

- **Rats may run free** in ORs and wards, leading to patient injuries and breaks in sterility.
- **Cockroaches, flies and other insects** are present in many hospitals and reflect the chances of infection after surgery.
- **Taps run dry** (especially when power fails): cases then get cancelled, or autoclaved water is poured from a bottle over the surgeon's forearms and hands while he scrubs up.
- **Central suction malfunction**: use power back-up or hydraulic suction.
- **Shortage of materials** like Betadine®, sutures, staplers, anesthetic medications (residents sometimes buy these for patients).
- **Operating lights may be inadequate** for major procedures, especially in obese patients. When you have an esophagogastric resection or a revision hepaticojejunostomy, the case will take no excuses!
- **Sterilization methods** like formalin chambers are used for lap instruments, or the glutaraldehyde (Cidex®) used may not cover all parts of the instruments.
- **Infection rates** are higher in clean cases like breast and hernia surgery as there is no laminar flow in the old theaters that have not seen any upgrade since inception. In these same places, vascular clamps would typically not be available, nor would defibrillators (what are those?).
- **Cautery contact burns** occur as the pads are reused and they do not stick to skin. This becomes severely embarrassing for the surgeon to explain in the postoperative visit.
- **Shortage of blood**: it is an anachronism for a postoperative patient to die of hemorrhage in this age, but blood is so scarce a resource that death from hemorrhagic shock is seen now and then.
- **No angiographic or interventional endoscopic services**: this leads to more reoperations. This is simply something for which one cannot do much. After all, there is much in the system that a surgeon cannot change. However, identifying a center with specific facilities for dire situations may be lifesaving.
- **Path results** arrive after patients are discharged and they are not easy to trace. Samples may be misplaced or misreported. Report credibility is a major problem for patients and doctors alike, and getting slide reviews from other pathologists or centers is daily work, especially in cancer.

- **Lack of supervision** by experienced surgeons during nights leaves the juniors to decide and perform on operative surgical emergencies.
- In rare instances, an **(ancient) operating table may break** down whilst a surgery is in progress (this has happened to me, unfortunately), with the intubated patient crashing to the floor.
- **During a laparoscopic procedure**, the monitor may die off mysteriously, or the CO_2 cylinder may dry up, with no replacement in sight. Ideally, there should be back-ups for everything, but in real life, who checks? Answer: the once-bitten surgeon!

It is imperative to add that in many locations, **relatives turn violent at the hint of a complication or, God forbid, death.** The classic escape method for the surgical team has been the creation of a 'back door' through which the good doctors escape the mob gathered at the front of the hospital. However, it is far more sensible to exercise discretion, wisdom and maturity before taking up a case and pre-empt this kind of ugliness.

Specific third-world complications

Atypical mycobacterial infections

This is a dreaded complication of laparoscopic surgery, though it may also strike the patient with an orthopedic or other implant. You may call it the fatal flaw of third-world surgery. You can't see it, and you may try your best to eradicate and prevent it, but it may still bite you.

This cousin of the TB germ (*M. chelonae* is by far the most notorious) is an unforgiving marker of breakdown of sterility. In lap surgery, the incidence of **chronic port sinuses and abscesses** has come down significantly, but a lot remains to be done. Some of the reasons for improvement in its incidence include:

- Awareness amongst surgeons of the need to be sharply focused on sterility (not traditionally the surgeon's job).
- Thorough cleansing of trocars.
- Autoclaving and ethylene oxide sterilization techniques, rather than chemical disinfection of lap (and general) instruments.
- Use of enzymes to reduce organic burden (tissue fragment, blood, clot, stone debris, etc.) in the nooks and crevices of trocars and other instruments.
- Abandoning reuse of disposable trocars.

Cases may continue to pile up while the surgeon is struggling with a rash of chronic port infections. This is a sinister mechanism: while the surgeon is focused on his own instruments and the autoclaving, in reality the problem may be different. The autoclave itself may be malfunctioning or derelict, or the nurses may be immersing scissors, needle holders and forceps (used in port creation or closure) in Cidex®, perhaps to manage successive cases. Few people in rural centers understand that disinfection and sterilization are not the same! Whatever be the source, this disease is enough to destroy any benefit of lap surgery that may be thought of in treating a patient.

Abdominal dehiscence

In rural centers, catgut is still used for abdominal closure, setting up a mechanical cause for abdominal dehiscence. Lack of awareness amongst surgeons about **intra-abdominal hypertension** may lead to closure under tension or continuing conservative management in the setting of abdominal compartment syndrome.

Gastrointestinal fistulas

External GI fistulas may devastate not just patients but their families, often from the financial implications of managing the same. **Very few people would have the wherewithal to pay for prolonged TPN, antibiotics, hospital stay and reoperations**. Cost becomes the defining issue more often than not. Some ways to reduce the impact in a given case are:

- Use jejunal access for feeding where possible (a no-brainer, of course).
- Hire a suction machine and institute continuous or intermittent suction of the wound to keep it dry. Fistula management is labor intensive. To make it happen and help the patient, use someone in the family who could be trained to do simple things like switch the suction off or on, apply Karaya gum on skin, etc. In desperate cases, hire someone at your own expense and get him or her to take care of the patient. The return of your investment is when the patient dries up and becomes a normal person. And no member of the family tries to decapitate you...
- Avoid unnecessary antibiotic use, and remember that a cheaper antibiotic is not always the most economic choice. The opposite may be true as well ☺.

Postoperative fevers

Remember that malaria may be the actual cause of fever, especially in specific areas and seasons! A simple blood test for the parasite may give you the answer while an expensive CT scan would not. **Otherwise use the 6Ws mnemonic below**.

The 6Ws mnemonic:

■ **What the f***?** Has temperature been measured properly?

■ **Wound** infection?

■ **Water** — urinary tract infection?

■ **Wind** — respiratory infection?

■ **Walk** — DVT/PE (yes, I know this rarely produces fever).

■ **Wonder** — if caused by drug fever, anesthesia (malignant hyperthermia) or even withdrawal of a drug (neuroleptic malignant syndrome).

[Disclaimer: I am not the originator of the above. Don't know who was.]

Friendly fire

In the third-world hospital, the surgeon is often called upon by his gynecologist colleague for help. Nothing much different from the other worlds, except that you should keep some points in mind:

- Many general surgeons actually do the laparoscopic part of a hysterectomy, with most gynecologists outside of big city hospitals not trained in the procedure.
- **Uterine perforations from D&C** (dilatation and curettage) may be associated with multiple intestinal perforations (as they are often done by poorly trained people who have no idea of their instruments going through the full thickness of the uterus). In many cases of advanced pregnancies where abortions are medically done, mishaps occur. Be very suspicious of post-abortion fevers or abdominal distension.
- Be familiar with **ureteric, rectal and bladder injuries** management: this is not a cliché, but reality. In an ideal world, this would happen rarely. In the context we are in, this is not uncommon. Along with the

retained mops after a messy C-section or other, you should be well trained in damage control, and learn to be tactful about it!

- Rarely, you may be called upon to **ligate the internal iliac arteries** (for uncontrollable uterine bleeding): be prepared with the anatomical exposure!
- In the rarest of rare cases, I have been called for an injury to the **inferior vena cava during a neurosurgical lumbar disc surgery** (the surgeon mistakenly gouged out through-and-through the disc). In the prone position, they could not make out the blood collecting inside the abdomen and retroperitoneum. By the time the patient was turned so I could open his abdomen, he was dead.
- **Urological emergency** calls may be for post-suprapubic cystostomy abdominal distension (urinary peritonitis/ascites or bowel injury), or duodenal/bowel injury during or after nephrectomy, etc. While these are rare, the general surgeon in the developing country should know that many people do venture outside their zone of competence, and complications arise. It is a tricky job to handle the searching questions from the patient's relatives without giving away the family jewels of the original culprit!

Final advice

It is assumed now that we are highlighting the challenges of handling difficult situations in third-world surgery. Every place is not the same, and every situation could well be unique. Once you have a bad result to deal with, you would give anything to get out of it. In the course of this desperation, don't make mistakes! In my experience of over 20 years, some thoughts may be worth your while:

- **Fess up to operative difficulties**. Learn to speak truthfully but tactfully. Sometimes, confessing to a mistake you managed competently may backfire in violent communities. This may appear to be contradictory advice, but life is complex, as are my teachings! Live with it (insert evil laugh here).
- **Never treat your patient any differently than you would your own family member**. This is obvious, you say, but own this principle. You will find that your confidence while dealing with people is powerful and decisive. No contradictions, no ifs and buts. Just say, "If this were my family, I would do this".
- Try and find points of agreement with the aggrieved family, and address them. **Humbly apologize when wrong or when under threat of physical danger**. I once lost a patient while doing a hepatectomy

(from air embolism) and the relatives came to me later, all prepared to launch an attack on me. I met them all in my room, apologized for their loss, and gave them the operative videos so that they could substantiate their case against me. I pleaded guilty and asked them to proceed legally. This very act melted them, and the emotional closure of the death was achieved. **The lesson here (at least for me) is to be scrupulously honest in your dealings with all people, not just patients.** People sense a good person, even if they think the surgery was not done well. Hostile acts of violence (e.g. lynching of doctors), rife in the Third World, are often (not always) the result of doctors and staff being impatient or secretive in their version of what happened.

- **Intra-operative deaths** can be nasty, not just tragic. Many a mature surgeon has called for police back-up in this scenario.
- **Waiving off costs** is sometimes an effective way to cool off violent people. Often their violence is a ploy to ensure the same (in cases where patients die in spite of appropriate treatment), so play their way!
- **At all times, document everything in detail!** What does not exist on the file did not happen, and the lawyers will make sure everyone knows that!

"Whenever you are confronted with an opponent, conquer him with love."

Mahatma Gandhi

"Or with money. Lots of it."

B. Ramana

Chapter 12

Going to the country: the rural situation

Moshe Schein

> *The small town needs the best and not the worst doctor procurable. For the country doctor has only himself to rely on: he cannot in every pinch hail specialist, expert, and nurse. On his own skill, knowledge, resourcefulness, the welfare of his patient altogether depends. The rural district is therefore entitled to the best-trained physician that can be induced to go there.*
>
> **Abraham Flexner**

What exactly defines a surgical practice as "rural"? Is it the (small) size of the location, its geographic remoteness, and the low ratio of surgeon(s) to inhabitants; or is it the limited facilities which make it rural? The specific setting varies from country to country and place to place but usually some or all of these factors coexist — a rural surgeon knows that he is a rural surgeon whether in Afghanistan or Switzerland (or on a small Pacific island); whether there are cows or camels walking around or lions roaring.

The spectrum of rural practice across the world is wide (■ Figure 12.1). For example, the facilities available in what is considered a rural practice in northern Wisconsin (e.g. CT/MRI imaging day and night) are probably lacking even in midsize towns in the Ukraine or central Asia. What is considered rural in Sweden may appear to the Indian rural surgeon like a temple of science. However, humans are humans everywhere and so are surgeons — we have met them all over the world — there is much more in common between a rural surgeon in Portugal and Poland than between you and your next door internist...

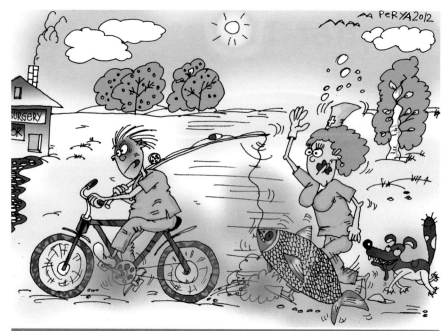

Figure 12.1. OR nurse: "Doc, who is the patient?"

Country life, small town circumstances, remoteness, isolation, all combine to create a unique situation which provides a unified narrative applicable anywhere. **What we will try to bring to this brief chapter is this: principles and truths which are valid universally.**

"Happy families are all alike; every unhappy family is unhappy in its own way", wrote Tolstoy. Similarly, in a good rural ('happy') practice, surgical quality should not be different or inferior to that available in the Ivory Tower — if you cannot do it as well locally then you better refer out! However, when the 'family' becomes 'unhappy' — when complications develop — each rural situation becomes unique and complicated in its own way. And this is the focus of this chapter.

General considerations

What makes rural surgical practice distinctive is evident to any surgeon who has moved from town to country or — this is a much less common passage — from country to town.

The 'lonely surgeon'

In a small town you are relatively 'lonely'. Even if you have a partner he may be out of town or enjoying (finally) his glass of *vino rosso* exactly when you desperately need his help. This is usually not a problem when things go smoothly. But when disaster strikes, a second brain could be helpful to open up your tunnel vision, a second pair of watchful eyes could spot the intra-operative problem that yours have missed, and obviously, a second pair of trained hands could be invaluable in critical moments. The characteristic loneliness of any surgeon faced with serious postoperative complications is much more acute in the rural setting, when he is all alone, with nobody (who *understands*) to talk with or to confess to. In order to survive and excel, you have to wrap your practice in adaptive mechanisms.

There is no immediate feedback

When working with other doctors, even very junior colleagues, you always have somebody to talk to. When you decide to operate, or during the operation, you speak constantly to your juniors — you explain and teach and this helps your own thinking process (clearly uttered is clearly thought). They ask questions and (we hope) challenge you: Why do you want to operate? Shouldn't we wait? Why don't you do what the other surgeon did last week? You explain — you think and it keeps you alert. Should you become crazy and decide to do something really stupid, the chief resident would ask: what are you doing? But here in the country you can do whatever you choose — no one will stop you. Of course some OR nurses are excellent and do understand what you are doing and what should be done, but often they won't confront or challenge you directly. You can speak and explain but the feedback from the nurses and scrub techs will always be supportive and positive. **You have to learn to rely only on yourself!**

You do a little of everything

In a small town, with a limited catchment area, one is rarely able to develop a high-volume interest in a specific field; instead, one has to do a little of everything. Therefore, preferably, you should arrive in such a practice with significant experience because the existing volume can support a learning curve in almost nothing. And even if in your previous incarnation you were doing a large volume of major cancer surgery, this does not mean that you can, or should continue to do it in the rural setting. **You have to recognize that some of the old skills undergo attrition over time**.

Limited resources

In the country your practice is limited in that there are things that you may not be well trained to do, or believe that others can do them better, but there are other constraints. **Here there are also things you can do very well, but should not do, because the system can't support you in doing them safely.** Gone are the days when you leave the OR and hit your bed while others work on the patient in the intensive care unit, trying to keep him alive. Now it is your job to stay up and attend to the multiple details of supportive care — day and night. But frequently, it is simply not doable and it is better to ship the patient away. You will have to familiarize yourself with the ability of your hospital — the intensive care, nursing, OR team and the other docs. You must even know exactly what instruments the OR keeps and which are missing. Do you wish to attempt repair of an injured femoral artery if your OR lacks vascular clamps and/or Fogarty balloon catheters? That your little hospital boasts a state-of-the-art spiral CT and MRI technology doesn't mean that there will be always a radiologist to drain your patient's intra-abdominal abscess on the weekend. You have to plan in advance.

Geographic remoteness

The location of your rural center and how far it is from tertiary referral centers has to be factored into your decision-making. Most patients (but not all) are not charmed by the large marble-clad hospitals and prefer to be treated *locally*, staying near their homes and families. **But learning when not to tackle a case locally is perhaps more important for your reputation than even your own operative skills for, as you know, in surgery the selection of patients is the key to outcome.** Therefore, you have to learn and master the local referral and evacuation pathways — in elective situations as well as emergency ones. The wise rural surgeon develops trustworthy ties and referral channels with surgeons in the regional centers, surgeons he trusts and respects and who would be willing to accept, without any questions, his referral — the 'good cases' as well as the 'disasters'.

Emergency 'shipping' out

You have to develop **protocols of emergency evacuation**: knowing when, where to and by which route to ship away the patient, facilitates the process in the middle of the night. You should think about multiple potential case scenarios in advance: do you want to do a laparotomy on the hypotensive blunt trauma patient in your 'single-surgeon center' when the chopper could deliver him to the regional trauma center within 45 minutes? What to do if a snow storm is raging and the chopper cannot fly? Are you ready to deal with him?

Obviously, an Ivory Tower only fifty miles down the highway is very different from one that is hundreds of miles away across the mountains. You have to be creative in utilizing limited resources to achieve the best possible outcomes under your specific circumstances.

Complications are more visible

In a little town and the surrounding county, everybody knows each other. Each patient that you see is somehow related to somebody that you may know (the nurse), you need (the bank clerk), you depend on (hospital director) or you will soon meet or need (your hairdresser or dentist). Rumors, alleged or true, of your complications or alleged (or true) arrogance, impatience, and negative attitude, spread around rapidly and are unforgiving — destroying your standing. Thus, you have to be 'nice' all the time, 'positive' and at eye level with the local population of *all social strata*. In brief: **like the local politician or the sheriff you have to be popular and trusted — this is handy if and when complications occur.**

You can't take chances

Even a single major complication in a small town may seriously harm your reputation. **The common perception is that mortality or complications after an operation in a rural hospital are *because* of the "inexperienced surgeon or poor care", while if the patient dies in the Ivory Tower then he dies *despite* "the best efforts of the excellent doctors in a great hospital" — an act of God!** Thus, when performing 12 emergency colon resections per year in a large center you can select ten for primary anastomosis and accept one leak. But in the country, if you do three such procedures per year, you will opt for a *colostomy*, which precludes leakage. Nobody will ask you why did you do a colostomy, but if the patient leaks and dies they may ask: "why did you not do a colostomy?" Although a one-stage procedure is based on 'good evidence', in the country good evidence often stops at the doors of the library or the local tavern — where your case is being discussed. Surgical complications occurring in a large hospital are easily 'diluted' and rapidly forgotten; but when you are the only surgeon in the county everybody will hear about your major bile duct injury and people will remember it forever. **You can't take chances!**

Rural patients are different

Rural communities worldwide have much in common. While they want to take pride in their local hospital and trust their doctors, they tend to be shrewd, practical and suspicious. Many are aware of the following 'rural law': "**As long as the patient has an appendix, a gallbladder, a uterus and two ovaries you refer him to the local surgeon. Once these organs are gone you refer to the University**." Last year on a vacation in Switzerland, an alpine farmer, after hearing that I'm a surgeon in a small town in Wisconsin asked me: "Are you an appendix surgeon?" He explained: "in our district hospital here, anything bigger than an appendix goes to the big town…"

A young internist who has recently relocated from our little center to a tertiary care center (within the same state) told me that the patients he encounters now are 'different' — not only representing a different socio-economic mix but also "less stressed, less suspicious… more accepting". No wonder: at the back of the minds of patients seeking care in rural centers there is always the worry (sometimes justified) that their problems are beyond the skills and capabilities of the local health system to deal with. On the other hand, the Ivory Tower is for them the "ultimate house of medicine" — when they arrive there, there is nowhere else to go. This is the different attitude that we as rural surgeons have to recognize. Always give the patient an option to be referred elsewhere. For example: "I would be glad to do your mastectomy here but if you wish, I could refer you to the breast center in Chicago." Most patients will stay with you but by giving them another option you have reassured them.

Pre-operative considerations

Pre-operative considerations in the rural environment should be exactly the same as in the best of academic centers. But there are a few points to emphasize, as outlined below.

CT

The CT is your friend. Today, when most rural hospitals (at least in the developed world) possess a modern CT scanner, you should use it as an extension to your palpating hands and stethoscope — timely CT images and a good radiologist (often looking at the images from his home) provide the 'balance' or second opinion that the partner you do not have could provide. The negative CTs — showing that there is 'no problem' — help you to sleep well. "No appendicitis, no free gas, no free fluid, no intestinal obstruction": now you know that rather than spending the night re-evaluating the patient you can safely send him home, to be seen in the office the next day. Forget about the literature and evidence — who cares that allegedly "overall, routine CT scanning has no advantage"? The only 'evidence' a country surgeon wants is to play it safely, solve problems instantly and avoid complications and satisfy referring doctors and patients. You have, however, to make yourself an expert in evaluating the CT and to talk directly with the radiologist on call. **Never trust a CT 'report' without looking at the images yourself, preferably together with the radiologist!**

Should I do the operation here?

Always ask: should I do the operation here? Think: What if the patient with grade IV chronic obstructive lung disease develops respiratory failure after the colectomy? Will I be able to ventilate him here? How good is our ICU? **Remember**: the guys at the tertiary care center resent having to treat complications *after* your operations; they would rather do so following procedures performed in their own house. The mere thought that the patient could develop a complication which you won't be able to handle is a reason to consider referring him out. **It is better (for your coronaries and reputation... and the patient) to transfer him *before* the operation (for an operation) than *after* the operation with a complication.**

Transfer and shipping

That you have to master the methodology of referral/transfer and shipping we emphasized above. But even if you have decided to ship out an emergency surgical case, it is still your job to *stabilize* him — to optimize his physiology so he'll tolerate the journey. In rare cases this may involve 'damage control' surgery (e.g. clamping or shunting an injured artery, packing the liver). **You must not lose touch with the patient awaiting transfer**: during the 30 minutes before the chopper arrives he may crash — calling for your action: endotracheal intubation, chest tube, laparotomy. And of course you have to communicate effectively with the surgeon on the 'other side'. Talk to him on the phone in person. Send a detailed written note with the patient.

Obviously, some of you who live and practice in the most desolate corners of the world have nowhere to send the patient, nor is there a chopper or ambulance at your disposal. In that case you have to rely on yourself. But **please try not to play the role of God**. Under certain circumstances a non-operative approach makes more sense than a desperate or futile operation. **And remember this aphorism — in my opinion one of the most useful in surgery and especially relevant to the rural situation: "Never operate on a patient who is getting rapidly better or rapidly worse." [Francis D. Moore].**

Politics

Finally, when referring out you also have to think about your local rural 'politics'. **There is always a 'fine line' in the treatment of acute surgical patients in the rural hospital**: if you ship them away some may accuse you of laziness, cowardice, or losing income for the hospital; but if you treat them locally they'll accuse you of being a 'cowboy' or endangering the patient. The hallmark of an astute rural surgeon is that he can dance effectively between those lines!

Intra-operative considerations

Assistants

The crucial difference between operating at a rural hospital and the Ivory Tower is not the size and number of operating rooms, or the laparoscopic 'plasma' screens, but the **quality and number of assistants** — unless you have a dedicated partner to scrub with you whenever necessary. If you are in solo practice your assistants in the OR will be nurses or scrub 'techs'. In general they tend to assist in a 'passive mode'. Most of them will know how to remove the clamp when you tie the knot; they will be able to 'fry' the tissue between the jaws of your dissecting clamp with the diathermy. But they will rarely have the guts or impetus to take initiative — they'll reposition their hands or shift a retractor from site to site only when told to do so. They will start sucking the blood away only if told "suck!" Operating with partners or (good) residents is different: they take the initiative and move their hands spontaneously and do things — sometimes too much. But the change from active resident-assistants to passive nurse-assistants can be painful. Slowly you'll realize that you cannot wait for the assistants to read your mind; you'll have to stop, reposition the retractor and say "would you please…".

If you want your operations to be pleasurable and not irritating nightmares you will have to pick up, train and support at least one or two solid assistants. Their actual degree or qualifications does not really matter (Ken, one of my best scrub techs, is a logger). But they have to be able to read your mind, understand what you are doing, assist actively (but not too actively so that they don't interfere with your movements or cause more damage), and show interest and empathy. You, in return, must show them appreciation and treat them like 'partners' or brothers (sisters) in arms. A good assistant is crucial for the safe conduct of the operation.

Gradually, you will adjust to operating 'solo'. You will learn effective employment of 'mechanical assistants' and develop technical tricks that make operating alone possible. And, at the end of the day, old country surgeons are well accustomed to 'doing it all alone', so much so that they cannot tolerate being assisted by active colleagues, preferring the good old OR girls, who are always agreeable and supportive, and who will always laugh at their jokes.

There is no one around to clean the s**t after you

When you become a rural surgeon it may take a few weeks or months to realize that everything, however minor it might be, depends on you! No hospitalists, interns, residents or physician assistants to solve even the smallest, silliest problem. **Do you want to sleep well, avoiding problems that develop as soon as the patient reaches the ICU?** Then think about the tiny details before finishing the operation or leaving the OR. So, forget about being a big shot, putting in the last stitch and leaving the operating room — if you forget to tape the chest tube to the drainage system, then 12 hours later, at three o'clock in the morning, you will be driving through the ice to treat the collapsed lung.

Postoperative considerations

Trust only yourself

The key to early diagnosis and management of postoperative complications in the rural setting is to trust only yourself. Trust nobody! Yes, it's a cliché… but how true it is! Of course, every small hospital has a few good nurses who actually tend to look at the patients and not only at the EMR screens. They are your best allies and have to be cultivated and pampered. **But still: trust only yourself!**

Last week a day three post-laparotomy patient started vomiting late at night.

"Please insert a nasogastric tube", I instructed the experienced night nurse, "and call me back after it is in".

She called half an hour later: "It went in easily. We got some 500cc of bile-stained fluid. Yes, I am sure it lies deep within the stomach. I checked it together with Joanna…"

Next morning on the abdominal X-ray the tip of the NG tube was seen at the lower esophagus. **Trust only yourself!**

There are numerous similar examples relevant to any aspect of your patient care. **To avoid postoperative complications you have to loiter around your postop patients like a mother hen around her chicks**.

Dealing with complications

When complications develop you must, yet again, consider which ones you can and want to deal with locally and which would be better managed elsewhere. Oh yes, we are sure that you know how to treat surgically and medically a complex abdominal catastrophe. **But what about your system**: will it be able to cope with a case of an open abdomen and high-output intestinal fistula? And who will look after the patient two weeks later, when you have to attend that out of town meeting?

Listen to the family's opinion (and the patient's even more, if he is not too sick to express his opinion). Provide full disclosure of what happened. Suppress your pride. Acknowledge their anxieties, it is only natural for them to want their loved one to be transferred to a 'higher-level' center. **Again: stay with the patient and family until they leave the door**.

Follow-up

Do not lose touch with the patient the moment the weight of responsibility has dropped off your shoulder (what a relief!). Call the family and ask how the patient is doing after the transfer — procure the mobile phone number of the patient's spouse before they leave — they will appreciate it immensely! Getting up-to-date follow-up from the referral center — if you do not share an EMR system — can be tasking (you will appreciate why some people refer to the "centers of excellence" as the "centers of arrogance"). But for the sake of your patients and your own sake, you have to develop reliable referring channels to the specialists you trust. (More about **rural surgeons and ivory towers** can be read here: http://www.docschein.com/ivorytower.pdf.)

If the complicated patient continues to be managed by you, treat him like a VIP. When he goes home, see him at the office as frequently as possible, dress his wounds by yourself — show him that you care, that the complication has upset you not less than him — or perhaps more! This is called *empathy* ☺.

Remember: complications can impose considerable financial cost on the patient and family. Even if they are fully insured, there is 'co-pay' to pay, and other expenses, let alone loss of earnings. If you can, try to alleviate their financial burden as much as you can. Overbilling (not always your fault) of a patient who has developed an infected mesh is a recipe for litigation.

In a small town, many people will know about your recent complication: that Mr. Jones, the octogenarian who managed the feed store for many years, has passed away after your operation. Some will even read it on his granddaughter's *Facebook* account. But if you act along the aforementioned lines you will be 'forgiven', provided of course that this does not happen every week ☺.

In conclusion: be extremely careful and cautious in your practice — do as much as you can as long as you know what you are doing and you can do it safely. In brief: be the same good old surgeon you have been in the big city, but get rid of your 'attitude'. Dark suit, fancy cars and arrogance do not work on your behalf in the country. **Remember: a big fish in a small pond is exposed to many dangers. Try to blend in...**

> **Read the "21 commandments for the new surgeon in a small town"** by Paul Zaveruha
>
> (*World J Surg* 2005; 29: 1200. http://www.docschein.com/21commandments.pdf.)

PART II

Specific considerations

Chapter 13

The Intensive Care Unit (ICU)

Ronald V. Maier

I did not include the term "complications" in the title of this chapter because the **ICU means complications** — non-complicated patients do not need the ICU! And, as depicted in ■ Figure 13.1, the ICU itself can be a dangerous

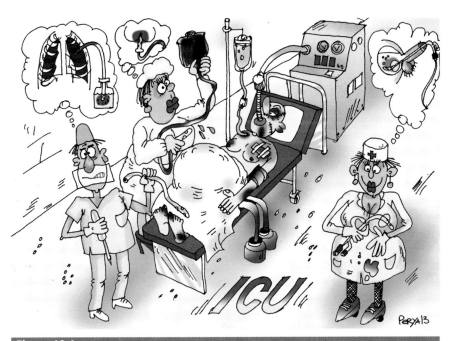

Figure 13.1.

place — a small factory of iatrogenic complications. Now let me advise you on how to prevent, mitigate and treat ICU complications.

Background

The surgical ICU setting combines most of the elements for a maximal risk of complications. Patients in the ICU are severely physiologically deranged, with established or imminent organ failure. Simultaneously, in an attempt to avoid complications, extensive, and frequently invasive, monitoring is required. In contrast to our typical, operating room, surgical mindset of "reaction to disease", **the primary purpose of the surgical ICU, in the majority of patients, is to prevent disease, organ dysfunction, or complications from occurring or worsening**. Early intervention, even when modest, has been shown to have major incremental effects over the duration of care. **However, despite our efforts, the combination of high-risk underlying disease, significant physiologic derangement, increasing age, baseline comorbidity and loss of functional reserves leads to a 50-100% complication rate in the critically ill surgical patient**.

This unique set of challenges requires a team approach to patient care, and the surgeon, whether a surgical critical care intensivist or the operating general surgeon, needs to be intimately involved in the care of the surgical patient, and versed in the common predictors and risks, in order to contribute to the avoidance of complications.

Surgical complications in the ICU

> *Principles of intensive care: air goes in and out; blood goes round and round; oxygen is good.*
>
> **Robert Matz**

Matz has a point, but in real life things are a little more complicated ☺. **Here I will deal with the most common complications and those with the greatest risk of significant morbidity in the surgical patient**. While this chapter is by no means exhaustive, the focus is on important complications which the general surgeon or surgical intensivist has a potential impact in preventing or, at least minimizing, to limit morbidity and optimize recovery and ultimate function. A list of common complications is shown in ■ Table 13.1.

In general, and supported by a good evidence base, several principles underpin optimized care in the ICU. The complex clinical interactions involved require a team of specialists under the coordination of a dedicated intensivist,

Table 13.1. Surgical ICU complications.

Hypovolemia:
- Ischemia — reperfusion.
- Coagulopathy — consumptive.
- Traumatic brain injury (TBI).
- Multiple organ failure (MOF).

Hypervolemia:
- Cardiac failure.
- Abdominal compartment syndrome (ACS).
- Intracranial hypertension (ICH).
- Adult respiratory distress syndrome (ARDS).
- Coagulopathy — dilutional.

Resuscitation fluids:
- Renal failure with hetastarch.
- Hyperchloremic acidosis with normal saline (NS).

Pulmonary failure:
- Adult respiratory distress syndrome (ARDS).
- Ventilator-associated pneumonia (VAP).

Blood transfusion:
- Immune suppression.
- Infections.
- Multiple organ failure (MOF).

Central venous catheters:
- Pneumothorax (PTX).
- Line infection.

Venothromboembolism (VTE):
- Pulmonary emboli (PE).

Hypoglycemia:
- CNS dysfunction/injury.

Hyperglycemia:
- Infections.

Antibiotic misuse:
- Resistant organisms.
- *Clostridium difficile* colitis (CDC).

Malnutrition/TPN:
- GI bleed.
- Infections.
- Wound breakdown.

Over-sedation:
- Respiratory failure.
- Aspiration.
- Withdrawal/delirium.

Urinary tract infection (UTI)

not unlike the trauma surgeon as a 'captain of the ship' during an initial resuscitation. Increasingly, evidence-based protocols and standardized approaches to care minimize complications and enhance recovery. **To ensure consistency, the daily use of check lists, usually based on a standardized evaluation of each organ system, identifies physiologic trends and risks to be addressed and corrected.** The use of these 'systems' produces consistent, progressive improvement in care and a decrease in complications, thus improving outcomes.

> # Remember — general concepts of care in the surgical ICU patient are:
>
> ■ Return to baseline as quickly as possible.
> ■ The critically ill patient does not tolerate rapid swings in physiology (the patient is not a 'yo yo'...).
> ■ Do not over-treat (better is the enemy of good...).
> ■ Care in the ICU is a team event, requiring coordination of multiple specialists (caveat: someone, preferably a surgeon, has to take the lead and take the overall responsibility!).

Resuscitation

The challenge: not too little, not too much.

Virtually all critically ill surgical patients have an abnormal intravascular volume. The goal in therapy is adequate volume to support myocardial function, cardiac output, perfusion and oxygen delivery for cellular survival. This leads to support of end-organ function, minimizes organ dysfunction and improves survival of the patient.

Hypovolemia

Inadequate volume resuscitation, which is often 'occult', leads to numerous complications (see ■ Table 13.2). Frequently, the surgical patient is hypovolemic due to blood loss, 'third spacing' due to tissue damage, loss through exposed peritoneal surfaces during dissection, sepsis and, finally, inadequate replacement of intravascular volume by the anesthetist.

Table 13.2. Hypovolemia complications.

■ Tissue ischemia.
■ Enhanced inflammation.
■ Microvascular stasis.
■ Venous thromboembolism (VTE).
■ Trauma-induced coagulopathy (TIC).
■ Multiple organ dysfunction/failure syndrome (MODS/MOF).

Remember: the surgical patient entering the ICU should be considered to be hypovolemic unless proven otherwise! With pain control to eliminate autonomic stimulation, the patient should not only have stable hemodynamics — including heart rate and mean arterial pressure (MAP), but also be normal for age and baseline. So, for example, injury, including burns, should produce a *relative hyperdynamic state*, while comorbidities, including advanced age, would frequently require an elevated blood pressure at baseline for adequate perfusion. With 'occult' hypovolemia, MAP is maintained through compensatory splanchnic vasoconstriction (contributing 65-85% of the afterload) but this leads to significant intra-abdominal organ hypoperfusion, despite 'adequate' urine output. **Thus, in addition to vital signs and urine output, markers of adequate tissue perfusion should be monitored** — such as serial lactate and bicarbonate levels — to demonstrate progressive clearance of the metabolic load. Maintenance of adequate pulmonary ventilation clears CO_2 while adequate liver perfusion clears excess lactate (unless there coexists end-stage liver disease, severe liver injury or an acute ethanol liver poisoning).

An inability to clear lactate indicates the possibility of continuing hypoperfusion that requires increased invasive monitoring to ensure adequate resuscitation. The simplest form of invasive monitoring is insertion of a **central venous catheter**, through either the subclavian or internal jugular vein, which allows assessment of preload on the myocardium. While the correlation in the acutely ill patient between the central venous pressure (CVP) and overall intravascular volume is weak, the extremes and *trends of CVP* are valid and of significant benefit. So, for instance, a CVP of 2 supports a diagnosis of hypovolemia, while a CVP of 25 and worsening oxygenation is strongly indicative of excessive intravascular volume and primary pump failure, potentially requiring diuretics and/or inotropic cardiac support. In critically ill patients, particularly those with sepsis, with a **confusing response to apparently adequate volume**, I still advocate (yes, despite all the literature…) in selected patients the placement of a **pulmonary artery catheter** (PAC — also known to old farts as a *Swan-Ganz catheter*) to monitor more accurately the effects of altered preload and inotropic agents, and to ensure optimal cardiac output. An additional benefit of a PAC is the monitoring of **mixed venous oxygenation** to ensure adequate oxygen delivery which means maintaining a mixed venous oxygen tension of greater than 70%. One must remember, however, that with the progression of invasiveness, a careful risk-benefit assessment should be applied to avoid inappropriate utilization and unnecessary risk of the invasive monitoring. **The routine use of invasive intravascular monitoring produces more complications than benefit, and is to be avoided.**

Hypervolemia

The challenge of achieving euvolemia in patients that frequently have 'occult' hypovolemia highlights a major conceptual problem in the treatment of the critically ill patient. Due to the known detrimental effects of prolonged hypoperfusion on subsequent organ function, and the recognized difficulty in identifying persistent occult hypoperfusion, the tendency is to provide aggressive volume resuscitation to overcompensate through excessive preload. Allowing the pendulum to swing to this other side, however, may create another set of problems listed in ■ Table 13.3. Unfortunately, this 'rationale' of intentionally overloading the myocardium to drive oxygen delivery to compensate for prior insults of hypoperfusion and ischemia produced a significant increase in the incidence of tissue edema, elevated intra-abdominal pressures thus leading to a major surgical epidemic of iatrogenic **abdominal compartment syndrome** (ACS), **multiple organ failure** (MOF), **adult respiratory distress syndrome** (ARDS), and increased overall mortality. In addition, such an approach leads to a doubling of intracranial pressures and

Table 13.3. Hypervolemia complications.

- Tissue edema/organ dysfunction.
- Dilutional coagulopathy.
- Cardiac failure.
- Acute respiratory failure/ARDS.
- Intracranial hypertension (ICH).
- Intra-abdominal hypertension (IAH).
- Abdominal compartment syndrome (ACS).

mortality following **traumatic brain injury** (TBI). **So, while occult hypovolemia and hypoperfusion are to be avoided, inappropriate over-aggressive treatment with hypervolemia must also be avoided to prevent unnecessary morbidity and mortality.** Nowadays, with appropriate monitoring and resuscitation, along with damage control surgery, ACS has virtually disappeared as a complication (see ⊃ Chapter 24).

Which fluids?

The argument over which resuscitation fluid is ideal appears to continue indefinitely (see ■ Table 13.4). The debate about the value of oncotic agents,

Table 13.4. Resuscitation fluids.

- Lactated Ringer's solution → hyperkalemia.
  - D-lactate → inflammation.
- Normal saline (NS) → hyperchloremic acidosis.
- Hetastarch → renal injury.
- Albumin → increased interstitial fluid/organ dysfunction.
  - Immune response.
- Excess of each of the above → increased mortality.

such as *albumin* and *hetastarch*, in more efficiently increasing intravascular volume as opposed to standard *crystalloids* is longstanding. Multiple studies, including several prospective randomized trials and meta-analyses, confirm that there is no benefit in the use of oncotic agents and, in fact, in most studies a detrimental impact during the acute resuscitation phase has been suggested. Hetastarch has been shown recently not only to be not beneficial but also associated with a worse outcome, primarily due to renal dysfunction in the hypovolemic patient. Of the various crystalloid solutions, *normal saline* helps in restoring the sodium deficit frequently seen acutely; however, excess utilization leads to hyperchloremic acidosis that further complicates resuscitation and hinders elimination of any illness-induced acidosis. While the D-isomer of lactate has been shown to augment the excessive proinflammatory response in stress states, the standard use of the L-isomer of lactate is safe, so **lactated Ringer's (LR) solution remains the most common, and currently safest, agent used during the acute resuscitation phase**. The presence of potassium in LR requires monitoring of serum potassium levels to prevent hyperkalemia, particularly in the patient with either acute or chronic renal dysfunction. **However, the traditional use of crystalloid solutions has never included a recommendation of drowning the patient with salt water: the goal is euvolemia, not hypervolemia.**

Traumatic brain injury (TBI)

Traumatic brain injury (TBI) is a common component of severe injury. **Next to exsanguinating hemorrhage, traumatic brain injury is the most common cause for acute and sub-acute mortality, and a major contributor to long-term disability and dysfunction.** Since nothing can be done to restore lost CNS tissue, the primary purpose of ICU care is prevention of secondary injury in adjacent at-risk brain tissue. **The only confirmed major controllable factor in the ultimate extent of TBI is the avoidance of even**

brief episodes of hypotension or hypoxia. TBI, even minor, leads to loss of the normal vascular autoregulation to protect tissue perfusion. Thus, even brief episodes of hypotension produce a significant impact on ultimate functional outcome.

Monitoring of **intracranial pressure** (ICP), either via a subarachnoid bolt or a ventriculostomy, helps to ensure adequate volume resuscitation and tissue perfusion. In the patient with elevated ICP it is not illogical to maintain an increased mean arterial pressure to ensure an adequate **cerebral perfusion pressure** (CPP = MAP - ICP) of greater than 60mmHg — although the exact optimal level is unknown. I should mention, however, that recent studies show that attention to optimal overall perfusion, without direct measurement of ICP, produces a similar functional outcome. **Similarly, ischemia from hypoxia should be avoided**. The greatest risk to the injured patient is episodic hypotension or hypoxia during the course of intra-operative care, particularly during induction. Some advocate the use of prophylactic vasoactive agents to ensure that mean arterial pressure does not drop during induction of anesthesia. **Close attention to the maintenance of blood pressure and oxygenation during out-of-ICU episodes is mandatory**.

Optimize blood and fresh frozen plasma transfusion

Blood transfusion with packed red blood cells (pRBC) is frequently necessary for adequate oxygen delivery in patients with acute blood loss. Acutely, when the potential for continuing loss is present, treatment goals mandate a 'buffer' to compensate for possible delays in identification of life-threatening drops in blood volume. **During the acute bleeding phase, a hemoglobin of 10g/dL appears reasonable**. Unfortunately, in the past, this concept was extrapolated to the post-acute phase and transfusions were used to maintain a hemoglobin of 10g/dL in stable patients. Several studies have proved a deleterious effect of blood bank transfusion: a clear detrimental dose response effect of each unit of blood with multiple complications including infections, sepsis, MOF, lower functional CNS recovery and death. In addition, this negative effect is augmented by the age of the blood, particularly after 14 days. **I have no doubt that a transfusion trigger for hemoglobin of 7g/dL is safe and leads to improved outcomes compared to those transfused to higher levels**. It has been argued that selected patients (e.g. those with coronary artery disease or TBI) have increased oxygen needs and thus require higher hemoglobin levels. However, analysis of ICU subpopulations does not support higher levels in these groups, which like the overall population have a worse outcome with blood transfusion. **Only patients with concurrent ischemia, such as acute coronary syndrome, appear to benefit from a higher level of hemoglobin**.

As with pRBC, the use of **fresh frozen plasma (FFP) transfusions is associated with increased complications, including infections, organ failure and death**. FFP should be reserved for those with proven coagulopathy or in severely injured patients receiving a massive transfusion and at significant risk for **trauma-induced coagulopathy** (TIC) (⊃ Chapters 3 and 24).

> **Remember:** during acute bleeding episodes, maintain a hemoglobin of 10g/dL; after stabilization, transfusion should be limited to patients with a hemoglobin of less than 7g/dL. If possible, only 'fresh' less than 14-day-old bank blood should be used. Limit FFP transfusion to patients at proven risk for massive transfusion.

Infective complications

The most common complications in the surgical ICU are infectious, and these affect virtually every aspect of care. The cost in mortality, morbidity and resource consumption is enormous. Important infectious complications in the surgical patient include:

- **Surgical site infections** (SSI).
- **Ventilator-associated pneumonia** (VAP).
- **Line infections** (they want you to call it "line-associated bloodstream infections"…).
- **Urinary tract infections** (UTIs).
- **Atypical or resistant infections**, such as *Clostridium difficile* colitis.

Fortunately, changes in care giver behavior have been shown to have a major impact on the incidence of infectious complications. Many of these changes in habits are embarrassingly simple and inexpensive (e.g. wash your hands!). Several protocols package a group of activities together in what are referred to as 'bundles' to prevent unnecessary variability and optimize outcomes.

There are several generic principles to avoiding infections (■ Table 13.5):

- **Optimizing the patient's overall physiology is critical.**
- Appropriate, **early provision of adequate nutrition**, by the **enteral route** if at all possible, has a dramatic impact on reducing infectious complications.

Table 13.5. Prevention of infection.

- Resuscitation to euvolemia.
- Avoid unnecessary pRBC and FFP transfusions.
- Early enteral nutrition.
- Assess daily for extubation.
- Place invasive lines with full sterility.
- Assess and remove all indwelling tubes as soon as possible.
- Use contact barriers.
- Disinfect and wash hands before and after every contact.

- A major goal is to **remove indwelling devices as quickly as possible**. This includes endotracheal tubes, central venous lines, and urinary catheters. Maintaining any of these for 'convenience', as frequently occurs, is unacceptable! **Each device must be evaluated daily, and the reason for continuance confirmed or refuted**. Planned operative procedure, over-sedation or lack of adequate pain control should not be the reason for continuing an endotracheal tube. Easy access for fluids does not require retention of a central venous line. And the convenience of not having to use a urinal or bedpan is not an indication for a urinary catheter.

Notably, while recent studies testing various components of prevention bundles have failed to demonstrate an individual impact, these results do not negate the benefits achieved in combination — now you understand why they invented the term 'bundle' ☺. While total elimination of the problem is probably not achievable, with implementation of the concepts iterated throughout this chapter, infectious complications can be reduced greatly. In addition, once the environment of care is modified, the patient benefits continue even if not controlled by strict protocol compliance.

The commonly employed bundles are protocols that most consistently have a beneficial impact on infectious complications. The practice of monitoring wounds for colonization with resistant organisms, and using such data for isolation of patients to prevent spread, has become a well-accepted standard. In addition, contact precautions for all open wounds or procedures with exposure to secretions prevent dissemination through clothing or body transfer. The simple measure of frequent hand washing to remove clostridial spores and using sanitizing agents to reduce nosocomial organisms, is highly effective in preventing transfer from patient to patient, stopping outbreaks and decreasing the overall incidence of

nosocomial infections. All invasive devices should be placed as a surgical procedure, with full draping and skin preparation during insertion.

The appropriate use of antibiotics is critical to prevent selection and overgrowth of resistant organisms. The use of peri-operative prophylactic antibiotics should be limited to 24 hours of maximum dosing. In general, the selection of antibiotics should be adequate, but not overly broad, and driven by culture results. Empiric antibiotic treatment of infection should be limited to those with acute, life-threatening conditions and modified based on culture results when available. Stopping antibiotics when evidence of the infection has resolved (afebrile with normal WBC for 24-48 hours), rather than treat for prolonged, arbitrary time intervals, is rational. The only exceptions to this are the occasional bacterial or fungal infections that are known to have a high recurrence rate unless treated for prolonged intervals.

A recent study of the **entire genomic response in severely injured patients** identified a '**genomic storm**', where greater than 75% of the entire genome was significantly altered. Importantly, there was a major impact on the innate and adaptive immune responses, with an excessive increase in proinflammatory innate immune responses and a prolonged suppression of the adaptive immune response. **The clinical impact of these changes produces a markedly enhanced risk of infection and complications of organ injury and failure leading to MOF, and death**. In addition, the genomic response in those with a complicated clinical course demonstrated a prolongation in the genomic derangements compared to those without complications, whose genomic activity quickly returned to baseline. Ultimately, to control and prevent associated complications, we will need to identify the genomic state of the patient and individualize therapy based on the specific genomic dysfunction present. These findings also highlight that the earlier any necessary intervention occurs, the better the long-term course of the illness.

Remember: to minimize infectious risk, practice contact precautions, wash and sanitize hands frequently, insert all invasive devices with full sterile precautions and remove them as soon as possible. Treat only proven infections and limit duration and broad-spectrum antibiotics by daily assessment.

Pulmonary complications — ventilator-associated pneumonia (VAP)

A frequent condition in the surgical ICU patient is ventilator dependence due to pulmonary insufficiency (usually due to acute respiratory distress syndrome [ARDS]). This is commonly associated with a major infectious complication — VAP.

VAP typically develops in the critically ill, immunocompromised patient, with an incidence of over 30-40% following major illness. Previously, this rate was accepted as being unavoidable; however, **close attention to management of the ventilated patient can lead to a significant decrease in VAP and its complications, including death** (■ Table 13.6). While specific components of *ventilator care bundles* do not have a significant impact, this does not negate the overall benefits that attention to ventilator management has on minimizing infectious complications.

Table 13.6. Ventilator 'bundle'.

- Elevate head of bed (30-45°).
- Oral hygiene with chlorhexidine.
- Daily sedation vacation/assess for extubation.
- Limit use of acid suppression (H_2 blocker/PPI).
- VTE prophylaxis.

It is the pooling of secretions in the posterior pharynx with continuous chronic microaspiration, despite the presence of a cuff on the endotracheal tube, that leads to VAP.

Therefore, to prevent VAP:

- Maintain the patient as upright as possible (>45°) to allow gravity drainage into the esophagus.
- Suction the oropharyngeal secretions frequently, along with constant suctioning of the trachea just proximal to the cuff.
- Apply oral care with chlorhexidine.
- Avoid as much as possible tubes that cross the lower esophageal sphincter causing incompetence and increased reflux leading to microaspiration. (BTW: distal tube feeding into the jejunum provides no benefit over gastric feeding.)
- Limit the use of acid-suppressing agents to prevent gastric bacterial overgrowth. Sucralfate or H_2 blockers may be preferable to PPI.
- **Most importantly** — since VAP is a time-dependent complication — **minimize the number of days of intubation**. Formal *sedation vacations* to prevent over-sedation allow patient contribution to respiratory efforts, and assessment of adequate spontaneous ventilation expedites extubation.

Management of VAP

Once an intubated patient develops VAP, aggressive empiric treatment must be implemented early to optimize survival. However, the diagnosis is not straightforward: these patients frequently have microaspiration-associated underlying pulmonary changes and/or direct lung injury on chest radiography that makes detection of a new infection difficult. Sampling tracheal aspirates will always produce positive cultures, which may lead to inappropriate treatment with antibiotics.

However, in the face of an increasing white count, fever and new chest X-ray changes, empiric antibiotic therapy should be started immediately following bronchoalveolar lavage (BAL) or brush-directed sampling, as any delay in therapy leads to a high mortality. If the cultures refute infection, the antibiotics should be stopped to prevent the development of multi-resistant organisms in both the individual patient, and the overall milieu of the ICU. The ultimate duration of antibiotics with culture-proven pneumonia is still undefined. Most argue for a fixed duration — either 7 or 10 days, with 14 days for difficult gram-negative infections, such as *Pseudomonas*, to prevent recurrence. Others utilize a return to normal white cell count, an afebrile state and a decrease in sputum production as indicative of resolution of the infection, and if present for 24-48 hours, will stop antibiotic therapy, thus minimizing the impact on the bacterial environment in the ICU.

Remember: utilize a *ventilator bundle* to decrease the incidence of VAP; elevate the HOB (try to guess what it means ☺) [1], optimize oral hygiene and practice a daily *sedation vacation* to assess whether extubation is possible. Treat based on BAL or brush biopsy-proven disease.

Adult respiratory distress syndrome (ARDS)

The major life-threatening pulmonary complication is development of adult respiratory distress syndrome (ARDS), induced by an excessive proinflammatory immune response. In the past, this process had a mortality rate of up to 70%. The disease is, in part, caused by and worsened by over-resuscitation during a massive capillary leak, leading to interstitial edema and flooding of alveoli; this results in fulminant hypoxia requiring excessively high ventilator pressures, which in turn cause barotrauma to the lung parenchyma.

---

[1] HOB = head of bed.

From a **prevention standpoint**, early reduction in the excessive inflammatory response is best achieved by limiting the duration and repeated episodes of ischemia-inducing inflammation. In addition, avoidance of proinflammatory stimuli, such as transfusion of old blood, is also beneficial. **By minimizing the insult, and carefully avoiding over-resuscitation and flooding of the damaged alveoli, even though acute pulmonary dysfunction occurs, the disease has become less severe and more short-lived with a lesser impact than in the past** — see ■ Table 13.7.

Table 13.7. ARDS treatment.

- Avoid under-/over-resuscitation.
- Avoid unnecessary pRBC and FFP.
- Avoid large tidal volumes (TV >8cc/kg).
- Utilize PEEP to increase PaO_2/recruit FRC.
- Decrease TV to 6cc/kg with a P/F (PaO_2/FiO_2) ratio <300.

In the past, attempts to improve oxygenation were dependent on increasing lung volumes to recruit alveolar and functional reserve capacity (FRC) volumes, even though this needed high ventilatory pressures. Subsequently, CT scans demonstrated dishomogeneity of the process and the remaining normal alveolar units were being grossly over-distended and directly damaged by the high tidal volumes, while collapsed and fluid-filled alveoli resisted attempts at ventilation; all this contributed to the increased shunt fraction and worsened hypoxia. This ventilator-induced lung injury is also a major cause of the excessive inflammatory response leading to additional local and systemic damage. **To break this cycle, the use of increased levels of positive end-expiratory pressure (PEEP) (10+ mmHg) — apply Maier's Rule: FIO_2/PEEP should be five or less — recruits and maintains alveolar and FRC volumes, while simultaneously decreasing the tidal volume (6cc/kg) prevents over-distension and damage in the remaining functional alveolar units.** The ARDSnet prospective RCT Trial proved that low tidal volumes (which produce lower ventilator pressures) led to a significant decrease in mortality related to ARDS, and this has become the standard of care. Low-volume ventilation, with volume being a surrogate for low pressure, prevents over-distension-induced injury and progression of ARDS.

Remember: avoid over-resuscitation and 'salt water drowning' and utilize low-volume protective ventilation for diffuse lung injury to prevent worsening ventilator-induced lung damage.

Nutrition and GI bleeding

Nutrition is an important component of recovery from critical surgical illness. **Current goals routinely involve achieving a caloric intake of 25-30 calories per kilogram per day, while ingesting approximately 1.5g of protein per kilogram per day.** It is thought that this level of nutrition is needed to reverse the deleterious effects of the stress response to illness — which include insulin resistance, hyperglycemia, increased glycolysis and breakdown of structural protein — and to provide basic nutrition, primarily for the CNS and heart. **Unfortunately, the majority of patients do not achieve this level due to multiple interruptions for operations, radiographic testing, rehabilitation and other activities. The enteral route is preferable for nutrition. In fact, repeated studies have shown that the early institution of total parenteral nutrition (TPN) is not only of no benefit, but also increases significantly the risk for central line infection, pneumonia and other complications, including increased mortality. For up to seven days post-insult, there is no need for the initiation of parenteral nutrition.** During this period, attempts should be made to obtain enteral access, preferably via the stomach (directly or through the nose...) and to increase tube feeding as tolerated to reach the stated goals. Enteral feeding, even if unable to achieve the goal levels of nutrition, has a demonstrated significant benefit on the incidence of infectious complications and mortality. Thus, to assist in avoiding these complications, aggressive early feeding should be attempted. **However, recent studies show that even in the patient without gross aspiration, the incidence of VAP in the intubated patient appears to increase with aggressive feeding in the first several days post-ICU admission.** The risk must be carefully balanced, and with significant gastric residual volumes, and risk of aspiration, the tube feeding volume must be titrated to tolerance.

A major benefit of early enteral nutrition is prevention of gastric bleeding. At one time nearly ubiquitous, GI bleeding has been largely eliminated in the ICU patient. With enteral feeding there is an increase in gastric mucosal blood flow, with subsequent increase in function, particularly mucus production that prevents back diffusion and mucosal damage from endogenous gastric acid. The occurrence of gastric bleeding after burns, referred to as *Curling ulcers*, has dramatically decreased with a protocol of enteral tube feeding in the burn patient within the first 18-24 hours post-insult. **Similarly, in the severely injured or critically ill surgical patient, any amount of tube feeding, even trickle feeds, appears to be protective,** allows the discontinuation of proton pump inhibitors (PPI) and H_2 blocker acid suppression, and simultaneously reduces episodes of potentially lethal gastric hemorrhage.

Contraindications to enteral feeding are extremely limited, consisting of non-continuity of the GI tract, complete obstruction, or repeated non-tolerance to tube feeding despite gastric and enteral stimulants such as metoclopramide

(Reglan®) and erythromycin. **Tube feeding can begin within 24 hours of surgery in virtually all patients**. Anastomoses do not need to be 'protected' — the liver and pancreas produce far more volume than the tube feeding will be providing, and the vast majority of patients have tolerance of tube feeding, even those with an open abdomen. **A caveat**: there have been reports of small bowel necrosis associated with early postoperative jejunal tube feeding administered to severely traumatized or septic patients; thus, delay the feeds until the patient is stable and his splanchnic vasculature is no longer constricted.

> **Remember:** early (<24 hours) initiation of enteral (preferably intragastric) feeding reduces complications, primarily infectious. TPN increases infections and possibly death, and should rarely be started unless unable to feed for at least for seven days. Enteral feeding prevents GI bleeding. If not possible to feed use an acid suppressant, preferably a PPI, until intake is initiated.

Line complications

Critical illness requires monitoring to prevent complications. Unfortunately, monitoring still requires invasive venous cannulation in many circumstances — mainly utilization of central venous catheters as discussed above. **The two major complications of these interventions are infections and pneumothorax** — see ■ Table 13.8.

Table 13.8. Prevention of line complications.

- Treat as major procedure.
- Pre-procedure education and simulation training.
- Surgical procedure 'time-out'.
- Complete sterile technique.
- Chlorhexidine site prep.
- Ultrasound location if possible.
- Three attempts only per provider.
- Post-placement chest X-ray.
- Daily site evaluation.

Pneumothorax

Pneumothorax (PTX) is a recognized complication in 2-5% of all central line placements. This incidence goes up in the hands of the novice, with a fairly steep learning curve, and a dramatic decrease in incidence in the hands of the experienced clinician. To minimize this complication I recommend pre-training using both didactics and simulation until proven facile because these lessons have a significant impact on the practitioner's skill set. **In addition, there is a direct correlation between the number of attempts at placement and the incidence of PTX. Most institutions utilize a rule of three: any individual should not attempt more than three passes at any vessel, and if cannulation is not achieved then a more seasoned clinician should attempt placement**. Utilization of **handheld ultrasonic devices** for location of the vein dramatically increases success rates and decreases the incidence of false passage, arterial cannulation and other complications. Ultrasonic guidance is highly recommended for all internal jugular vein access, and, as appropriate but less usefully, with subclavian veins. Placement of all central lines should be confirmed by chest X-ray. PTX will need close monitoring with follow-up chest X-ray, with or without (for very small PTX) chest tube placement. Occasionally, a pig-tail catheter is adequate for drainage.

Line infection

Infection of central venous lines is a major complication in surgical ICUs. While met with great resistance, implementation of care protocols have had a major impact on the incidence of line infections. **The procedure must be approached as any other major intervention** with a time-out check list immediately pre-procedure, complete aseptic preparation — with *chlorhexidine* rather than iodine solutions — with draping and rigorous attention to sterile technique. Daily care with permeable coverage and observation for purulence or increasing redness, leads to either early replacement over a wire or via an alternative site if systemic infection appears to be present.

Remember: central line placement should be treated as any major sterile procedure. Pre-training, including simulation, use of ultrasound guidance and limitation of number of attempts decrease complications.

Venous thromboembolism (VTE)

The risk of venous thromboembolism (VTE) depends on the type of operation or injury, along with numerous other patient risk factors (see ■ Table 13.9). **Without prophylaxis, the risk of developing deep venous thrombosis**

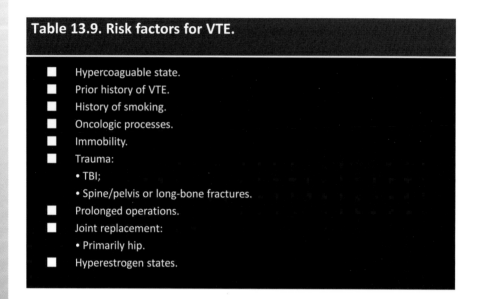

Table 13.9. Risk factors for VTE.

- Hypercoaguable state.
- Prior history of VTE.
- History of smoking.
- Oncologic processes.
- Immobility.
- Trauma:
  - TBI;
  - Spine/pelvis or long-bone fractures.
- Prolonged operations.
- Joint replacement:
  - Primarily hip.
- Hyperestrogen states.

in the ICU patient ranges from 20-80%. VTE prophylaxis relies on graded compression devices, such as stockings, intermittent sequential compression devices, or pharmacologic interventions, most commonly unfractionated or low-molecular-weight heparin. **Early ambulation should be remembered as an overall excellent prophylaxis for VTE and many other postoperative complications.** These approaches affect two of the three phases of increased risk, prevention of stasis and endogenous and exogenous treatment of hypercoagulability. With short cases, and otherwise low-risk patients, particularly in the out-patient setting, the risks outweigh the benefits of prophylaxis.

Optimal utilization of anticoagulants is still unclear. The risk of bleeding must be balanced against the risk of thrombosis. **Again, factors in surgical patients such as:** duration of the procedure, history of smoking, cancer, hypercoagulable state and/or, importantly, prior history of VTE, presence of trauma with immobility and hyperestrogen states all contribute to risk. Joint replacement or fracture reduction therapy also puts the patient at significant VTE risk. Several national organizations, using primarily consensus and evidence-based medicine when possible, have established **guidelines for VTE prophylaxis**. High-risk operations usually require some form of chemical VTE prophylaxis, whereas low-risk procedures, including endoscopic and/or high-risk hemorrhage-associated procedures such as some urologic procedures, argue against prophylaxis. If VTE prophylaxis is to be given, low-molecular-weight heparins are more effective; however, the half-life of effect is significantly greater and therefore the potential bleeding risk is increased. When bleeding risks are high, low-dose unfractionated heparin, given three times daily, is preferable.

An **additional risk for complication is erratic or intermittent implementation of therapy**. Once risk is determined to warrant intervention, therapy should be started as rapidly as safely possible and interruptions avoided. There appears to be an enhanced 'rebound' effect, which subjects the patient to even greater risk of thrombosis. In fact, with elective procedures prophylaxis should be started before the insult. Most orthopedic and general surgical procedures can be performed while receiving a standard unfractionated heparin for prophylaxis. **In the setting of the injured patient, once the patient has demonstrated stabilization for 24-36 hours, and there is a confirmed lack of progression of intracranial bleeds or other evidence of continuing bleeding, heparin prophylaxis can be instituted with close monitoring.** Our institution has moved to every evening dosing with unfractionated heparin to prevent interruption of prophylaxis due to multiple surgical procedures in our injured patients.

Remember: critically ill patients are at high risk for VTE, and some form of prophylaxis is indicated in all patients. Low-molecular-weight heparin is preferred but must be balanced against the risk of bleeding. Unfractionated heparin is short-lived and can be continued through most procedures. Interruption of dosing leads to a rebound increased risk of thrombosis and should be avoided.

Glucose control

Diabetes is a risk factor for morbidity and mortality in surgical patients. **Even in the non-diabetic patient, stress-induced hyperglycemia increases the risk of complications, primarily infectious, and is a biomarker for severe stress and systemic inflammation.** Hyperglycemia stimulates the innate immune inflammatory response, and potentially contributes to the dysregulation leading to infectious complications and multiple organ failure (MOF).

Numerous studies, initially in the cardiac surgical literature, demonstrated that lowering glucose levels from the 250+ mg/dL (14.0mmol/L) range, to the mid-100s, had a dramatic impact on infectious complications. Subsequently, tighter glucose control, between 80-110mg/dL (4.4-6.2mmol/L), also appeared to benefit the patient. However, recent studies comparing tight control of 80-100mg/dL (4.4-5.6mmol/L) with levels of 130-150mg/dL (7.2-8.3mmol/L), have shown no benefit, but are associated with a detrimental impact due to frequent hypoglycemia, particularly CNS risk, and an increase in mortality. Using composite data, the break point for an increase in infectious complications occurs at approximately 150mg/dL (8.3mmol/L). **Thus, to prevent episodes of hypoglycemia, maintaining glucose levels between approximately 120 and 150mg/dL achieves the benefit of minimizing inflammation and immune dysregulation while avoiding detrimental hypoglycemia**. Importantly, early intervention during the peri-operative phase is critical to avoid complications. Protocols should ensure close glucose control intra-operatively and continue throughout the critical-care course of the patient. **Again, rapid swings in glucose level are particularly harmful**.

Remember: baseline diabetes and stress-induced glucose intolerance increase risks, particularly infectious. Monitor glucose early and frequently, and treat intra-operatively and as necessary to keep glucose at an appropriate level — 120 to 150mg/dL; utilize monitoring and treatment protocols to avoid inadvertent hypoglycemia.

Clostridium difficile colitis

A prime example of iatrogenic disease is *Clostridium difficile* (*C. diff*) colitis. It represents the most rapidly increasing infectious complication in the hospital setting. **The primary cause is misuse and overuse of broad-spectrum antibiotics**. While the use of clindamycin is most frequently associated with the onset of *C. diff*. colitis, the disease has been associated with most broad-spectrum agents. Thus, the use of antibiotics that are excessive in scope or duration for any indication increases the risk. **Prolonged or excessively broad coverage for prophylaxis of surgical procedures or treatment of infections after source control is a common error**. *C. diff* colitis is ubiquitous in the environment, and the endogenous barrier to colonization is gastric acidity. Inappropriate use of acid suppressants augments the incidence of *C. diff.* colitis, in a dose response matching the effectiveness in blocking acid production, with PPIs producing a greater risk than H_2 blockers. To both interrupt *C. diff.* colitis outbreaks and to prevent spread of colonization, identify and isolate the patient using PCR (polymerase chain reaction) antigen screening, provide universal barrier protection during direct contact, and use soap and water to decontaminate hands after every contact. Hand contamination is the primary source of transfer and colonization. Notably, clostridial spores are not killed by usual hand disinfectants; see ■ Table 13.10. I hope that you know how to treat *C.diff.* colitis.

Table 13.10. Prevent or stop *C. difficile* colitis outbreak.

- Limit duration and spectrum of antibiotics.
- Avoid acid blockers:
  - PPIs worse than H_2 blockers.
- Monitor diarrhea with PCR antigen testing.
- Utilize contact barriers and isolation.
- Wash hands with soap:
  - Spores resistant to disinfectants.

Remember: avoid unnecessarily broad and excessive duration antibiotic therapy, avoid gastric acid inhibitors, isolate and use barrier protection for care of infected individuals and wash hands after every exposure.

Drug continuity

Acute changes in baseline levels of therapeutics are a significant risk for complications in the surgical patient (see ■ Table 13.11). As mentioned, both anticoagulants and glycemic agents should be continued or restarted as soon as possible. **Two other common treatments that need to be continued to avoid complications are beta-blockade and statin therapy**.

Table 13.11. Continue/restart chronic medications.

- ASA, anticoagulants (particularly heparin).
- Beta-blockers (adrenergic receptor antagonists).
- Statins (HMG-CoA reductase inhibitors).
- Insulin.
- Anti-hypertensives.
- Diuretics.
- Anti-depressants/anti-psychotics.
- EtOH withdrawal protocol.

Beta-blockade therapy

These agents are frequently present in patients admitted to the ICU. Beta-blockade has been shown to be of benefit in reducing subsequent cardiac events in patients sustaining acute myocardial ischemia. Unfortunately, this was inappropriately extrapolated to other patient populations at presumed risk for CAD: *if good for MI, then beta-blockers should also be beneficial for the stress of an ICU or planned major operation.* Pursuit of this rationale substantially increases mortality, primarily due to an increase in stroke incidence. In contrast, **patients currently on beta-blocker therapy should have therapy continued through the operation and in the ICU setting**. Sudden changes in baseline physiology are poorly tolerated, particularly in combination with the stress of ICU care. **Do not start nor stop beta-blockers 'prophylactically' in the ICU!**

Statins

Statin therapy has become one of the most commonly used chronic therapies. The modern high-fat diet and concomitant dyslipidemias are a common cause for vascular disease. To control the hyperlipidemia, statins are used to block excess cholesterol and LDL synthesis in the liver and presumably decrease the deposition of atheroma and blockage of the vasculature. In addition, while the exact mechanism of protection is unknown, it is clear that these agents have many biochemical functions, including antioxidant and cellular stabilizing effects. **In addition, a 'reset homeostasis' occurs similar to beta-blockers, aspirin, CNS medications and other chronic therapies, which produces a rebound response when therapy is discontinued. Injured patients chronically on statin therapy fare much worse when the statin therapy is discontinued** compared to patients who have the therapy reinstituted as rapidly as possible post-injury or surgery.

Reinstitute all chronic medications to prevent rebound dysfunction and significant morbidity.

> **Remember:** do not start beta-blockers or statins prophylactically, continue or restart both peri-operatively to avoid 'rebound effects'. Reinstitute or continue all longstanding therapeutics.

Sedation and pain control

Pain control and sedation are major components of care. For recovery and minimizing complications, adequate pain control to participate in procedures, such as wound care, respiratory function and rehabilitation, is mandatory. **Pain control should be titrated to achieve analgesia and control agitation**. While previously debated, currently **i.v. bolus administration is considered superior to continuous high-level intravenous infusion**. Bolus infusion allows continuous assessment of pain and agitation, allowing the bedside provider the opportunity to rapidly titrate medications and thus prevent overt overuse. However, low-level use of adjuncts to therapy, including baseline use of agents such as acetaminophen or ketamine, may reduce the overall narcotic requirements, and thus minimize the potential side effects. Similarly, sedative medications should be administered to treat agitation, tolerate extreme ventilator modes, including low-volume protective ventilation, and to complement pain control as required for safe and humane care.

Overuse of pain and sedative medications produces a calm patient with increased ease of care, but leads to multiple complications. In non-intubated patients, overuse of both pain and sedative medications can lead to respiratory depression and aspiration requiring mechanical ventilation, and in intubated patients can lead to a prolonged need for mechanical ventilation. As a result, these patients, due to their treatment, are at increased risk for the development of hospital-acquired pneumonia. Additionally, accumulation of sedative drugs or active metabolites is common, especially in adipose tissue of the obese patient or when hepatic and renal dysfunction occur. This leads to over-sedation, greater hemodynamic instability, and prolonged duration of intubation and ICU stay. This is especially problematic in drugs with a low clearance, when given as continuous infusions that are more prone to accumulate, leading to over-sedation.

Over-sedation and ongoing release leads to prolonged alterations in mentation and delirium in up to 80% of critically ill patients. Prolonged dissociation in mentation and loss of normal sleep patterns leads to hallucinations and confusion. **The best approach to avoid overdosing is to provide daily 'sedation holidays'**, allowing the patient to awaken to baseline function and to optimize trials of spontaneous breathing to gauge ability to tolerate extubation. Careful assessment for delirium is tracked, sedation is minimized, and alternative agents, such as haloperidol or quetiapine (Seroquel®) are used to control hallucinations and dissociation, while restoring normal sleep cycling. In addition, alternative agents have been developed that minimize the potential effects of narcotics and sedatives. Agents such as dexmedetomidine (Precedex®) and propofol have less risk of delirium, and their short half-life increases the ability to assess a patient's neurological status. However, both drugs have significant potential side effects, with Precedex-induced hypotension and propofol-induced cardiac collapse.

Remember: do not over-prescribe sedatives or narcotics, ensure a daily 'sedation vacation'. Monitor for hallucinations and delirium daily, and treat appropriately with anti-psychotic agents.

Communication and professionalism

Communication is crucial!

The challenges of optimal communication and professionalism could easily be the most critical factors in preventing unnecessary complications in the ICU setting. Similar to the child's game of telephone, where a message is passed from one child to the next by whispering, the rapidity of distortion of the message could be comical, unless it is a message to add a critical antibiotic or decrease the dose of drug due to renal dysfunction. **No longer comical, the outcome is a common cause for complications in the complex world of ICU care, which is increasingly complicated by more frequent handovers by health care teams**. Each must strive to provide timely, accurate and complete information for the care of the patient. Use of confusing initials, such as POA[2], BAL, etc., to ease the volume of the communication only leads to further problems. The object is not to keep secrets from the next care giver during handover or to test their acuity or knowledge, but to provide all pertinent knowledge for appropriate care. This is magnified in the ICU setting where trips to radiology for imaging to rule out PE, abscess or other drainable fluid or progression of disease, such as brain infarct, are frequent and often involve

---

[2] Present on admission.

several handovers in the care of the patient. Similarly, frequent operative interventions to stabilize fractures, wash out open abdomens, and further debride devitalized or infected/ischemic tissue, while providing optimal resuscitation monitoring, ventilator support and correction of coagulopathy/hypothermia and acidosis, are a test of team function in complex care. **Remember to stay with the patient until the handover is complete and pass on all pertinent information to the receiving care giver**.

Professionalism is not a gimmick

Professionalism refers to setting the expectations for oneself and all other members of the team. Care of the critically ill patient requires input from an increasingly complex medical team. **The surgeon in the ICU is frequently in the position of overall team leader or primary consultant**. As such, the surgeon must set the tenor and expectations for the interactions of the team. Each member is considered important to the decision-making process and worthy of input. Respect for each member of the team and reasoned discussion by all members as appropriate to synthesize the optimal plan for care is the model set by the surgeon as a true professional. **Disregard of a team member's opinion and arrogance or a condescending attitude can be lethal for the patient**. The system must ensure mechanisms for feedback and recognition of dysfunctional teams and means to intervene with required education and counseling or even dismissal if any individual, including the surgeon, is unable to interact appropriately with the medical care team.

Remember: critical illness requires a team approach to care but also involves an increasing number of handovers. Mechanisms to ensure accurate and adequate information at transfer are critical. All members of the team are crucial and each must be involved and respected. The surgeon must set the professional standards expected of the position.

A note to those of you who do not have a modern ICU at their disposition. In this chapter, Dr. Maier, a leading surgical intensivist, preaches from the pulpit of his state-of-the art ivory tower ICU — a unit with facilities that most of us can only dream of. However, this does not decrease the importance of his message to those of you in the 'periphery' or the developing world. With care, dedication and improvisation, you can apply most of his recommendations even in your rural, one-bed 'high-care' area in the 'bush'. **The Editors**

Selected reading list [3]

1. Artinian V, Krayem H, DiGiovine B. Effects of early enteral feeding on the outcome of critically ill mechanically ventilated medical patients. *Chest* 2006; 129: 960-7.
2. Attia J, Ray JG, Cook DJ, *et al*. Deep vein thrombosis and its prevention in critically ill adults. *Arch Intern Med* 2001; 161: 1268-79.
3. Chesnut RM, Marshall LF, Klauber MR, *et al*. The role of secondary brain injury in determining outcome from severe head injury. *J Trauma* 1993; 34: 216-22.
4. Dong Y, Chbat NW, Gupta A, *et al*. Systems modeling and simulation applications for critical care medicine. *Ann Intensive Care* 2012; 2: 18.
5. Gentile LF, Cuenca AG, Efron PA, *et al*. Persistent inflammation and immunosuppression: a common syndrome and new horizon for surgical intensive care. *J Trauma Acute Care Surg* 2012; 72: 1491-501.
6. Gruen RL, Brohi K, Schreiber M, *et al*. Haemorrhage control in severely injured patients. *Lancet* 2012; 380: 1099-108.
7. Herbert PC, Wells G, Blajchman MA, *et al*. A multicenter, randomized, controlled clinical trial of transfusion requirements in critical care. *N Engl J Med* 1999; 340: 409-17.
8. Howell MD, Novack V, Grgurich P, *et al*. Iatrogenic gastric acid suppression and the risk of nosocomial *Clostridium difficile* infection. *Arch Intern Med* 2010; 170(9): 784-90.
9. Khan H, Belsher J, Yilmaz M, *et al*. Fresh-frozen plasma and platelet transfusions are associated with development of acute lung injury in critically ill medical patients. *Chest* 2007; 131: 1308-14.
10. Kress JP, Pohlman AS, Hall JB. Sedation and analgesia in the intensive care unit. *Am J Respir Crit Care Med* 2002; 166(8): 1024-8.
11. Loo VG, Bourgault AM, Poirier L, *et al*. Host and pathogen factors for *Clostridium difficile* infection and colonization. *N Engl J Med* 2011; 365(18): 1693-703.
12. Marik PE, Preiser JC. Toward understanding tight glycemic control in the ICU: a systemic review and meta-analysis. *Chest* 2010; 137(3): 544-51.
13. Marik PE, Zaloga GP. Early enteral nutrition in acutely ill patients: a systemic review. *Crit Care Med* 2001; 29(12): 2264-70.
14. McLeod AG, Geerts W. Venous thromboembolism prophylaxis in critically ill patients. *Crit Care Clin* 2011; 27: 765-80.
15. Perel P, Roberts I, Ker K. Colloids versus crystalloids for fluid resuscitation in critically ill patients. *Cochrane Database Syst Rev* 2013; 2: February 28.
16. Reidenberg MM. Drug discontinuation effects are part of the pharmacology of a drug. *J Pharmacol Exp Ther* 2011; 339(2): 324-8.
17. Rivers EP. Fluid-management strategies in acute lung injury — liberal, conservative, or both? *N Engl J Med* 2006; 354: 2598-600.
18. Sebat F, Musthafa AA, Johnson D, *et al*. Effect of a rapid response system for patients in shock on time to treatment and mortality during 5 years. *Crit Care Med* 2007; 35: 2568-75.
19. Van den Berghe G, Wouters P, Weekers F, *et al*. Intensive insulin therapy in critically ill patients. *N Engl J Med* 2001; 345(19): 1359-67.
20. Ventilation with lower tidal volumes as compared with traditional tidal volumes for acute lung injury and the acute respiratory distress syndrome. The Acute Respiratory Distress Syndrome Network. *N Engl J Med* 2000; 342: 1301-8.
21. Villanueva C, Colomo A, Bosch A, *et al*. Transfusion strategies for acute upper gastrointestinal bleeding. *N Engl J Med* 2013; 368(1): 11-21.
22. Xiao W, Mindrinos MN, Seok J, *et al*. A genomic storm in critically injured humans. *J Exp Med* 2011; 208: 2581-90.

---

[3] Against the 'policy' of this book we have allowed Dr. Maier to include this long list of references. The reasons for our decision are confidential ☺ [The Editors].

Chapter 14

Colon and rectum (and the humble anus)

Mark Cheetham

This chapter has been subdivided into the following two sections:

1. Colon and rectum.
2. The anus.

1   Colon and rectum

> *A good reliable set of bowels is worth more to a man than any quantity of brain.*
>
> *If you don't eat — you don't shit.*
> *If you don't shit — you die!*
>
> **Baz**

A 76-year-old woman is referred to you with a newly diagnosed rectal cancer; it goes without saying that you are the *local guru* in laparoscopic colorectal surgery (isn't everyone nowadays?). How can you ensure that she has a complication-free operation?

Colorectal surgery is notorious for the frequency of complications — not surprisingly there are some risks innate to operating on a muscular tube stuffed full of Gram-negative and anaerobic bacteria. In this chapter I will discuss strategies to reduce the risk of complications and how to recognize and manage common calamities and misadventures should they occur.

Pre-operative considerations

First of all: avoid pointless operations. One sure way of avoiding complications is not to operate at all. Some surgeons take this to the extreme and find any excuse not to operate (funnily enough this does not seem to be a problem in fee-for-service systems! In the USA, for example, where the opposite seems to be true…). Some patients will have incurable cancer at presentation; in such circumstances the role of surgery is to **palliate** symptoms; **remember that it is not possible to palliate a patient who has no symptoms**.

A few more points:

- **I would routinely stage all patients with newly diagnosed colorectal cancer with a CT scan of the chest, abdomen and pelvis**. In some patients the burden of metastases could suggest that only palliative measures may be indicated.
- Nowadays, of course, a **colonoscopically placed stent** can palliate many patients with obstructive symptoms due to a left colonic lesion. Whether the stent is placed by yourself or 'the competition' is related largely to the local politics in your hospital (suffice it to say that most gastroenterologists would be quite happy for your children to go to the 'poor school').
- **Remember: a stoma is not a disaster** — in selected patients a well-constructed colostomy may improve a patient's quality of life. If a stoma is likely in a planned operation, I always ask our **stomatherapist** to see the patient before surgery. This allows the patient to be better prepared psychologically and will also cut the length of postoperative stay by allowing stoma training to begin before the operation.
- Other patients may **not be fit for surgery at all**. Traditionally the operating surgeon has made a 'gut-based', 'eye-balling' decision about fitness for surgery — nowadays you may be lucky enough to have access to CPEX (cardiopulmonary exercise testing). **Resist the urge for blanket consultations with other doctors** — most other specialties have little idea of the risks of major colorectal surgery: how often has the cardiologist, who 'cleared' the patient for surgery, been seen in the hospital at a 2 a.m. reoperation on the leak?

Special considerations in inflammatory bowel disease

Patients with **Crohn's** and **ulcerative colitis** present some particular challenges pre-operatively. These are often young people with jobs and dependent children. They may have been ill for some time prior to seeing a surgeon and are frequently taking steroids and immunosuppressants. **A key point is the timing of surgery**: leave the patient too long and they may become so ill that complications are inevitable. Conversely, if you operate before the patient is psychologically prepared for surgery, they will tolerate complications poorly and complaints are inevitable.

I am fortunate to work with a skilled and enlightened group of gastroenterologists who recognize that surgery is just another treatment for inflammatory bowel disease. They refer patients early if they may need surgery — allowing the patients and surgeon time to establish a therapeutic relationship. Elsewhere things may not be so rosy: I know some gastroenterologists who are so convinced that surgery is a bad thing that they use this as the primary endpoint in trials!!

Locating the tumor

Commonly, in modern surgical practice, **the target lesion (large polyp/small cancer) for a colectomy is small and non-palpable**. If you perform the operation laparoscopically you will lose the ability to feel the colon in any case. Can you trust the pre-operative colonoscopy to locate the lesion? If the local turf wars allow you to perform colonoscopy, you will know that tumor location at colonoscopy is an imprecise science (as an aside, I believe that there is great merit to surgeon-performed colonoscopy — this improves the relationship between gastroenterologists and surgeons and ultimately benefits patients). If you are not in the rectum or within sight of the ileocecal valve, you may not be able to correctly identify the appropriate colonic segment. **I now insist on tattooing of all lesions pre-operatively** — unless they are palpable at rectal examination or are visible adjacent to the ileocecal valve. This prevents that awful sinking feeling of not being able to identify the cancer at surgery.

I also insist on personally **performing a rigid sigmoidoscopy before any left-sided resection** (it is amazing how often a gastroenterologist reports a "tumor at 20cm at the rectosigmoid junction" only for a low rectal cancer to be felt at rectal examination! In surgery, unlike 'blind dates', surprises are never fun!

To prep or not to prep?

Traditionally it was considered mandatory to purge the gut before any colorectal resection. Of course, as a modern surgeon, you will know that **oral bowel prep is largely pointless**; doesn't the Cochrane Collaboration say so? Does that mean you completely abandon bowel prep? I did for a while, but after a couple of nasty surprises, I now use bowel prep selectively. It is certainly true that oral bowel preparation is unnecessary for colonic resections. Indeed it seems that oral bowel preparation may actually increase the risk of wound infection. What about tumors in the rectum? I would treat cancers of the rectosigmoid junction/upper rectum as for colonic resections — no oral bowel preparation needed.

However, it would seem illogical to perform a low colorectal anastomosis and a proximal defunctioning stoma if the intervening colon is full of s**t; thus, now I routinely give oral bowel prep to patients who may need a diverting stoma. Anecdotally, oral bowel prep in this situation seems to mitigate some of the effects of an anastomotic leak; there is a reduced need to reoperate for a leak if the bowel has been prepped (as is the case with colonoscopic bowel perforations) and a better chance of avoiding a permanent stoma.

American surgeons are still fond of adding **oral antibiotics** to their mechanical colonic prep (⮌ Chapter 6, section 5). I, on the other side of the pond, however, believe that i.v. antibiotic prophylaxis suffices. This is not dissimilar to a much more important controversy: which is better? **Scotch or Bourbon?** (I trust that most readers of this book will know the correct answer!).

Make a plan

I ensure that I have a detailed plan for the operation prior to surgery — would you set off on a road trip without looking at a map? (Until the day there is an operative GPS ☺). I share the plan with the theatre team in a briefing before the operating list starts — this makes sure that the team all know what I am planning to do and that all the necessary kit is available. However, I do not stick irrationally to the plan — rather I'm prepared to be flexible and adapt the plan to any changing circumstances. In your mind, during the drive (or preferably the bike ride) to the hospital — if not during the previous evening — go over the detailed operative plan (■ Table 14.1). And while you scrub, ask again: prophylactic antibiotics given? What about DVT prophylaxis? Check each and every detail yourself — even 'administrative check lists' are not fool proof!

Table 14.1. The operative plan for a colorectal operation.

✓ Have I reviewed the staging, imaging and colonoscopy?
✓ Where is the tumor?
✓ Has it been tattooed pre-operatively?
✓ Can I resect it?
✓ Can or should I perform an anastomosis?
✓ Will I need to make a diverting stoma?
✓ Can I do this case laparoscopically?
✓ Do I need a second video monitor?
✓ Lateral or medial approach?
✓ What will I use for dissection?
✓ How to divide the vessels?
✓ Where will I make the specimen extraction site?
✓ How will I do the anastomosis? What stapling devices are needed?
✓ Where will the patient be nursed postoperatively?

Intra-operative considerations

Reducing the risks of an anastomotic leak

Anastomotic leakage is a completely avoidable complication; providing you don't perform an anastomosis.

Brendan Moran

The principles of anastomotic technique are explained in ⮂ Chapter 6. Rather than repeat that advice here, I will discuss the decision-making surrounding an anastomosis. There are certainly situations where **you should definitely not perform an anastomosis** after a resection:

- Colectomy for **fecal peritonitis**.
- Relaparotomy for **anastomotic leak**.
- Colectomy for **fulminant colitis**.

At the other extreme are patients with a very low risk of anastomotic leakage (fit, well-nourished patients, with small cancers having an elective operation). In between these two extremes there is a continuum of risk and you will need to make a judgment call on a case by case basis. **You need to decide**:

- What is the chance of an anastomotic leak?
- What is the chance you would diagnose a leak early?
- If a leak occurs, what is the chance the patient would survive?

Important considerations are listed in ■ Table 14.2. In making your operative plan you will have decided whether to anastomose or not. Be prepared to adapt your plan as the operation proceeds; for instance, if there is a large volume of bleeding, perhaps you will avoid the anastomosis and stage the procedure.

Table 14.2. Risk factors for colorectal anastomotic leakage.

✓ Heavy intra-operative bleeding (greater than 500ml blood loss)
✓ Degree of contamination/peritonitis
✓ Systemic steroids
✓ Chronic debilitation/malnutrition (low albumin level)
✓ Chronic renal failure
✓ Crohn's disease
✓ Male sex
✓ Smoking
✓ Morbid obesity (would you notice a leak?)
✓ Severe comorbidity (would the patient survive a leak?)

Anastomotic leakage in particular is an issue with resections for **Crohn's disease**; these patients can be extremely ill, septic and malnourished. ■ Table 14.3 gives useful guidance as to risk factors for anastomotic leakage in this particular situation.

Table 14.3. When to avoid an anastomosis during resections for Crohn's disease.

✓ Intra-abdominal abscess/enterocutaneous fistula
✓ Poor nutrition
✓ Steroids
✓ Albumin less than 30g/dL

If more than two factors apply, consider a staged approach with resection and exteriorization (for example, as a double-barreled ileocolostomy) at the index operation and later restoration of intestinal continuity.

Diverting stomas

Diverting the fecal stream by placing a loop ileostomy or colostomy above a high-risk colorectal anastomosis is a time-honored way to reduce the risks of surgery. **A proximal stoma will not reduce the incidence of a leak, but it will mitigate the consequences of a leak**. So if a patient has a proximal stoma and the anastomosis leaks, the need for a relaparotomy is reduced and there is better chance of survival with good bowel function. Of course, patients will need a further procedure to close the stoma, and the risks of this should also be factored into your decision-making.

Iatrogenic splenic injury

Mobilizing the left colon to gain sufficient length may require the splenic flexure to be taken down. There is a small but finite risk of injuring the spleen during this maneuver. The risk of an iatrogenic splenic injury seems to vary according to the operating surgeon — I know a surgeon whose residents routinely seek informed consent for splenectomy for every anterior resection!

Avoiding iatrogenic splenic injury:

- Don't take the splenic flexure down unless you need to.
- Use gentle retraction on the left colon and omentum during mobilization.
- Don't try to move the splenic flexure to the incision; instead move the incision to the flexure.
- Divide adhesions to the splenic capsule early.
- **Attack from all directions**: the splenic flexure can be approached from laterally, inferiorly (under the descending colon) or from medially (via the lesser sac). Use and combine each of these approaches as necessary.

Managing an iatrogenic splenic injury:

- Most injuries are small capsular tears of the lower pole.
- Pack the left upper quadrant.
- Apply topical hemostatics.
- If this fails, then perform a splenectomy early. Like you, I have read the literature about various clever maneuvers to conserve the spleen; however, it is our experience that prolonged attempts at splenic conservation will cause more bleeding and risk further complications.

Ureteric injury

Recent data suggest that the rate of ureteric injury has increased with the widespread adoption of laparoscopic colorectal resections (think about laparoscopic cholecystectomy and bile duct injury). Seeing and preserving the ureter is an important step in any colorectal resection (whether open or laparoscopic).

Prevention

- **Visualize the ureter** (it should be posterior to the gonadal vessels) — if you see bare psoas muscle you are too deep. In patients with diverticulitis or in reoperative cases, beware: the ureter is often more medial than you would expect. In performing a laparoscopic resection, be careful not to tent up the ureter with the mesocolon; here it may be injured or even deliberately divided as an 'accessory inferior mesenteric vein'.
- **In selected patients mobilize the colon from superior to inferior**. In patients with hydronephrosis, I usually start the colonic mobilization high — exposing Gerota's fascia first and then exposing the upper ureter. Having found the normal ureter, dissection then proceeds inferiorly to do the difficult bit last with better exposure. This is useful in patients with diverticular disease, Crohn's disease and locally advanced cancers.
- **Peri-operative ureteric stenting** is useful if imaging suggests that dissection will be difficult. Fiber-optic 'glowing' ureteric stents are useful especially in laparoscopic surgery when the ability to feel a stent is lost. If you do use a peri-operative stent, remember (remind your urologist) to tie the end of the stent to the Foley catheter so you can remove it easily at the end of the case.

Treatment

Let's imagine a theoretical scenario in which you have accidentally transected the ureter (or if you would prefer let's imagine it's your worst enemy!). What should he do next? Recognizing the problem is half the battle — now you 'just' need to repair it. In most modern health care systems, you would call your best mate the urologist at this point (like him or loath him, at this point he is your best mate). In a rural setting you may have to repair this injury yourself — for details see ⊃ Chapter 26.

Bleeding in the pelvis

Massive pelvic bleeding is a rare, but problematic intra-operative complication of rectal surgery. The use of diathermy or other energy sources for dissection in the pelvis reduces the amount of bleeding and allows a much better view to avoid collateral damage to pelvic nerves, the ureters and blood vessels. Stop small bleeders as you go to keep your field of view clear. Major blood loss can occur quickly and if you do not act swiftly several units can disappear up the sucker.

Here is what to do if you cause major pelvic bleeding:

- Make sure you have **adequate access**; enlarge the incision (**time to convert to open surgery** if you are operating laparoscopically).

- Avoid the temptation to apply clips blindly — you may tear or injure other vessels.
- **Pack the pelvis** tightly with several large swabs or rolls of gauze: this will buy you time to get more kit, blood and other personnel together.
- **Cross-match** plenty of blood.
- **Get help** — another experienced pair of hands is invaluable as an assistant and to share decision-making.
- Now you may consider removing the packs and stopping the bleeding.
- **Don't use diathermy** in this setting: it will waste time and probably won't work. It may even burn a hole in a large vein.
- Stop bleeding from large veins (e.g. the iliacs) with fine vascular sutures (6/0 Prolene®) — using swabs on a stick (on both sides of the laceration) to maintain temporary control (applying vascular clamps to iliac veins is often difficult and risks tearing the vein). One trick to control the bleeding from major tears in the iliac veins is to insert a balloon catheter. Once the bleeding is controlled you can decide whether to try to repair the vein or just ligate it. The patient will tolerate the ligation, but will need postoperative measures to reduce swelling of the relevant extremity.
- If the bleeding is coming from the **pre-sacral veins**, then either **repack** the pelvis and leave the packs in for 48 hours or push sterile **drawing pins** into the sacrum to stop the bleeding (there are commercially available occlusion pins now). Oh yes, Americans would call them "thumbtacks".
- **Remember: resorting to packing early**, before the lethal triad of coagulopathy, hypothermia and acidosis sets in — not to speak about the adverse effect of blood transfusion on early (postoperative) and late (oncological) outcomes — is a mark of a mature surgeon! See also ⟳ Chapter 3.

Now that you have finally stopped the bleeding what to do? **Should you proceed with the resection and anastomosis?** This is a judgment call — but remember that major intra-operative bleeding is a factor in leakage of low pelvic anastomoses. For many surgeons it is easier to control the bleeding than their ego…

It won't reach…

I won't bore you again with details of the principles of performing an anastomosis (see ⟳ Chapter 6). You surely know that a key point is to avoid tension on an anastomosis. This can be a particular problem in rectal and left-sided resections — the anal side of the anastomosis is fixed and the **colonic side is limited by the attachments of the splenic flexure and the middle colic vessels**. You will read that some authorities believe it is mandatory to take the splenic flexure down in all left-sided colonic or rectal resections. **I would**

advocate a more flexible approach: if you can radically remove the tumor and create a tension-free anastomosis without mobilizing the splenic flexure — great! Why overcomplicate matters? Of course, when one operates on tumors in the descending colon or low rectum, splenic flexure mobilization is necessary, but it is rarely necessary for sigmoid cancers.

So what should you do if you are struggling to get well-vascularized colon to reach low enough to perform an anastomosis? This may occur because the patient has a congenitally short, or fatty (not only Americans are increasingly obese!) mesentery, poor blood flow in the marginal artery or for iatrogenic reasons (i.e. overgenerous resection or a mesenteric vascular injury). Here I would advocate a step-wise approach:

- Perform a high ligation and division of the inferior mesenteric vessels.
- Fully mobilize the splenic flexure.
- Pedicle the left side of the transverse colon based on the middle colic vessels.

These three steps are almost always enough and only rarely should further steps be needed — but if you are **still struggling** at this point then your further options are:

- Divide the right branch of the middle colic vessels.
- Mobilize the right colon and invert the cecum.
- Make a window through the small bowel mesentery between the ileocolic and superior mesenteric vessels. The transverse colon can then be passed through this shorter retro-ileal route.
- **Remember to check that there is pulsatile flow in the marginal artery before you finally perform your anastomosis**. If there is any doubt, I divide the marginal artery to observe the blood flow.

Finally if all else fails — and nothing would reach low enough for a safe anastomosis — or if the patient is frail — consider whether he would be better off with an ultra-low Hartmann's procedure. (A subtotal colectomy with ileorectal anastomosis would be an option if a good length of rectum remains; however, most of the difficulties relate to patients having a low anterior resection...).

Bubbles on air testing

Many surgeons 'test' their colorectal anastomoses prior to closing the abdomen (or port sites for you laparoscopic wizards). As with most technical aspects of surgery there are several ways of doing this. Here is what I do:

- Ensure that you have a good view of the anastomosis (using retractors and head-down tilt).

- Apply a soft bowel clamp/your fingers/atraumatic laparoscopic grasper across the colon upstream of the anastomosis.
- Fill the pelvis with saline.
- Have someone (I send the junior registrar crawling under the drapes…) insert a Foley catheter into the rectum and inflate the balloon, then inflate the rectum with air using a bladder syringe (you could use a sigmoidoscope and bellows instead).
- A hole in the anastomosis is visible as a steady stream of bubbles.

You will all recognize that sinking feeling after a long operation when a flurry of bubbles in the pelvis means that you have more to do. The first consideration is the size of the leak: is it so large that you may as well resect the anastomosis and redo it? In our experience this is rare: most commonly the leak is from a tiny area. If you have performed a double-stapled anastomosis, the leak is often at the junction of the circular staple line with the linear staple line used to close the rectal stump.

So this is what I would do:

- **For a high colorectal anastomosis** (following a sigmoid or rectosigmoid resection) the leak is often amenable to repair via the abdomen. I would use a figure-of-8 suture to close the leak (I have placed this laparoscopically on a couple of occasions). I would then repeat the air test. Assuming the second air test is normal the next question is **should you perform a diverting stoma?** I would say that this is not always necessary and providing there are no other risk factors for anastomotic leakage, I have done without diversion in some patients. This is yet another "damned if you do and damned if you don't" syndrome or 'gut-based medicine'!
- **Following a low anterior resection or ileo-anal pouch operation**, the anastomosis is below the peritoneal reflection and cannot be accessed from above. It is usually possible to access a low anastomosis transanally with careful and gentle retraction. Again if the defect is large, you may have to take down the anastomosis and redo it (this will commit you to a hand-sewn colo-anal or pouch-anal anastomosis — I hope you are up to this!!). In this situation I would always construct a proximal diverting stoma.

A stoma without complications?

A stoma should be considered as an anastomosis between the bowel and the skin. I will not insult you by telling you how to join the bowel together, but please remember the same principles when making a stoma. How often is the maturation of a stoma delegated to a junior surgeon while the senior surgeon drinks coffee in the surgeons' lounge?

In a planned setting, of course, the stoma site will be marked by a stoma therapist pre-operatively. Unfortunately for you, she will not be there when you resect a perforated colon in the middle of the night. That means that you need a working knowledge of how to site a stoma. **In simple terms, place the stoma in the 'triangle of safety' (bounded by lines drawn between the umbilicus to the midpoint of the costal margin and the anterior superior iliac spine).**

A few more key points:

- Avoid bony prominences.
- Avoid scars, wounds and the umbilicus ("Bringing a colostomy out through a laparotomy incision is like putting a toilet in the kitchen").
- Consider the type of clothing worn by the patient (skinny young girls with Crohn's always want a stoma in the groin).
- In 'fatties' place the stoma higher — if it is under the bulge ('fatty apron') the patient cannot see it without a mirror!

You should consider adding measures to **reduce the (significant) risk of a parastomal hernia**:

- **Implant a light-weight sublay mesh around the stoma site**: several centers now do this as a routine. Initial concerns about mesh infection and erosion into the bowel appear to be unfounded and there is good evidence of a reduction in the rate of parastomal hernia occurrence.
- **Lateral to rectus abdominis placed stoma (LRAPS)**: *traditionally* a cruciate incision is made in the anterior rectus sheath horizontally and posterior sheath with the rectus muscle split vertically. A variant is to incise the anterior sheath horizontally and then retract the rectus medially. The posterior sheath is then incised horizontally and the stoma matured. Extremely low rates of parastomal hernia are reported using this technique.

Avoiding wound infections

There are innate risks of infection when operating on a tube filled with crap. A detailed account of how to avoid wound infections can be found in ⮌ Chapter 5. Some particular matters are important in reducing the risk of wound infection following colorectal surgery:

- Give **prophylactic antibiotics**: a single dose of suitable antibiotics given within 60 minutes before the incision to cover both Gram-negative bacteria and anaerobes is all that is necessary.

- Avoid excessive **bleeding**.
- Use **meticulous clean/dirty techniques** (i.e. don't sew a colorectal anastomosis and then use the same instruments to close the skin).
- **Change gloves** as often as required to minimize contamination.
- **Protect the wound** using swabs or wound edge protectors when opening the bowel or constructing an anastomosis.
- **Warm the patient**: there is good evidence that avoiding peri-operative hypothermia cuts down the risk of wound infection (I use forced air heating for all patients having colorectal resections).
- **Cover the wound before maturing a stoma.** I liberally apply surgical glue over the wound if I am making a stoma. This acts as a dressing to protect the wound from contamination postoperatively.

It is hard to prove that each of the above steps is beneficial, but collectively (the 'bundle' concept) — they are!

Postoperative considerations

As you well know, the most comforting music to the ears of the colorectal surgeon is the sound of flatus passed by the post-colectomy patient. But while you wait for the bowel symphony (■ Figure 14.1) complications can develop…

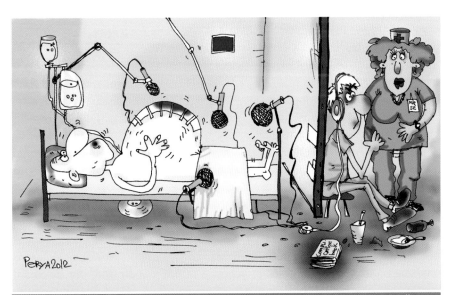

Figure 14.1. Nurse: "What are you doing Dr. Silberstein?" Surgeon: "I am waiting for him to fart!"

Rectal bleeding

I have occasionally encountered patients with profuse rectal bleeding after a colorectal resection. Anecdotally this seems to occur mainly after a **stapled anastomosis**. This may be recognized early on in the recovery room or some hours later back on the surgical ward. It can make for a worrisome time for the surgeon and the patient too. **Fortunately in almost all cases the bleeding stops without intervention, although blood transfusion will often be needed**.

If the bleeding does not stop after clotting abnormalities have been corrected (say after you have needed to transfuse two units of blood or the patient is hemodynamically unstable) consider this:

- Can you access the anastomosis transanally and suture the bleeder?
- If not, consider a cautious colonoscopy with minimal air insufflation and use endoscopic clips or adrenaline injections to stop the bleeding.
- Finally, consider reoperation with resection of the anastomosis. Whether to re-anastomose or not is a 'judgment call'…

Colonic ischemia

This is a rare situation mainly affecting patients after left colon or rectal surgery. It usually presents in the first day or two after surgery with an acutely ill patient with signs of sepsis and abdominal pain. Pain is often difficult to assess as a degree of pain is 'normal' at this point after surgery. **The diagnosis is mostly delayed because it is *too early for a leak***. The inevitable postoperative CT scan will often be normal (see "Recognizing and managing a leak" below). At reoperation — which often is delayed — you will find a gangrenous or even liquefied colon; the only option here is a Hartmann's procedure. The commonplace delay in diagnosis leads to a high mortality. *Charitably*, postoperative colonic ischemia may be thought to be due to inadequate flow in the marginal artery due to atheroma, vasopressors or anatomical variation — after all, a similar syndrome is recognized following abdominal aortic aneurysm surgery. *In practice*, however, it is most likely to be due to intra-operative injury to the marginal artery or ascending left colic artery during mobilization of the colon. A subacute variant of this situation has been observed and termed *devascularization colitis* (Thanks Angus G. Maciver!). In this entity (which anecdotally appears to be more common if the operation is performed laparoscopically or if the splenic flexure has been mobilized), the colonic ischemia is **not transmural**; the dominant symptoms are rectal bleeding and colonic ileus. Colonoscopy would demonstrate pale and ulcerated mucosa. As is the case with spontaneous ischemic colitis, this entity may resolve with supportive treatment plus broad-spectrum antibiotics. Devascularization colitis has also been observed in the mobilized colon distal to a diverting stoma. Obviously, if this is the case, then there is no need to rush to reoperate.

Recognizing and managing a leak

Yes, I know, Dr. Jon Efron has contributed an excellent chapter dedicated to this problem (⮑ Chapter 6, section 5). Nevertheless, my 'British version' of the remedy for such disasters may be of interest: if identified and treated early, a patient with an anastomotic leak has a good prospect of survival. Sadly, recognition is often delayed because symptoms are non-specific, they are blamed 'on the chest', or there is a reluctance to take down the anastomosis. Perhaps more than any other complication, anastomotic leaks are taken very personally by the responsible surgeon. This emotional attachment to the anastomosis can retard decision-making and is dangerous to your patient. **Remember: if a patient is ill after a colorectal resection, it is likely to be due to a leak**.

How to recognize a leak early

- **If a patient is ill** (i.e. has more SIRS than he should have) after a colorectal operation, assume that they have leaked.
- **Do not assume that sepsis** after a colorectal operation **is from the chest or urinary tract** without good evidence.
- New onset of **atrial fibrillation** after a colorectal resection is **due to a leak** (don't give the patient digoxin, he needs i.v. fluids, antibiotics and a stoma!). Well, not always ☺.
- **A CT scan in the first postoperative week is often misleading** (free air and fluid are normal findings at this time). Be prepared to operate without a CT scan or despite a reassuring CT scan if the clinical situation demands it.
- **A water-soluble contrast enema** may be useful in confirming a leak if the situation or other imaging is equivocal. This test may be more sensitive in proving a leak, but of course will give no information about intra-abdominal collections.
- **Drains can be falsely reassuring**. You know, of course, that a drain placed in the abdomen may be walled off within hours. This means that an empty drain bottle proves nothing. Conversely, do not assume that a drain will contain or localize a leak; if the patient is 'SIRSing' — he needs an operation to obtain source control.

Managing a leak

Having recognized the leak, the urgent priorities are to resuscitate the patient, treat the sepsis aggressively with antibiotics and **establish source control**.

Most patients with an anastomotic leak will need urgent surgery. The exceptions to this general rule are those patients with a low pelvic anastomosis and a proximal diverting stoma — here in the absence of severe sepsis or peritonitis, transanal drainage may salvage the situation and preserve the anastomosis. The late result will often be an anastomotic stricture and poor defecatory function. A recent variation to simple transanal drainage is to insert a sponge dressing connected to suction through the hole in the anastomosis (e.g. Endosponge™ — a commercially produced device). Anecdotally, this seems to reduce the degree of fibrosis around the anastomosis and improves late bowel function. However, this technique does require several sponge changes per week over a protracted time course and is labor intensive.

In a sick patient with generalized peritonitis, the best way to establish source control is to perform a laparotomy, take down the anastomosis, and exteriorize both ends as a double-barrel stoma or two separate stomas. For leaks following left sided-resections it is usually impossible to exteriorize the rectal side of the anastomosis; here it is better to close the rectal stump and perform an end colostomy (i.e. a Hartmann's). If you need to take down a low pelvic anastomosis, closure of the rectal stump will usually be impossible. Here I would insert a wide-bore Foley catheter (e.g. 30 French) through the rectal stump and leave this to drain any pelvic sepsis.

In selected patients who are systemically ill with a **localized leak**, it may be possible to preserve the anastomosis by draining any collection and performing a proximal diverting stoma. Washing out the distal bowel through the stoma (if possible) may help in controlling the sepsis. Use this option carefully; applying this to the wrong patient will fail to control the sepsis and result in a further risky and often 'too late to salvage' reoperation.

As everything in surgery, anastomotic leaks have a spectrum of severity and each case has to be managed individually. **Let us not forget that on the 'easy side' of the spectrum there are the so called 'mini' or 'contained' leaks — with minimal local and systemic repercussions — which can be managed expectantly with antibiotics.**

Fecal fistulas

A postoperative fecal fistula is a *forme fruste* of an anastomotic leak. It may present with a low-grade pyrexia which is shortly followed by a leakage of feculent fluid either though a drain or the wound. In this situation, the patient is not ill — there is minimal or no SIRS — and the abdomen is soft and non-tender. **Resist the primordial urge to reoperate.** Providing the fistula is controlled and there is no intra-abdominal collection, early reoperation is not needed. Use a stoma bag to collect any leakage — treat this as an 'unintended colostomy'. There is no need to starve the patient (would you place a patient with a colostomy on NPO?), as the metabolic and electrolyte disturbances seen with a small bowel fistula do not arise here. If there are signs of sepsis then a CT scan is mandatory in delineating any collection. In most cases, providing the colon is healthy, the fistula will heal spontaneously given sufficient time. If the fistula is via a drain, it is useful to shorten it progressively (i.e. gradually withdraw and resuture the drain) to allow the tract to collapse.

Complications of stomas

Complications of stomas are extremely common especially after emergency colorectal surgery. Because you took our advice earlier in this chapter, you will avoid many of the complications listed in ■ Table 14.4. Nevertheless, you may need to treat patients of other surgeons who have never read this book...

Table 14.4. Complications of stomas.

Early

✓ Psychological morbidity
✓ Stoma ischemia
✓ High-output stoma
✓ Dehydration
✓ Electrolyte imbalance
✓ Mucocutaneous separation

Late

✓ Parastomal hernia
✓ Stoma prolapse
✓ Skin irritation
✓ Body image and sexual dysfunction
✓ Stoma stenosis
✓ Stoma granulations
✓ Stoma retraction

Stoma ischemia

Stoma ischemia is usually evident early in the postoperative period. This may be caused by either a generalized state of hypotension or more commonly a technical problem during the construction of the stoma (for example, iatrogenic injury to the marginal artery — either during resection or when the colon is delivered through the abdominal wall). The severity of ischemia may vary from minor mucosal duskiness to a black, completely necrotic stoma.

All newly formed stomas should be inspected the day following surgery to assess their viability: don't be lazy — remove the colostomy bag and shine a torch (Americans call it a flashlight) onto the stoma! If the stoma looks dodgy (i.e. non-*kosher*), it can be useful to use either a proctoscope or a test tube inserted deeper to check the viability of the bowel under the fascia. **Urgent surgery to resect, mobilize more bowel, and refashion the stoma will be needed if the bowel leading up to the stoma is necrotic.** Conversely, if the bowel immediately under the stoma is viable, then an expectant approach should be taken. Often the ischemic mucosa will slough off the stoma and the late result will be a stenotic stoma. This can be dealt with on its merits later (see below) and is preferable to a difficult relaparotomy in the early postoperative period.

Stoma retraction

Retraction of a stoma is mostly a problem in obese patients when there is tension on the bowel or mesentery leading to the stoma orifice. In many ways this is the converse of a prolapsing stoma. Retraction is especially problematic if associated with an *ileostomy* when the liquid stoma effluent can cause severe skin reaction and problems with stoma appliance adherence. In most cases, the creative use of stoma appliances (e.g. a convex appliance) may allow the patient to cope without further surgery.

If surgery is necessary, the stoma will usually need to be revised; this can be a difficult undertaking in an obese patient. Although a local approach may be taken initially, you will often need to perform a laparotomy to gain sufficient length to correct the retraction. When revising an end colostomy in a fat patient, it may be necessary to take down the splenic flexure fully if sufficient length is to be obtained. Revising an ileostomy may be more troublesome; here the bowel is already fully mobile and the usual limiting factors are the depth of the abdominal wall and the mobility of the small bowel and its mesentery (neither being easy to correct surgically). In this situation, stapling the end ileostomy closed and performing a loop ileostomy immediately proximally (an **end-loop ileostomy**) may provide a solution.

Managing a high-output stoma

A fully adapted end ileostomy has a daily output of approximately 500ml. However, in the early postoperative period, ileostomy output is often greater than this (1000ml to 1800ml). This high output usually decreases in the first few postoperative days. Higher-output stomas (output greater than 2L/day) are associated with proximal stomas (i.e. jejunostomy), intra-abdominal sepsis and following resolution of postoperative ileus or small bowel obstruction. **If a stoma is producing more than 1000ml/day, then you will need to replace the losses of water and electrolytes with the appropriate i.v. solutions** (I would use Hartmann's — Ringer's Lactate). Often when oral feeding is established the stoma effluent will thicken up and its volume reduces dramatically. Restricting the patient's oral hypotonic fluids (e.g. water, tea, coffee, cola, whatever) to 500ml/day and replacing the rest of the oral intake with oral rehydration solution (e.g. WHO solution) will help reduce stoma output in some cases. Close monitoring of the patient's electrolytes and acid-base balance is crucial.

Other adjuncts to reduce a high-output stoma include:

- A low-fiber diet.
- Proton pump inhibitors (I use omeprazole 40mg a day).
- Antimotility agents such as loperamide (here the high dose of up to 8mg four times a day may be needed) or codeine phosphate (central nervous system side effects and dependence may limit the use of codeine).

In a patient with a persistently high output, it may occasionally be necessary to close a loop ileostomy early. Perform a water-soluble contrast study to check the integrity of the (distal) anastomosis, in case early ileostomy closure is needed.

Parastomal hernias

> *Some degree of herniation around the colostomy is so common that this complication may be regarded as virtually inevitable.*
>
> **John Goligher**

At the risk of being accused of sacrilege, I am not sure that I agree with the late Sir John Goligher here. Sure, parastomal hernias are common, but there are well-described steps which can reduce the risk of their occurrence — I have described these above.

Most parastomal hernias are unsightly, but do not cause much in the way of symptoms. I would usually treat these in conjunction with a stomatherapist (who will most often use a convex stoma appliance or a stoma belt). If it is possible to close the stoma (e.g. a loop diverting stoma or Hartmann's procedure), this has the best chance of curing the hernia (although there is an appreciable rate of incisional hernia after stoma closure).

If the stoma is permanent and the hernia is causing significant symptoms, you may need to consider surgical repair. The results of parastomal hernia repair are pretty dismal and I therefore have a high threshold for surgery. The details of surgical technique (laparoscopic, open, etc.) used for parastomal hernia repair is beyond the scope of this book; suffice it say that with so many options on offer, we do not currently know which technique is best.

Stoma prolapse

Stoma prolapse is more common in loop stomas and is a particular problem with **transverse loop colostomies**, presumably because the distal limb is so mobile. Prolapse of a stoma can be a dramatic and frightening experience for the patient — the first episode of prolapse will often result in the patient seeking emergency medical assistance. An acutely prolapsed stoma can usually be manually replaced; the use of ice packs or **topical sugar** (or honey) reduces the edema in the prolapsed stoma and facilitates less traumatic reduction.

If the prolapse is recurrent and causes problems with stoma care, a surgical solution is necessary. The most satisfactory surgical solution is to close the stoma, if this is feasible. If it is not possible to close a loop stoma then I would revise the stoma using a linear cutting stapler to divide the loop — effectively stapling off the distal limb and making an end stoma). This may be performed under local anesthesia and sedation if necessary.

Recurrent prolapse of an end stoma can be more difficult to correct. Options here include excising the redundant colon and revising the stoma (this may be done using a surgical stapler under intravenous sedation). Excision of redundant bowel is not useful for a prolapsing end ileostomy. Here revision of the stoma with several sutures fixing the bowel to the fascia may prevent the bowel from sliding through the fascia and initiating a prolapse. Rarely, if this does not work, I have used a *non-cutting* linear stapler to fix the stoma. This prevents the inner and outer layers of bowel in the spout from sliding on each other — stopping the initiation of prolapse. I use three firings of the stapler with one limb inside and one outside the stoma spout, taking care not to incorporate the mesentery in the staple line.

Stoma stenosis

Stenosis of a stoma is usually the late result of stomal ischemia or mucocutanenous separation leading to retraction of the stoma. Minor degrees of stenosis may be dealt with by dilatation using either a gloved finger or a suitably sized Hegar's or St Mark's pattern dilator. Teach the patient to pass a finger or dilator on a daily basis to prevent the stenosis recurring. If the stenosis is severe then it may be necessary to dilate the stoma under general anesthesia or intravenous sedation initially. More severe forms of stenosis will require revisional surgery; this may be performed using a local peristomal incision, but the need to gain sufficient bowel length will often necessitate a laparotomy, splenic flexure take down and refashioning of the stoma.

Stoma granulations

These are small inflammatory polyps of the stoma which usually present with bleeding. Histologically, these are composed of granulation tissue. These are usually caused by local trauma, often from cutting the stoma appliance too small, or due to stomal prolapse. Small granulations can be treated with silver nitrate cautery and attention to stoma care. Larger polyps should be excised and sent for histological analysis as these may be adenomas or, rarely, adenocarcinomas.

Closure ('take down') of a stoma

> *Failure of a colostomy closure is more due to the youth of the colostomy than the youth of the surgeon.*
>
> **Ivor Lewis**

It is easy to underestimate surgery to close or take down a stoma. Remember that this is an intestinal anastomosis with all the risks that this entails. Before undertaking surgery to close a stoma make sure that you understand the patient's anatomy — especially if you did not do the original operation. Are you confident that the distal anastomosis is healed and patent? I habitually request a water-soluble contrast enema before closing a loop stoma. I also examine the distal anastomosis under anesthesia (both digitally and with rigid sigmoidoscopy). The next thing is to mobilize the stoma widely using sharp dissection. **Take care not to damage the bowel wall or the mesenteric blood vessels: this is especially important with a loop colostomy when the marginal artery may be supplying the distal anastomosis!** It is important to continue the dissection into the peritoneal cavity to allow the bowel to be delivered outside. Once the stoma is fully mobilized, then I usually simply close the defect with a single layer of fine sutures (I use 3/0 PDS®). If closing a loop ileostomy, then resection/anastomosis may be performed — I only do this if the stoma has been traumatized during mobilization.

Take care during closure of the fascial defect that you do not injure any bowel loops and that good bites of fascia are taken to avoid a subsequent incisional hernia. I approximate the skin with a **subcuticular purse-string suture**. Tying this suture pulls the skin edges together leaving a small central hole, which offers some drainage. Such a wound heals surprisingly well and this technique avoids the dog ears that are often seen if simple skin sutures are used.

The danger of doing a 'trephine' sigmoid colostomy

'Trephine' sigmoid colostomy (fishing out the sigmoid colon and exteriorizing it through the same small incision where the colostomy is to be matured) is tempting when a diverting sigmoid colostomy is needed for conditions such as incontinence or advanced anal or rectal cancer. **However, this deceptively straightforward procedure could become a nightmare if you decide to create an end colostomy and close the distal loop**... as what you think is the distal loop may in fact be the proximal one — you staple it off and create a complete colonic obstruction. It happened to me once!

How to prevent such a disaster? Avoid trephine colostomy in the previously operated abdomen where the anatomy is distorted by adhesions. Always verify which loop is afferent and which is efferent: the simplest way is to insert a fiberoptic scope transanally. Inserting a laparoscope would, of course, require another incision. If you are in the bush just inject water into the fresh colostomy at the end of the procedure: if it comes out of the rectum you know that you have exteriorized the wrong loop. Re-do it immediately! It seems, however, that the safest way to avoid this disaster is to construct a LOOP colostomy — many, including me, believe it provides a complete diversion; the poop will not hop across. **Moshe**

And here as promised is the great encore to serve as the grand finale of my chapter. Ladies and gentlemen, please welcome the ANUS.

2   The anus

The anus is an intricate organ comprising highly innervated skin and a coordinated sphincter complex. As you must know, the ability to fart or defecate without pain is truly one of life's joys! Most anal surgery involves cutting through the anal skin and sometimes the sphincter muscles, with a risk of disrupting this ability and causing profound misery. The aim of all anal surgery should be to eradicate the disease process with minimal collateral damage to the anal skin and sphincters.

In this chapter I discuss common complications of anal operations, how to avoid them and how to deal with these complications as they arise.

Pre-operative considerations

The vast majority of patients with anal problems will seek your attention because of anal pain, bleeding from the anus, an anal lump or a combination of the above. This is not the place for a treatise on the diagnosis and treatment of anal conditions but please allow me a few words.

A **brief history** will lead to accurate diagnosis even *before* the patient takes off her underpants — for example:

- **Pain, intermittent**, associated with defecation and accompanied by fresh bleeding: **fissure**!
- **Pain, steady**, dull and increasing in severity for a few days: **peri-anal abscess**.
- **Pain has been improving** since yesterday plus the patient feels a lump: **thrombosed external hemorrhoid** (peri-anal hematomas).
- **Intermittent pain**, staining of underwear plus history of previous abscess: **fistula in ano**.
- **Prolapsing lump** which may need manual replacement: **hemorrhoids**.

Inspection of the anus, with gentle retraction of the 'cheeks', suffices to diagnose a fissure — in most cases no need for painful insertion of an anoscope.

When assessing an anal case don't ignore the colon and rectum: having to diagnose an advanced proximal sigmoid cancer six months after a painful hemorrhoidectomy is more than embarrassing! **Remember: colorectal cancer can develop in young patients also**. I know of a few such patients treated conservatively for many months for hemorrhoids. A fistulotomy on a patient with (undiagnosed) Crohn's disease may fail to heal…

There is little correlation between the cosmetic appearance of the anus and symptoms. Porn stars are the only occupational group needing cosmetic anal surgery. **Beware** the young (or older) lady not happy with the appearance of her anus — asking you to remove the 'excessive' mucosal folds around it. For she will be the one to develop anal stenosis or delayed wound healing. I remember a few of those... shudder...

In most cases, short of **colonoscopy** (or **flexible sigmoidoscopy**) when indicated, no other tests are needed before anal surgery. In *selected patients* and *clinical situations*, it is worth getting some further tests such as MRI for recurrent or complex anal fistulas; endo-anal ultrasound and/or anorectal physiology testing may be indicated if there are concerns about continence.

Clinical assessment of an anal fistula

The vast majority of anal fistulas have *low intersphincteric* or *low trans-sphincteric* tracts. In the main these can be treated by a straightforward **fistulotomy** with minimal risk of continence disturbance. Higher fistulas or those with secondary extensions (especially horseshoe fistulas) are more challenging.

In assessing an anal fistula, you need to determine the following:

- **Site of the external opening**.
- **Site of the internal opening**.
- **Primary track**.
- **Are there any secondary extensions?**

For simple anal fistulas, you may be able confidently to determine this by clinical examination alone — if so then great, crack on with the operation. Otherwise you may need further information. An **anal MRI scan** is the most useful test to assess an anal fistula; I have a low threshold for obtaining an MRI in a patient when I do not understand the anatomy and I request it always in a recurrent fistula. **In many ways the information obtained by examining the patient in clinic is complementary to that obtained at examination under anesthesia**. If there is significant anal sepsis, examination with the patient awake may be very uncomfortable and more information is gained intra-operatively. Conversely, the quality of the sphincters and the amount of sphincter muscle involved by a trans-sphincteric fistula is better assessed when the patient is awake. If the external opening is close to the anal margin and/or the tract is palpable, then this suggests either an intersphincteric or low trans-sphincteric fistula. **Ultimately, gently inserting a fistula probe through the tract during surgery is the most accurate clinical assessment of the primary tract.**

Which operation for anal fistula?

The degree of success of the operation in eradicating the fistula correlates with the risk of incontinence — as usual, the more you do, the more you cut, the higher is the risk of complications (■ Table 14.5).

Table 14.5. Risks and success of operations for anal fistulas.

Operation	Risk of fecal incontinence	Chance of success
Fistulotomy	+++	++++
Rectal advancement flap	+	+++
Anal fistula plug	0	++
Fibrin glue	0	+
LIFT *	0	?
VAAFT+	0	??

* LIFT = ligation of the intersphincteric track
+ VAAFT = video-assisted anal fistula treatment

So, for the **low fistula one would choose fistulotomy**. The more *fancy alternatives* should be reserved for situations in which fistulotomy would significantly endanger continence. That is unless, of course, you are developing a new treatment for anal fistula. Here one must take a different tack. First, design a new procedure which can only be done with special disposable equipment or an implant. You need to come up with a snappy name for your new procedure (preferably an acronym). Develop close links with the industry — you'll need their money to fund trips to conferences abroad. Now try your new technique on as many fistulas as you can, make sure you include plenty of low fistulas which could have been laid open by a simple fistulotomy and only include short-term outcomes. Next, publish and present at meetings in exotic locations; be quick though because someone else is right behind you and the gravy train won't run forever. Eventually someone will publish a large series of high fistulas with longer-term follow-up and the cure rate will be 50% or much less. Your promising new procedure will be consigned to history along with all the others. Oh yes, a few clips will remain on YouTube.

Which operation for hemorrhoids (■ Table 14.6)?

In choosing a procedure, consider the following factors:

- Type and degree of symptoms.
- Grade of internal piles and the amount of external hemorrhoids.
- Patient fitness.
- Patient preference.
- Any continence disturbance.

Table 14.6. Efficacy and risks of procedures for hemorrhoids.

Procedure	Efficacy	Degree of pain	Risk of complications
Injection sclerotherapy	+	+	+
Rubber band ligation	++	++	++
Hemorrhoidal artery ligation (HALO)	+++	+++	++
Stapled hemorrhoidectomy	++++	+++	+++
Excisional hemorrhoidectomy	+++++	+++++	++++

There is good evidence that **starting stool softeners pre-operatively reduces pain after surgery**. I use lactulose in a dose of 20ml twice a day started 24 hours before surgery; although any stool softener of your choice is OK.

I do not prescribe enemas before an anal operation such as hemorrhoidectomy (although this is a routine for any operation in the rectum). Although not 'wrong' I do not feel there are any benefits to emptying the rectum in this way.

Intra-operative considerations

There is a great desire to reduce the risks of pain and continence disturbance following anal surgery. This has led to the development of several new operations to treat anal disorders (stapled hemorrhoidectomy, HALO, LIFT, VAAFT, BBB [1]). These operations have in common the fact that they do not need incisions in the anal canal and there is good evidence that postoperative pain is less for these operations than for the traditional alternatives. However, the long-term results of these operations are uncertain. Some interesting new complications (not seen with traditional anal surgery) have been caused by these operations. Large bowel obstruction caused by inadvertent obliteration of the rectal lumen during stapled hemorrhoidectomy is a good example of this.

There is not space in this chapter to give detailed tips of how to perform each of these new operations, but here are some general words of advice regarding adoption of new techniques:

- Firstly, **do your due diligence** — is this procedure really a 'goer' or is it one which will vanish into the history books in a few years?
- Secondly, **be selective**. There is a trend to see all patients as candidates for a new technique. Be kind on yourself and your patients, start with easy cases and as your experience develops then gradually extend your indications for a given procedure.
- Thirdly, **get a mentor**. Scrub in with a more experienced surgeon first and ideally have them scrub in with you when you do your first few cases. Watching a DVD or having an industry rep in theatre (the OR) with you is simply not enough.
- Fourthly, that the company will fly you out to Vegas (food and drink included — but not the 'escort') to attend a two-day course is not a reason to adopt the new technique.

In the UK, most anal surgery is performed under general anesthesia; this compares with the situation in the USA where the majority of anal cases are performed under local anesthesia (plus/minus i.v. sedation) or regional anesthesia. There is little evidence of superiority of one technique over another; most of the differences in practice are cultural. Nevertheless, procedures which require prolonged anal retraction are probably more comfortable for the patient if performed under general anesthesia.

There is a similar cultural divide over positioning the patient for surgery. In the UK, most anal surgery is performed with the patient in the **lithotomy position**, while the **prone jack-knife position** is more commonly used in the USA. Again this difference is largely cultural, and relates to the differences in anesthesia discussed above — our anesthetists and nurses hate having the patients face down under anesthesia. (As to the Americans: perhaps they do not like to stand between the patient's legs in the so called "French position"? ☺.) However, the

---

[1] HALO = hemorrhoid artery ligation operation; LIFT: ligation of intersphincteric fistula tract; VAAFT = video-assisted anal fistula treatment; BBB = blah blah blah.

prone jack-knife position allows good access to the anus especially for anterior lesions which can be difficult to access in the lithotomy position. In addition, if there is bleeding, the blood will flow away from the operative field. The prone jack-knife position also allows your assistant to see the operation.

> Rectal surgery is a bit like sex. There are proponents of various positions and unique instances when some are much more enjoyable (anterior or posterior pathology). Most people experiment with a variety of approaches, but generally stick to the one which offers them consistently predictable and satisfying results.
>
> **Angus G. Maciver**

Here is some advice on 'safe' but 'curative' anal procedures.

Tailor a lateral sphincterotomy

In recent years lateral anal sphincterotomy has had some bad press. However, the high historical rates of incontinence in the literature relate to division of the entire length of the internal anal sphincter, sometimes even performed bilaterally. There is certainly a small risk of continence disturbance, but in practice, if performed properly, the risk is low: perhaps a 5% chance of difficulty in holding wind or occasional minor skidmarks — for many patients this represents the status quo.

Tips to reduce the risk of incontinence:

- Don't perform a sphincterotomy in patients with pre-existing continence problems (here I would use an anal advancement flap).
- Keep the internal sphincter on a stretch using an anal retractor.
- Divide the internal sphincter under direct vision — not blindly as in the 'closed' sphincterotomy.
- Only cut what you need to cut; **stop the sphincterotomy at the level of the top of the fissure — not, as has been recommended, up to the level of the dentate line.** This is why it's called a "tailored sphincterotomy".

How much is too much — safe hemorrhoidectomy?

> When it looks like a clover you know that it's over. If it looks like a dahlia you know it's a failure.

In the right patient an excisional hemorrhoidectomy is an excellent long-term solution to their hemorrhoidal problems. The most worrying complications of excisional hemorrhoidectomy are anal stenosis and fecal incontinence. Anal stenosis relates exclusively to the excision of too much anoderm. Fecal incontinence after hemorrhoidectomy relates to either an injury to the internal anal sphincter or over-enthusiastic excision of anal cushions.

Tips for safe hemorrhoidectomy:

- Stop the bleeding as you go to keep the anatomy clear.
- **Be careful in patients with circumferential hemorrhoids** (where do you stop?). I would often use a stapled hemorrhoidectomy for these patients. Other alternatives are HALO (accepting that the long-term results are uncertain) or to excise the largest hemorrhoids (two groups) and use a whip stitch to under-run intervening residual hemorrhoidal tissue.
- Keep the internal anal sphincter on the stretch to avoid a sphincter injury.
- Remember **this is not a cancer operation** — no need to ruthlessly destroy all hemorrhoidal tissue. Leave some anal cushions to preserve continence.
- Leave a minimum of 1cm skin bridges between excision sites. **Let the anus look like a clover!**

Much effort has been put into developing ever more complicated ways to excise piles. I usually use a standard hand-held diathermy unit (costing about $5). This has the benefit of good hemostasis allowing accurate visualization of the internal anal sphincter. The literature has reported the use of LASER dissection, LigaSure™ and the Harmonic Scalpel®. Whilst some of these methods have shown a small statistical benefit in terms of postoperative pain, the cost effectiveness of using a $500 disposable instrument for straightforward anal surgery is questionable! Besides, accusations of naivety may follow uncritical acceptance of such (industry supported) studies...

Safe surgery for anal fistula

Fecal incontinence after fistula is the result of aggressive surgeons, not progressive disease.

John Alexander-Williams

An inexperienced surgeon with a fistula probe is more dangerous than a gorilla with a machine gun.

Robin Phillips

Again: most anal fistulas are either intersphincteric or low trans-sphincteric. These are usually straightforward to manage with a fistulotomy. Higher fistulas or those with complex secondary extensions are more difficult to manage and a degree of caution is needed here. **The main problems with these complex**

fistulas relate to the risk of iatrogenic incontinence and failure to eradicate peri-anal sepsis permanently.

A few tips for how to stay on the safe side:

- **Don't operate until you understand the anatomy of the fistula.** Selectively use imaging (MRI or endo-anal ultrasound scanning) if you are unsure.
- **If you cannot confidently identify the internal opening of a fistula,** inject dilute hydrogen peroxide through an i.v. cannula inserted through the external opening. Foam will then appear through the internal opening of the fistula. If you have access to intra-operative endo-anal ultrasound scanning, the H_2O_2 will act as a simple contrast agent allowing you to see the whole fistula track. If peroxide is not available, then **UHT milk** may be used as an alternative.
- **Don't force a fistula probe** through the track.
- If a probe seems to go superiorly, *parallel to the rectal wall* rather than into the anus proceed with caution. Is this an **extra-sphincteric fistula?**
- **If you are unsure if it is safe to lay open a fistula — then don't. Instead insert a loose *seton* and live to fight another day.**
- Be cautious in laying open a fistula in the **presence of acute anal sepsis** (abscess). This is safe in selected patients with an experienced surgeon, but be aware that the anatomy may be distorted.
- Don't attempt complex sphincter-preserving operations in the presence of acute anal sepsis — they will inevitably fail. Instead drain any extensions and leave a loose *seton* for at least three months.
- **Remember, many of the 'high' or 'complex' fistulas treated in specialized colorectal units are not 'naturally-occurring' but are produced by humble surgeons like you who 'forced' a false passage through the fistula's tract...**

Anal dilatation

In years gone by anal dilatation was a common operation performed for anal fissures and hemorrhoids. In general terms anal dilatation is now thought of as passé; most surgeons feel that the risks of damaging the internal anal sphincter considerably outweigh the benefits. In my humble opinion, a tailored lateral sphincterotomy allows a controlled division of the lower internal anal sphincter with a smaller risk to continence.

The end of the operation

Before finishing any anal operation, check that the bleeding is controlled using diathermy or fine absorbable sutures. **Anal packing increases** postoperative pain and should be used selectively. I use cellulose-based anal sponges if there is any minor oozing, but the majority of patients will have no packing at all (cotton gauze swabs are very painful to remove and I never use them). **Remember to infiltrate the wound with a long-acting local anesthetic** (the theoretical risks of local sepsis are not seen in practice).

Postoperative considerations

> *The only time human beings wish they could defecate and fart is when they are not able to do so.*

Pain!

Pain is a constant concern after anal surgery and historically this led to most patients staying in hospital after surgery, crying for morphine. The fear of pain keeps some patients away from the surgeon and prevents them from having the best treatment.

Pain following anal surgery relates to:

- Cuts in the anoderm.
- Increased tissue tension (edema, inflammation or hematoma).
- Local sepsis.
- Internal anal sphincter spasm.

It is possible to perform almost all anal surgery as a day case providing that attention to detail is paid before, during and after the operation. For example:

- I advise patients to start taking laxatives 48 hours before their operation. I usually use lactulose, but any osmotic laxative would be fine — **the important point is that the first postop crap is a soft one!**
- As described above I infiltrate all anal wounds with **bupivacaine** and avoid anal packing unless absolutely necessary.
- **If there are significant open wounds in the anus, I also give the patient a week's course of oral metronidazole and topical glyceryl trinitrate ointment.**
- Give the patient a good selection of oral analgesics (I use paracetamol and an NSAID).
- Try to avoid opiate analgesics if possible because of the risks of constipation.
- The use of **warm sitz baths** relaxes the anal sphincter and reduces pain for the first postoperative week.

Bleeding after hemorrhoidectomy (and other anal surgery)

Minor degrees of bleeding are common after anal surgery, but significant bleeding needing blood transfusion or further surgery should be rare. There is a comparatively high pressure within the anal canal and this can result in blood pooling in the lower rectum with no signs of external bleeding. The classical presentation of bleeding after hemorrhoid surgery is of a pale, tachycardic patient who then suddenly passes a large volume of blood per anum.

Most patients who are hemodynamically compromised in the immediate postop period will need resuscitation and an urgent return to the operating room to stop the bleeding. Whilst making arrangements for surgery, it can be useful to pass a **large-bore Foley catheter** into the rectum and inflate the balloon; this will allow more accurate estimation of the amount of blood loss and with gentle traction on the balloon may tamponade the bleeding.

At surgery (I would always do this under general anesthesia), usually all that is needed is a figure-of-8 stitch to under-run a bleeding point. If the patient had a stapled hemorrhoidectomy, it may be difficult to see the bleeding point as the piles are still present and the bleeding will always be from the staple line above the piles. In this situation, simply open another stapled hemorrhoidectomy set; the transparent anoscope and suture guide will retract the piles, allowing good access to the bleeding point.

The unhealed hemorrhoidectomy wound

Most anal wounds heal completely within 6-8 weeks of surgery. Occasionally you will come across a patient whose wound(s) take longer. The best treatment for these patients is MICLO (masterly inactivity with cat-like observation), i.e. do nothing but try to keep the patient happy. With time and patience all wounds will heal; try to avoid the temptation to do something when doing nothing is the best option.

The persistent anal fissure

Lateral anal sphincterotomy is one of those rare operations which is both straightforward to perform and has an excellent cure rate. Only rarely will a patient return for follow-up with an unhealed fissure. So, how do you handle this situation?

Consider the following:

- **How much internal anal sphincter has been divided?** This can really only be assessed by performing an endo-anal ultrasound scan. It will easily confirm the presence of a sphincterotomy, but to measure the extent of a sphincterotomy a 3D endo-anal ultrasound scan is needed.
- **Is this a 'high-pressure' anal fissure?** Most idiopathic anal fissures are associated with an elevated anal canal resting pressure and reducing this pressure with a lateral anal sphincterotomy should heal the fissure. However, there are some situations where an anal fissure is associated with normal or subnormal anal canal resting pressure (often associated with an obstetric trauma). It is illogical to perform a sphincterotomy in these patients (which would risk incontinence). If a fissure has not healed following an adequate sphincterotomy consider this a low-pressure fissure — arranging for anorectal physiology to be performed should clarify the situation.
- **Is this an anal fissure?** I have seen low anal fistulas, posterior intersphincteric abscesses, small anal cancers and even syphillis *misdiagnosed* as an anal fissure. If the patient is in a lot of pain, it may be necessary to examine the patient under anesthesia to establish a diagnosis. At this procedure consider taking a **biopsy** from the fissure.

After this assessment you will be left with three situations:

- A **high-pressure fissure** with an **inadequate sphincterotomy**. Here you could consider using **botulinum toxin** injections or even a cautious **repeat sphincterotomy** (I would advocate performing the repeat sphincterotomy on the **other side** to avoid the scarred area within the intersphincteric plane).
- A **low-pressure anal fissure** with or without a **significant sphincterotomy**. In this situation, I would usually excise the fissure and reconstruct the defect with an anal advancement flap.
- **It's not an anal fissure** — here treat the underlying cause. A posterior chronic intersphincteric abscess may be misdiagnosed as an anal fissure; the treatment for this is a dorsal sphincterotomy through the abscess cavity.

Recurrent anal fistula

More accurately this should be called a *persistent* anal fistula — only rarely in Crohn's disease, for example, may a fistula recur after truly being eradicated. Scarring from previous sepsis and surgery makes clinical assessment difficult and inaccurate. MRI scanning is extremely valuable in this situation.

Considerations in evaluating a recurrent anal fistula:

- Is this simple cryptoglandular sepsis or is there another underlying disorder?
- Why did the fistula recur?
- Common reasons are failure to identify the primary track, failure to drain extensions adequately or failure to eradicate the primary track.

Treating anal stenosis

In the hands of an experienced surgeon, anal stenosis should be rare following hemorrhoid surgery. It can be diagnosed clinically by the inability to insert a finger into the anus. Initially it should be treated by dilating the anal canal using **Hegar** dilators under anesthesia. After the initial dilatation, restenosis is common — prevent this by repeat dilatation under topical anesthesia — you may be able to persuade your patient to do this at home. I would also advocate adding fiber supplements to give the stools added bulk. In most patients this approach will work; dilatation for more than four weeks or so should not be necessary.

In difficult cases where dilatation has been performed for more than four weeks or when the stenosis recurs, surgery is needed. I would treat this by incising the scar within the anal canal, taking care to preserve the anal sphincter. Perform an **anoplasty** by advancing a supple, well-vascularized flap of peri-anal skin into the resulting defect to prevent restenosis. Here I would use a 'house advancement flap'.

In conclusion, anal surgery is often thought of as a minor surgery (by surgeons), but probably not by the patient whose anus is being cut open! The anus is a complex organ with a highly organized nerve supply and a coordinated sphincter complex. We surgeons disrupt this organ at our (or rather our patient's) peril. I urge you to have respect for the humble anus and particularly its sphincters.

> "We suffer and die through the defects that arise in our sewerage and drainage systems."
>
> **William A. Lane**

Chapter 15

Hernias

Danny Rosin

You can judge the worth of a surgeon by the way he does a hernia.

Thomas Fairbank

For many years, hernia surgery was considered to be a "simple, first-year resident" procedure, and in busy centers it was commonly left to the end of the surgery list — with obvious results (■ Figure 15.1). But actually, hernia surgery was never simple, as the 3D anatomy of a hernia is difficult to grasp, and the great variability in hernia types and repair options makes it relatively complicated. We currently see the flourishing of 'hernia surgeons' and 'hernia centers', and in many places hernia operations are mostly done by 'experts'.

Being a very prevalent condition, complications are frequently seen. Although most complications will be considered 'minor', new approaches and techniques have brought with them novel and sometimes major complications.

General considerations

Objectives in hernia surgery

Analyzing results, and defining complications, depend on our (and the patients') expectations. **For a hernia operation to be considered 'successful', we will want the patient to recover with minimum difficulties, and achieve a durable repair that will last a lifetime.**

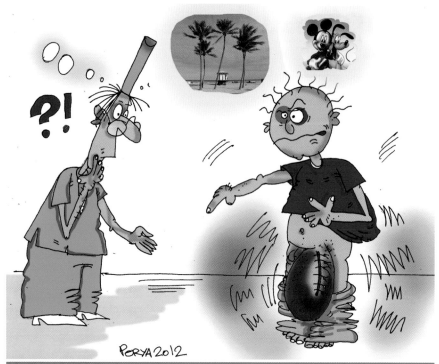

Figure 15.1. "Doc, you promised that I would be able to take the family to Disney a week after such a minor procedure..."

Complications after hernia repairs thus include both short-term intervention-related complications, and long-term problems, including chronic pain, late infection, and failure of the repair to pass the test of time. **Remember**: what may seem to us as a minor, or even an expected postoperative condition, may be conceived by the patient to be a significant, disabling or even disastrous complication. **And in our efforts to make hernia surgery as trouble-free as we can by introducing new materials and techniques, we should beware of creating new complications unknown to our surgical grandfathers.**

Variability in hernia surgery

It is somewhat misleading to use the term "hernia surgery" as the variability enclosed within this term is immense. Indications, techniques, and of course complications vary widely based on hernia location, size and other characteristics. For the sake of simplicity the discussion will be kept general when possible, but some situations will merit specific consideration.

Site of hernia

The vast majority of hernias occur in the **inguinal** region, but surgeons often deal with midline hernias such as **umbilical** and **epigastric** or **incisional** hernias, and lateral hernias such as **lumbar** or **Spigelian** hernias. The differences in approach, technique and materials used are necessarily associated with wide differences in the resultant complications, both in type and severity.

Prosthetics

Prosthetic materials are the cornerstone of modern hernia repair. While primary tissue repair is still widely practiced in specific situations like in an infected surgical field, or due to financial constraints, **recurrence rates are invariably higher for *meshless* repairs** — this is even true for the tiny umbilical hernias! The use of mesh is, however, associated with specific complications, the most common of which is infection. Mesh contraction (*meshoma*), chronic pain (*meshalgia*) and erosion of mesh into adjacent structures such as the urinary bladder or the bowel (with resultant infection and fistulization) are significant complications that frequently necessitate reoperation. Mesh removal may be needed and this is usually a major undertaking. When mesh is placed intraperitoneally — as commonly practiced in laparoscopic repair of incisional/ventral hernias — 'adhesion-resisting' meshes are used, **but the real value of the different adhesion barriers appears to be much less than advertised**.

Approach

The approaches available to repair exactly the same hernia vary widely. The armamentarium of the versatile hernia surgeon could include variations in the surgical approach like open and laparoscopic, transabdominal and extraperitoneal, anterior and posterior (preperitoneal) repairs, and within each variation one can find different tactics such as mesh-bridging, tissue mobilization and hernia defect closure, and of course different levels of mesh placement relative to the abdominal wall structures. **It should be obvious that complications will vary widely based on the selected approach**. Bowel injury, which may be diagnosed during or — go unnoticed — after laparoscopic incisional hernia repair, is a dangerous complication that is virtually never seen after open extraperitoneal repairs. On the other hand, large collections and hematomas are more common after the latter than the former. **A selective approach, based on the hernia itself (size, location) as well as the surgeon's expertise, should help keep the risk of complications to the minimum**.

Pre-operative considerations

The simple hernia

While never really 'simple', repairing the primary, unilateral, small to medium sized inguinal hernia in a young and fit patient is the prototype of low-risk surgery that should result in a good outcome with minimal complications and a high success rate. Avoiding wound-related complications, and achieving a durable repair through a safe procedure that will allow early return to normal daily activity, is our goal.

Laparoscopic or open?

Probably one of the most debatable questions in modern hernia surgery, this choice is not an easy one. Multiple factors are involved in the decision, **assuming that the surgeon has the capability of successfully performing both**. Risk vs. benefit analysis is not always easy to make. **Remember**: numbers cited in the literature rarely represent 'real life' results. While laparoscopy may result in 'easier' recovery, the advantage over open surgery may be negligible, especially if compared to the potential disasters. Familiarity with local and personal results and expertise is mandatory in making the correct selection.

> *Laparoscopic umbilical hernia repair is like going to the centre of the earth to plant a seed near the surface.*
>
> **Rolando Ramos**

Primary or mesh repair?

While mesh repair is the key to reducing the hernia recurrence rate, there are some specific complications associated with its use, and at times (e.g. in a contaminated field) it is preferable to complete the operation safely without mesh and accept the increased risk of hernia recurrence. **The main risk with the use of foreign material is infection. Using prophylactic antibiotics is the standard of care (!)**, especially if the incision is immediately over the site of the implanted mesh. When surgical site infection is likely to occur — as when operating on an incarcerated hernia with strangulated bowel requiring resection — most surgeons will avoid the use of a prosthetic mesh; especially if there are signs of active inflammation in the surrounding tissues.

The recurrent hernia

Sadly, no one has yet devised the perfect hernia operation (despite not just a few claims for a 0% recurrence rate by some authors — **never believe a zero rate of anything!**). Recurrences are possible after any open or laparoscopic repair, after tissue or mesh repair, early after surgery or many years later. Some patients present with multiple recurrences and pose a significant surgical challenge.

When compared to primary surgery, operating on a recurrent hernia is always more difficult and prone to complications — and to yet another failure. **Remember: not every recurrent hernia needs to be fixed: an asymptomatic small bulge in an old and frail patient may be better left alone**. (This is of course true also for primary hernias…).

Operating through a previous scar results in more difficult delineation of the anatomy, a higher risk of injury to the spermatic cord structures (vas deferens transection, spermatic vessel injury), and a lack of strong supporting tissues to hold the repair. **Choosing a different approach, to avoid the previously scarred tissue, or a previously placed mesh, is recommended**. This may be achieved by laparoscopy after a previous open repair, but also by open surgery after previous laparoscopy.

The huge hernia

Giant hernias are the result of longstanding hernias that were not repaired earlier, and the original reasons for avoiding surgery are why complications are expected. Recurrent hernias, old age and multiple comorbidities are common characteristics of patients suffering from these gigantic bulges. Apart from the need to repair large abdominal wall defects, the surgeon must also reduce the herniated contents back into the abdominal cavity, usually years after they have lost their domain. **Increased intra-abdominal pressure, and resultant respiratory insufficiency, are often the limiting factors in performing these difficult procedures**. Heroic measures, such as stretching the abdominal wall using pre-operative pneumoperitoneum, or even resecting viscera (e.g redundant colon) have been described — but beware! These may result in catastrophic complications which you better avoid. **Some hernias are simply inoperable**, and you have the right to resist the patient's insistence, and refer him to your adventurous friend (or better an enemy).

Anesthesia — local, regional, general?

Anesthesia considerations may direct the surgeon into choosing the hernia repair procedure. Laparoscopic repair of inguinal hernias usually requires general anesthesia. The choice of anesthesia is commonly based on local and personal preferences, as modern general anesthesia is considered safe in most patients. Financial factors may also affect the anesthetic choice. Significant cardiovascular and respiratory diseases may make the choice of regional or local anesthesia (with or without sedation) more appealing. **It is sometimes not easy to calculate the risk vs. benefit equation**: is the risk of testicular ischemia in a third-recurrence inguinal hernia repaired again by an open approach worth taking just to avoid the general anesthesia needed for a laparoscopic repair in a patient with ischemic heart disease? Complicated, isn't it?

The old and frail

While hernia is a disease of all ages, it is not uncommon for an old and sick patient to present with a hernia that poses a major disturbance to the quality of life, usually to ambulation. Automatic rejection of such a patient due to fear from complications may not be the wise and correct decision. **Optimization of medical conditions, and choosing a simple procedure probably under regional or local anesthesia, may provide the patient with a significant boost to his well-being**.

The painful hernia, the 'sportsman's hernia'

The association between the presence of a hernia and pain resulting from it is complicated. Many patients will describe discomfort in the area, but severe pain is not that common. However, small hernias in young patients are more likely to present as a painful disorder, even without a bulge. The diagnosis of a painful groin is not always straightforward, and ultrasound or other imaging modalities are frequently used to prove the existence of a hernia. As opposed to larger hernias evident on physical examination, with a clear peritoneal sac and protrusion of abdominal contents, these small hernias are often only protrusion of preperitoneal fat through the inguinal ring. **The condition is commonly seen in young athletic patients, and is not easy to differentiate from other, sports-related injuries of the lower abdomen, groin and pelvis (also confusingly termed "groin strain" or "pubalgia"), resulting from heavy lifting in labourers**.

The diagnosis, the decision to operate, and the procedure to perform are all under great debate and far from any consensus among surgeons. While many patients will eventually benefit from intervention, some will continue to suffer from chronic pain (now sometimes attributed to the operation itself), and be a source of frustration to the surgeon.

The incarcerated/strangulated hernia

Emergency operations for an incarcerated or strangulated hernia are associated with specific difficulties and complications. Firstly, the urgency limits your ability to prepare the patient for surgery, and one often needs to operate on a sick and frail patient who, if not at immediate risk, would have been sent for multiple tests and consultations — if not rejected altogether. Accordingly, the risk for postoperative, anesthesia- and procedure-related complications is significantly higher. On top of that, the **local conditions are hostile**: the tissues are edematous, the anatomy is unclear, and the risk of infection, especially if bowel ischemia is present, is higher — often excluding the possibility of mesh repair. In addition, the operation is conducted after-hours, commonly by less experienced surgeons and so the increased risk of complications, as well as a higher recurrence rate, is obvious.

Elevated intra-abdominal pressure

Some pre-existing conditions increase the risk of hernia development, and also increase the risk of surgical complications and failure. The resultant hernia may be considered a 'symptomatic' (or 'secondary') hernia — being a symptom of another pathology!

High intra-abdominal pressure may result from constipation. **You should never forget the possibility of a latent, partially-obstructing colonic carcinoma**. You surely don't want to fix a hernia and leave the cancer behind, for your smart colleague to operate on, a month later. While routine colonoscopy before hernia surgery is obviously unnecessary, never forget to ask about bowel habit (and any change…).

Benign prostatic hypertrophy (BPH) and obstructive urinary symptoms are also important to diagnose before hernia surgery. Apart from increasing the risk of recurrence, there's a higher likelihood of postoperative urinary retention (see ⊃ Chapter 26). If symptoms are suggestive, or the diagnosis of BPH is known already, make sure the medical treatment is optimized, and always ask the urologist whether prostatic surgery is planned. If yes — it may be better performed before the hernia repair (or sometimes as a combined procedure).

Chronic cough probably leads to the highest levels of intra-abdominal pressure, and has been implicated as a major cause for hernia recurrence.

Optimization of medical treatment, and smoking cessation, are important measures but are only partially effective — do you know any smoker who would really quit smoking prior to his hernia operation?

Chronic ascites is of major concern. It frequently leads to hernia formation (an umbilical bulge is common). It is usually a manifestation of a major disease like end-stage heart failure or advanced cirrhosis, so the patient is considered high risk for surgery. Hernia repair may result in infection of the ascitic fluid (and in turn liver failure) and a high recurrence rate is expected — that is if the patient is not dead! **Medical optimization of the patient's condition and 'drying' of the ascites are mandatory before any surgical attempt is even considered**. An extreme bulge leading to **skin bursting and ascites leak is a dangerous complication that often leads to ascites infection and may result in death**. The temptation to repair the hernia at this point is difficult to resist, but without medical optimization (ask for a transjugular intrahepatic portosystemic shunt [TIPS] if necessary), the 'simple' hernia operation may only contribute to the patient's demise.

Obesity — there is no need to remind you that **obesity produces a chronic elevation in intra-abdominal pressure** (junk food-induced ACS ☺) and thus is a huge risk factor for the development of hernias, their recurrence and the morbidity of surgery. "I'll fix your hernia only if you lose 15kg", we often say but eventually give up…

Non-operative approach

The best way to avoid postop complications is to avoid the operation altogether (at the price of complications related to the pathology itself, like incarceration). **Remember: not all hernias need to be operated upon**. Evidence exists that the risk of incarceration for a small, asymptomatic inguinal hernia is very small, and is actually lower than the risk of the operation itself. Therefore, a small hernia detected 'by chance', during a routine physical examination is not necessarily an indication for surgery. Planned follow-up, to detect enlargement of the swelling, or the onset of symptoms, is a reasonable approach in this situation.

However, some asymptomatic hernias are more prone to incarceration (e.g. **femoral hernias**) and an expectant approach may not be the best choice. For other hernias the data are not clear, and some experience and common sense is needed to assess the risk/benefit ratio in the individual case. A wide-based incisional or lumbar hernia may have a small risk of incarceration, but the decision should be patient-specific and include the patient's desire — guidelines are not easy to provide.

Intra-operative considerations

The distinction between an intra-operative difficulty, a mishap and a complication is often blurred. Some operations are more complex, some have a 'bad' starting point (like a very big or incarcerated hernia), and some call for decisions and solutions that, in other situations may be conceived as complications (like excision of the umbilicus in umbilical hernia repair, or performing a planned orchiectomy as part of a large, recurrent, hernia repair). **Expecting difficulties**, including them in the informed consent, and openly and honestly explaining the operative decisions, and the conditions that led to these decisions, will allow the patient and the family to accept what has been done, and may reduce anger that might otherwise lead to litigation.

Irreducible hernia

The definition of hernias with 'stuck' contents is somewhat confusing. When the contents cannot be easily reduced back into the abdominal cavity, the condition may be **acute** (*incarcerated*) or **chronic** (*irreducible*), and the contents may suffer vascular compromise ('strangulated') or not. The contents, bulging out through the hernia defect, may be dangerous if left untreated (bowel, leading to obstruction or perforation), or just painful (preperitoneal fat or omentum). **Therefore, the decision to operate should be quick enough to avoid complications resulting from the incarcerated contents, but not too hasty — as a small umbilical hernia with incarcerated fat in a pregnant woman, or a large, chronically irreducible hernia in an old and frail patient, may be better dealt with at a more appropriate time than the middle of the night, if at all.**

Emergency surgery on an incarcerated hernia may lead to complications associated with the contents and with the repair itself. The contents of an incarcerated hernia should be examined for ischemic injury, which may require bowel resection if not recovered after release of the incarceration. However, occasionally (during emergency operations for inguinal hernias) the contents can slip back into the abdominal cavity before the surgeon has the chance to inspect them — and this often happens after the muscle relaxation at induction of anesthesia. **In order to avoid missing an ischemic bowel, especially in high-risk situations like prolonged incarceration, or the presence of bloody fluid in the hernia sac, an effort should be made to retrieve and examine the bowel, through the opened peritoneal sac.** If difficult or unsuccessful, laparoscopy (through the opened sac in the groin or through the umbilicus) has been used to examine the bowel before completing the repair. Otherwise, a **mini-laparotomy** is usually adequate to deal with the 'missed' bowel. **Remember: missing an ischemic loop of bowel may lead to an ischemic stricture or even a catastrophic perforation a few days later.**

When bowel ischemia with the associated inflammatory process is encountered, and the need for bowel resection arises, the use of mesh is usually avoided for fear of mesh infection. However, primary meshless hernia repair, especially with swollen and edematous tissues, carries a higher incidence of hernia **recurrence**. While the debate regarding the use of mesh in the acute setting is heated, and far from resolution, it is not a taboo to use mesh in properly selected patients, especially if no bowel resection was required. On the other hand, be aware that most patients undergoing primary repair without mesh never suffer a recurrence. **We hope that you know how to do a proper non-mesh repair of any hernia! One day you will need to do it...**

Reduction of incarcerated contents, if not necrotic, should be gentle. Enlarging the hernia defect is often needed, and is much preferred to an inadvertent tear and spillage of bowel contents. **Reduction en masse** is the term used to describe what happens when the contents are reduced together with the hernia sac, with its constriction ring still compressing the contents after being replaced into the abdominal cavity. This uncommon complication is more likely to occur when repairing large, multiloculated incisional hernias. It was more common in the old days when surgeons attempted reducing acutely incarcerated inguinal hernias under sedation. **Nowadays, we know that a painful, acutely incarcerated inguinal hernia belongs in the OR!**

Sliding hernia

Sliding hernias have a wall of an adjacent viscus, like large bowel or the urinary bladder, as part of the hernia 'sac'. The parietal peritoneum, protruding through the hernia opening, may pull with it viscera that are partially extraperitoneal. Understanding this concept is not easy, and neither is identification of a sliding viscus during surgery, as it is often covered by fat, and the exact transition point between it and the 'pure' sac is never clear. The risk of opening the viscus or suturing through its wall (and the resultant contamination in the case of bowel) may be avoided if extra care is used when the sac looks too thick or fatty. Of more concern is the risk of missed injury. **Remember: it is better to leave part of the hernia sac and reduce it if the possibility of a sliding hernia exists.** This is perhaps an opportunity to remind you that excision of the hernial sac, and/or its 'high ligation' is not a requisite of any hernia repair: **the repair is as solid if the (now empty) sac is simply pushed back to where it belongs followed by closure/repair of the defect.**

Injury to large vessels: the femoral vein and inferior epigastric vessels

While the hernia repair is considered 'minor surgery', vascular injuries — which fortunately are very rare — may transform it to a major catastrophe. The proximity of major vessels warrants knowledge of the relevant anatomy, care in tissue handling and suture passing and, should hemorrhage develop, the surgical maturity to do what is necessary: stop the operation, apply pressure to control the bleeding, and — if you do not know how to fix it — call for assistance. Here is some advice:

- **The inferior epigastric vessels** mark the medial border of the internal ring, and are therefore a constant feature in the surgical field of inguinal hernia repair. While injury and bleeding are not too hard to control (suture-ligating the vessel is harmless), retraction of a severed epigastric artery and initial spasm may lead to delayed bleeding, usually resulting in significant hematomas. **The key to prevention lies in careful blunt dissection at the neck of the indirect sac until the vessels are visualized**.

- The **femoral vein** borders the femoral canal, and is therefore more at risk in *femoral hernia repair*. Injury during dissection may result in significant blood loss and is not easy to repair. Sometimes the tear is small, and is only enlarged by attempts at repair — when all that is needed is local pressure, waiting for the natural coagulation process to do its magic. Injury to the femoral vein by including it in the stitch used to repair the hernia may lead to a stricture, and even **thrombosis**. If the latter is diagnosed after surgery, anticoagulation should be started, and insertion of a vena cava filter should be considered, especially if surgical repair is planned. Failure to do so may result in a shower of emboli and even a fatal pulmonary embolism. A late complication would be post-phlebitic syndrome of the affected lower extremity. Note that also during operations for *inguinal hernias* — especially in thin patients — the femoral vessels, coursing just below the inguinal ligament, could be injured by excessively 'deep bites' taken during suturing of the mesh (or conjoint tendon) to the lower edge of the inguinal ligament. A preventive 'trick' is to draw on the skin, with a sterile marker, the outline of the palpable femoral artery, and the femoral vein medial to it. This serves as a reminder to be careful when placing sutures just above those vessels. Finally, anyone who has placed a **mesh plug** into the internal ring knows how close the femoral artery can be — so easily felt by the index finger placed deep into the ring. **Think about this when inserting a plug: use a soft one or avoid it altogether in the very thin patient!**

- **Special care should be given to the iliofemoral vessels during laparoscopic inguinal hernia repair**. The proximity of these vascular structures to the cord structures is even greater 'from within', and attempts to 'reduce' the femoral vein instead of the hernia sac may happen if knowledge of the anatomy is lacking. The resultant possible catastrophe is obvious.

Injury to testicular vessels

The paradox of inguinal hernia repair in a male is the attempt to close a defect, while nevertheless leaving an opening through it (for the cord structures). **This internal struggle may sometimes lead to injury to the spermatic vessels by two mechanisms**: a too tight closure of the internal spermatic ring (rare), and overly enthusiastic clearing of the cord — with inadvertent injury to the artery or the veins (the chief cause of testicular ischemia). Vascular injury is also more likely to happen with large hernias, and when repairing recurrent hernias — especially following previous mesh repairs — having to mobilize the cord buried in scar tissue.

Compromised venous outflow will commonly lead to extremely painful and tender testicular swelling, and to venous ischemia which is often reversible and improves over a few weeks. **It may, however, lead to pressures that will compromise arterial flow, resulting in irreversible testicular ischemia and necrosis**. Testicular vascular flow can be imaged using Doppler ultrasound, and conservative measures (analgesics, scrotal elevation) should be enough when blood flow exists. When no testicular perfusion is noted testicular atrophy is expected. Whether to perform early orchiectomy (which may reduce suffering), or wait for the symptoms to subside spontaneously is never an easy decision.

Remember always to warn the patient about the dangers of testicular ischemia and emphasize it even more before operations for recurrent hernia. In addition, it is not unreasonable to recommend a **prophylactic orchiectomy** in a small, selected group of patients; for example, the nonagenarian with a large incarcerated hernia who already had three mesh repairs… An orchiectomy would greatly simplify the operation and repair, and avoid the prolonged morbidity of testicular ischemia. After all, at some stage of our lives we can function reasonably well with a single testicle.

'Surface' bleeding

The amount of dissection needed to complete a hernia repair varies widely, based mainly on the size of the hernia, the need to separate the hernia sac from the surrounding structures, and the dissection needed to mobilize tissues in order to complete the repair. In **open incisional hernia** repair, typically large flaps are created, and abdominal wall musculature is mobilized, resulting in wide areas of exposed tissue and a higher risk of hematomas and fluid collections. Drains are commonly used in these situations, but they may fail to eliminate collections altogether.

In **inguinal hernia** repair, such hematomas are less frequent and drainage is very rarely indicated (**remember: drains increase the risk of infection!**). Swelling of the cord and scrotum, creating a tender, swollen, purple 'eggplant' (*aubergine syndrome*), are a major source of concern (and pain) for patients, but, fortunately, nothing more than reassurance and some local measures are needed (or possible). An organized hematoma may take weeks or months to be absorbed, and aspiration of the liquefied hematoma can hasten recovery (at the slight, added risk of secondary infection — so always do it under strict sterile conditions). Prevention: be obsessive about hemostasis during hernia surgery, especially in high-risk patients treated by antiplatelets and anticoagulants. **Even the smallest capillary left oozing on the surface of the spermatic cord can compromise your otherwise perfect repair!**

Vas deferens transection

Ouch! Just the thought of dividing the vas deferens during inguinal hernia repair makes me sweat profusely. Fortunately or not, male fertility is never over, and the last thing we will want to do as surgeons is to prematurely terminate it, even in a 70-year-old patient... who may be more sexually active than we are! Of course it is especially important to avoid injuries to the vas deferens in patients who are in their most fertile years — despite the fact that only one side is enough for adequate function.

The risk of injury to the vas deferens is higher with large inguinoscrotal hernias, where more dissection is needed to separate the cord structures from the sac. Even more difficult is avoiding injury during repair of a recurrent hernia, where the cord may be embedded in scar tissue or adherent to old mesh (shudder!). **It is important to know the type of previous repair**, and whether the cord was left subcutaneously or placed back into the inguinal canal. This will assist in expecting the cord in its correct place and meticulously dissecting it. **Always read the old operative reports!** Obviously, during each repair, feel for the vas deferens, identify and safeguard it.

> **Op notes may lie!** Recently I had to operate on a recurrent hernia: the op note described "Lichtenstein repair", but at operation I found a huge patch of Marlex® mesh *covering* the cord! Beware: op notes are not always "non-fiction"! **Moshe**

Bowel injury

Bowel injury in hernia surgery may be the result of the primary pathology (incarceration-strangulation), or manipulation during the operation.

Strangulated contents

The incarcerated contents may suffer frank necrosis at the time of surgery, with or (more commonly) without perforation. Even if the fate of the strangulated bowel is doomed, efforts should be made to reduce the chance of resulting complications. Gentle handling and avoidance of rupture and spillage will reduce the already higher chances of wound (or mesh) infections. When survival of the bowel is in doubt, release of the compression at the hernia ring and warming the bowel are the usual measures to try and revive it, but much patience is needed. **Leaving the bowel to recover for 10-15 minutes, without peeking every minute, may eventually prevent the need for bowel resection**. However, in doubtful cases — resect! — to avoid the risk of perforation a few days later, and the resultant peritonitis. **Remember: the risks you take are the patient's, not yours**.

Iatrogenic injuries

Gentle handling of the bowel, and attention to the possibility of a sliding hernia, as mentioned above, are essential to avoid injury to the bowel in the hernia sac. One specific condition which merits special notice is the risk of bowel injury during **laparoscopic incisional hernia repair**. While open incisional hernia repair is often completed extraperitoneally, laparoscopic repair is always accomplished transabdominally, and therefore lysis of adhesions from the abdominal wall is almost always a part of the procedure. Laparoscopic dexterity is needed to accomplish this adhesiolysis safely, but even in 'good' hands the risk of bowel injury is not negligible. **Sharp and *cold* dissection is needed to prevent thermal injuries, and accurate visualization is compulsory. If an enterotomy is created and detected, the surgeon has a decision tree before him**: To convert or repair laparoscopically? To continue with hernia repair or abort the procedure? And if a repair is being performed — should a mesh be used or not? **Despite the heated debate in the literature, playing it safe is the wise thing to do in most cases: conversion to achieve a safe bowel repair (a limited incision may suffice, but use one that allows an easy access), and completion of the procedure at a later date**. Occasionally, a non-mesh repair would suffice. After all, the recurrence rate of non-mesh repair was never 100%!

Urinary bladder injury

In open inguinal hernia repair, injury to the bladder is extremely rare and is usually related to the presence of a sliding hernia with the bladder wall as part of the hernia sac. Recognizing this is the key to prevention, as mentioned above. The bladder may be at a higher risk of injury **during laparoscopic inguinal hernia repair**, and especially during total extraperitoneal (TEP) repair, if a previous scar adheres to the bladder anteriorly. Previous lower abdominal

Table 15.1. Common controversies in hernia surgery. *Continued overleaf.*

Question	On one hand...		On the other...	
	Pro	**Con**	**Pro**	**Con**
Lap or open?	**Lap:** • Less tissue trauma • Preferred for recurrent or bilateral! • Less acute (yes) and chronic (?) pain	• Difficult technique • Learning curve • General anesthesia • Unique complications	**Open:** • Relatively simple • Cheaper • Local anesthesia	• More pain • Recurrence makes it difficult
Mesh or primary repair?	**Mesh:** • Lower recurrence rate! • The 'tension-free' concept	• Risk of infection • Delayed mesh complications • Lower sperm count?	**Primary suture:** • No foreign body • Cheap	• Recurrence rate!
Light or heavy mesh?	**Light:** • Less pain? • Less stiffness • Less prone to infections?	• Not 'strong' enough? • Price • Unproven advantages	**Heavy:** • Easier to work with	• More foreign body • Contract and get stiff (e.g. forming 'meshomas')
Mesh tack-fixation in lap hernia?	**Tacks:** • Prevent mesh migration • May be absorbable	• Painful • May injure nerves • Expensive	**No tacks:** • Not really needed? • Alternatives exist — glue?	• Early mesh folding/migration?
Nerve division in inguinal hernia?	**Divide:** • Best chance to avoid neuralgia	• If well identified — why cut?	**Keep intact:** • Keep sensation	• If neuralgia does happen — a major problem!

Table 15.1. Common controversies in hernia surgery.

Question	On one hand...		On the other...	
	Pro	Con	Pro	Con
Defect closure or mesh-bridging in ventral hernia?	Close defect above mesh: • Better abdominal wall physiology • More mesh interface — less recurrence?	• More dissection • More tension	Bridge: • Less tension (?) • Simpler	• Postoperative bulge • Higher recurrence at the periphery of the repair?
Position of mesh in ventral or incisional hernia?	Retromuscular/pre-peritoneal: • Less adhesions • Less visceral complications	• Technically more demanding	Intraperitoneal: • Easy!	• Adhesions to viscera • Hazardous reoperations • Intestinal injury
	Underlay: • 'Physiologic' • Less recurrence	• Technically more demanding	Onlay: • Easier	• More recurrence • More wound complications
Biologic mesh?	Use: • 'Natural' matrix for native tissue • Infection-resistant (?)	• Very expensive! • Higher recurrence rate!	Avoid: • Non-proven benefit • Can use absorbable mesh	• May lose company support for your next trip!
Drains?	Use: • Prevents seromas • Prevents infection?	• More infections!	Avoid: • Unnecessary	• Against the department's dogma...

surgery, like open prostatectomy or Cesarean section, are considered by most as contraindications to this approach, and the transabdominal (TAPP) repair, or an open repair, should be preferred. Fortunately, urine is sterile and bladder injuries are usually easily repaired (see ⮕ Chapter 26). A missed injury, though, may lead to peritonitis or a urinoma and significant morbidity.

To summarize, when fixing any hernia you encounter multiple dilemmas and decision points, some technical (how many tacks to use to fix the mesh?) and others fundamental (am I experienced enough to offer laparoscopic repair?); some are based on judgment and experience (will this loop of bowel recover or will the ischemia lead to perforation?) and some are based on probabilities or luck (will the prophylactic antibiotics really prevent infection in this low-risk patient or is he the one that will develop pseudomembranous colitis?).

Table ■ 15.1 mentions some of the issues in debate, and a few associated pros and cons. **Eventually — it is you who will have to balance the factors and decide, based on your experience and understanding of the literature! This is not the place to tell you my personal preferences but if you have any questions please email me.**

Postoperative considerations

Swelling and hematoma

The most common complication after hernia repair (mainly but not only after the open approach) is local swelling. Located in a dependent area, and having a spongiform consistency, the scrotum frequently gets swollen in response to injury. While expected, and considered 'minor' by most surgeons, the various types of swelling are a major source of concern for the patient. On top of the local pain and disfigurement it is frequently associated with anxiety and fear that the repair has failed, since "it bulges as it was before".

Local edema is the commonest cause of swelling. **Seroma** is occasionally seen, and depends on the amount of dissection needed to complete the procedure. Separating a large hernia sac from the spermatic cord structures may cause **cord edema**, felt in the upper part of the scrotum. **Swelling of the scrotum**, and of the testis itself, may develop after repair of large inguinoscrotal hernias.

As mentioned above, vascular compromise of the testis may result from venous compression if the repair is too tight around the cord, resulting in venous congestion. Arterial injury, causing **ischemic orchitis**, may cause initial (painful, tender!) swelling before the end result (atrophy) is seen. **Remember: with inguinoscrotal hernias, it is preferable to avoid major dissection by transecting the hernia sac proximally within the inguinal canal, leaving the distal sac in place**. Usually the distal peritoneal sac will cause no harm, unless the surgeon ties its cut end leading to a **residual hydrocele**. So please just leave the distal sac wide open!

Hematoma of the inguinal area may result from injury to a named vessel, like the inferior epigastric or the testicular vessels. However, in most cases the dissection of the cord and the hernia sac results in 'surface bleeding', which is less easy to control. Not uncommonly the surgical field is dry at the conclusion of the procedure, only for the next morning to reveal a significant hematoma or ecchymosis, especially in patients treated by anti-aggregation and anticoagulation medications. While most such hematomas are self-limiting and will be absorbed within 2-4 weeks, some will become organized within a 'capsule' and create a residual inguinal mass, often mistaken for a recurrent hernia. Secondary infection of the hematoma may happen, but even without infection, a local inflammatory reaction (redness, swelling, pain) and a systemic reaction (fever) are frequent.

Management

Reassurance is of the utmost importance, as the above conditions are self-limiting in most instances. Symptomatic measures include NSAIDs to reduce pain and inflammatory response, scrotal elevation at night, and supporting underwear during the day. Ultrasound examination of the inguinal area is occasionally ordered by the (inexperienced) doctor for the (concerned) patient but is rarely of any significant help, apart from reassurance. If ischemic orchitis is suspected, Doppler ultrasound will confirm the presence (or lack) of testicular perfusion, but even then expectant treatment is the rule in most cases (see below).

Surgical site infection (SSI)

The proximity to the 'dirty' inguinal area, and the implantation of mesh, are reason enough for most surgeons to give a single dose of prophylactic antibiotic before surgery. Whether such a practice is justified also in laparoscopic inguinal hernia repair is a question that should be examined. However, operations for ventral hernias (incisional and also umbilical!) involve wider dissection, creation of flaps and dead spaces, and insertion of larger pieces of mesh, and thus are associated with higher rates of infection. **Therefore, in these cases, antibiotic prophylaxis is considered the standard of care**. Despite all prophylactic measures, SSI still happens, and may range from mild wound erythema to catastrophic suppuration (see also ⤳ Chapter 5).

Wound infection

Wound infection is usually caused by skin commensals, mainly *Staphylococci*, and is treated like anywhere else by drainage of wound collections and administration of antibiotics in selected cases. *Early*, spreading, necrotizing infections, usually caused by *Streptococci*, are uncommon but should be diagnosed and treated promptly as they are associated with significant morbidity and even mortality. The presence of mesh underneath the wound is always of concern, but avoiding wound opening and drainage of pus, in order not to expose the mesh, is an error. You should remember that **suboptimal treatment of the superficial wound infection may actually increase the risk of deep infection involving the mesh. Preventive note: layered closure of the wound is important — keep the mesh well covered by viable tissues (fascia, subcutaneous fat) and far from the skin!**

Mesh infection

As most hernias today are fixed with the aid of synthetic mesh, there is an added risk of infection due to the presence of a foreign body. It appears, however, that the concern which caused (and is still causing) many surgeons to avoid the use of mesh, is exaggerated. Most modern synthetic meshes are porous, allowing ingrowth of tissue and enough access to the cells responsible for immune response and tissue repair. Therefore, even if wound infection or a deep infected collection causes the mesh to be involved in the process, proper drainage and antibiotic treatment are usually enough to 'save' the mesh and avoid the need for mesh removal. **Non-porous mesh materials, like PTFE, are not infection-resistant, and therefore commonly require early explantation. Avoid them!**

Persistent/chronic mesh infections

In some cases, persistent suppuration, or specific infectious agents (MRSA, acid fast bacteria), leave the surgeon no choice but to reoperate and remove the foreign body. The resulting hernia should therefore be repaired primarily, and the wound properly drained or left open for secondary healing. The chances of hernia recurrence, after primary repair in a septic field, are of course increased. Acute mesh infections, treated conservatively, may at times lead to persistent, chronic infection, usually presenting with chronic discharge, formation of sinus tracts, and recurrent 'acute exacerbations' with cellulitis. While in the occasional case the process can be controlled with repeated courses of antibiotics, drainage of collections and much, much patience (of the patient as well as of the surgeon), **most such infections will end only after**

removal of the mesh, or at least the parts that are not well incorporated into the surrounding tissues.

Late mesh infection

Do note that mesh infection can appear even years after the original surgery. Blood-borne bacteria can land on the foreign material and infect it, and sometimes stay dormant for years 'waiting for a chance' — probably some immunologic changes — that let it propagate. Such late infections may respond to non-operative treatment, but commonly will turn into a chronic infection that mandates mesh removal. When late mesh infection occurs, a thorough investigation should be made (e.g. CT), **as deep-seated mesh may erode into nearby viscera such as the small bowel, the colon or the urinary bladder**. Intraperitoneal placement of the mesh is the main risk factor for such a complication — it could happen even with the use of modern 'protected' mesh material. Removing such an infected, eroding mesh is a major undertaking, commonly associated with bowel resection and secondary complications. **Think about it when implanting intraperitoneal mesh!**

Testicular damage

Mentioned briefly above, testicular complications merit some elaboration, as they are often associated with patient dissatisfaction and even litigation.

Ischemia and atrophy

Testicular ischemia can result from injury to the arterial blood supply, although mere transection of the testicular artery does not necessarily lead to ischemic necrosis, due to the presence of collaterals along the vas deferens. More common than transection is vascular compression due to a 'tight' repair, which constricts the spermatic cord, compromising the venous return. Testicular ischemia tends to develop in recurrent hernia surgery (where the cord may be buried in scar tissue), or when repairing large inguinoscrotal hernias with distorted anatomy. **Immediate testicular necrosis is rare**. The more common presentation is that of testicular swelling and extreme tenderness, frequently associated with fever. Expectant therapy, which includes NSAIDs (and commonly antibiotics... without much supporting evidence) usually leads to resolution of symptoms, over a period of several weeks. The end result, if the testis is indeed ischemic, is an atrophic testicle that may be small and hard (the eggplant turns into an olive...). In a minority of cases, necrosis with ongoing fever, swelling and pain will lead to an early intervention, by completion orchiectomy.

Secondary hydrocele

When dealing with inguinoscrotal hernias, complete separation of the hernia sac from the cord structures is often tedious, and requires extensive dissection that may cause edema, hematoma or injury to the vas deferens or the testicular vessels. Therefore, as stated above, proximal transection and ligation of the sac, leaving its distal part open and intact, is a common practice. **At times, however, the distal peritoneal sac rearranges as a closed sac around the testis, secretes fluid and a secondary hydrocele is created**. A different kind of fluid collection around the testis may occur when a scrotal hematoma gets organized, forming a pseudo-capsule which contains the liquefied hematoma. Both conditions result in a fluid-filled scrotal mass that can be quite large and disabling, and may look similar on ultrasound examination. However, a **scrotal organized hematoma usually resolves with needle aspiration, while a secondary hydrocele will often recur after aspiration, and if symptomatic may warrant hydrocelectomy**.

Postoperative pain

Early

In general, hernia repair is a painful operation. Although acute postoperative pain is not considered a complication, its implications on the well-being of the patient are significant and much thought and effort have been invested in measures to reduce postoperative pain. **Avoiding tension** on the tissues, with the use of mesh, not only results in a lowered incidence of failure, but is implicated in reduced postoperative pain. Avoiding the inguinal incision and limiting the dissection and the tissue injury is accomplished by laparoscopic repair. While the debate is not over whether laparoscopic inguinal hernia repair is 'justified', when all aspects are taken into consideration, it is quite clear, and supported by many studies, that postoperative pain is less compared to the open procedure. **Remember: limiting the size of the incision, and amount of dissection, during open repair is facilitated by the use of 'fancy' mesh techniques such as the 'plug and patch': the less you cut — the less pain you produce!**

Neuralgic-type pain may result from catching sensory nerves within the sutures used to repair the hernia defect, most commonly the *ilio-inguinal nerve* running within the inguinal canal on top of the spermatic cord. Some surgeons advocate intentional transection of this nerve, preferring a tiny area of numbness over the risk of neuralgia. Most others just pay attention not to injure it or even ignore those nerves altogether and do not have any problems.

During **laparoscopic repair** direct nerve entrapment may be caused by the spiral tacks used to fix the mesh. Avoidance of areas where the nerves run is imperative, and the use of more delicate, or absorbable tacks may further reduce the incidence of this complication. Many laparoscopic surgeons now use minimal fixation of the mesh, or none at all. **There is no doubt that the risk of nerve entrapment is higher during laparoscopic repairs, if multiple tacks are used**.

In cases when the main indication for hernia repair was a 'painful groin', and especially when the diagnosis of hernia was made *only* by ultrasound, there is a higher risk that the pain will persist after the operation. As mentioned above, when the diagnosis of a hernia as the cause of pain is doubtful, other possible diagnoses should be investigated, and a period of physical rest and anti-inflammatory medications should be tried before the final decision to operate. **Remember: rushing to operate on a painful groin may leave both the patient and the surgeon dissatisfied and frustrated. Pain in the groin for the patient = pain in the ass for the surgeon...**

Chronic

While acute pain after hernia repair is destined to resolve within a few weeks, chronic pain, lasting for months and even years, may actually 'drive the patient crazy', and have significant implications regarding the quality of life and functional capacity. A chronic inflammatory process, often related to the presence of mesh (and even called *meshalgia*), is manifested by ongoing pain, and local tenderness – sometimes the shrunken/scarred mesh is felt (or seen on CT) at the operative site (*meshoma*). Nerve entrapment, within a stitch, a tack or scar tissue, leads to a characteristic type of burning, shooting or radiating pain, often produced by a specific movement or tapping on a certain spot.

Treatment is protracted and frustrating, and better conducted under the care of a specialized pain clinic. It involves the use of medications including analgesics and other pain modulating agents like antidepressants, local injections of local anesthetics and steroids, and less conventional modalities like acupuncture. While many patients will respond sufficiently to return to their previous activity, even if some residual pain remains, some will declare failure and return to the surgeon (more commonly to another surgeon, which is a relief... ha ha...) for possible surgical intervention. Always consider issues of 'second gain' — be it 'insuritis' or 'litigatitis'.

Surgery for post-hernia-repair pain could entail the removal of the mesh, which is found contracted, folded, and with much scar and inflammatory tissue around it, and may be quite traumatic to remove. Transection of the inguinal nerves, if found embedded in the scar tissue, should be added, especially if the pain is of the 'neuralgic' type. Through the retroperitoneal approach it is possible to transect the offending nerves, without returning to the hernia repair site. This **triple neurectomy** operation (transecting the ilioinguinal, iliohypogastric, and genitofemoral nerves), which can also be accomplished laparoscopically (and even through the anterior approach — through the old scar), requires thorough familiarity with the involved anatomy, but is considered to be the ultimate solution to this frustrating complication. Notably, even patients in whom the pain does not respond to nerve blocks can benefit from the surgery! Let the 'specialist' do it! Refer!!!

Hernia recurrence

Failure of the hernia repair may be considered the ultimate complication, and most of the efforts in the history of hernia repair have been focused on reducing the recurrence rate — sometimes at the price of creating new complications! Currently, the acceptable rate of recurrence after elective inguinal hernia repair is considered to be 1% or less (much higher for incisional hernias), but many factors are associated with still higher recurrence rates in different hernias, repaired under different conditions, by different surgeons, at different locations and on different times of the day... which is beyond the scope of this chapter.

Immediate and early recurrences

'Recurrence on the table' ("recidivo a tavola" is the Italian source) is a derogatory term, used to describe a hernia recurrence that actually represents a technical failure to correctly identify and fix the defect. It may result from misdiagnosis, like performing a perfect inguinal repair when the actual femoral hernia is completely missed. Sutures in feeble and edematous tissue, frequently found when incarceration was present, may quickly fail to hold, especially if elevated abdominal pressure (e.g. bowel distension, severe cough) continues after surgery. Recurrence may happen quickly, even during postoperative hospitalization. In laparoscopic hernia repair, failure to identify and reduce an indirect sac, or failure to keep the mesh nicely spread at the desufflation phase (just at the conclusion of the operation), may leave the hernia actually unfixed.

Rarely, a misinformed patient decides to engage in strenuous activity immediately after the operation (e.g. *schlepping* a refrigerator from the kitchen to the pickup...). It is easy to imagine (shudder, shudder...) what this could do to your otherwise beautiful repair. **While mesh repair, and especially laparoscopic mesh repair, usually entails less limitations on physical activity than the classic suture repair, educate your patients on what they can or cannot do after the operation!**

Since the vast majority of, if not ALL, cases of very early recurrence are the result of technical failure, prevention is usually achieved by attention to detail and familiarity with the 'disease': the relevant anatomy, the possible variations and the various ways to confront the problem. **Leaving hernia surgery to the untrained is a common cause of failure. Unfortunately, it is still the common practice worldwide**. If this happens to you — review what you did, and if you have a video — watch it! And consider more supervision in your next cases…

Late recurrence

Late hernia recurrences can develop months or years after the original repair. While primary tissue repair may seem solid to the satisfied surgeon at the end of the procedure — self-satisfaction often conveyed to the admiring junior resident — the resultant scar will never gain the original strength of the healthy tissue. And although the strength of a primary tissue repair will, in most cases, suffice to keep the hernia closed for life, **there is no doubt that the way to reduce recurrence is not by making the repair more sophisticated, but to reinforce the original tissue with a supporting material**.

Before repairing a recurrent hernia, familiarity with the details of the previous operation, investigating possible causes for the recurrence (like elevated intra-abdominal pressure), and proper planning of the next procedure, choosing the best of all possible options, are mandatory. **Remember: the chance for hernia recurrence is higher when a previous repair has already failed**. Recurrent hernias may never cease to provide us with occupation and frustration. Hopefully, the combination of knowledge of the relevant anatomy, adequate dissection, avoidance of a missed hernia, using physical forces to our advantage, and properly reinforcing the repair with strong and lasting material, will all combine to bring us nearer to the goal of a perfect and lasting hernia repair — and free of complications.

> "Hernia repairs are like sex… you have to do what works best for you, with the minimum of complaints afterwards."
>
> **Angus G. Maciver**

Chapter 16

The gallbladder and bile ducts

Danny Rosin, Paul N. Rogers and Moshe Schein

You may want to think this way:

The main aim in laparoscopic cholecystectomy is not to remove the gallbladder but to avoid an injury to the bile duct.

The complications of gallbladder and bile duct surgery are as old as the history of biliary surgery itself, but with the advent of laparoscopic surgery there was a 'revival' of their incidence, and, if you wish, 'importance'. **The combination of more operations (they are now considered 'easier'), a new technique (with its infamous *learning curve*) and the ever increasing reliance on complicated technology have led to an increased rate of complications when compared to the 'open era'.**

We will not bore you with incidence and prevalence figures, but it is enough to say that a ten-fold increase in bile duct injury was observed in the early days of laparoscopic cholecystectomy (LC), and the number has never returned to that of the open era. Criticism of laparoscopy revolves mainly around complications related to the technique, and biliary complications have become the focus of attention. Likewise, you will likely become the focus of attention as the surgeon who "has a biliary complication" and particularly so if the operation was laparoscopic.

Today's public perceives LC to be a 'piece of cake' — after all, any general surgeon, even in a small hospital, is doing it and patients are expected to go home immediately and back to work after only a few days. So any deviation from such a perfect scenario is surprising and traumatic to the patient and is even more traumatic and humbling to you — without considering any associated legal ramifications.

Prevention, early recognition and proper management — the triumvirate in surgical complications — are the components of this chapter. Naturally, most of the focus will be given to stone disease, LC and bile duct problems, as the potential scope of this topic (e.g. choledochal cyst, cholangiocarcinoma, etc.) is much greater than the capacity of this chapter.

Pre-operative considerations

There are multiple surgeon- and patient-related factors that contribute to the complexity of the operation and increase the risk of complications.

General factors

You've probably heard the term "learning curve" more than once, and maybe even read about it in one of this book's chapters. **The analogy of climbing a steep mountain is appealing, but unfortunately the peak is never reached in surgery, and you will continue climbing throughout your career, as new techniques and technology never cease to appear**... until you get old... then you'll climb no more! In fact, not a few start to fall down...

Yes, you have to be conscious of the stage of training you are at, your level of expertise and dexterity, and recognize the fact that complications are more likely to happen early on the learning curve. But please note that even experienced surgeons have complications, and one can cut the common bile duct (CBD) for the first time at the 1000th laparoscopic cholecystectomy. **It is important to avoid the HUBRIS of "it will never happen to me", and never lose the sense of danger when stepping into the minefield of biliary surgery. Remember: many CBDs have been cut during simple and 'easy' cholecystectomies, and avoiding this disaster requires attention to detail in every single case!**

Other general factors that contribute to the risk of complications are related to the **patient himself**. There are of course general factors like age, health status and associated diseases that increase the general risk of surgery and anesthesia, but these factors also have a specific impact on the biliary pathology:

- **Age**: older patients tend to have more 'difficult' gallbladders, probably related to longstanding disease, repeated attacks of (acute-on-chronic) inflammation and fibrotic changes.
- **Gender**: as much as we wish to keep this book gender-free and politically correct, a multitude of evidence shows that male gallbladders are more difficult.
- **Associated diseases** may have specific effects on the risk of complications. **Cirrhosis and its associated portal hypertension** were once considered as absolute contraindications for cholecystectomy due to the significant risks of bleeding, liver failure and postoperative mortality. **However, multiple studies have confirmed the relative safety of LC in Child A and even Child B — but not Child C — cirrhotic patients**, but still, the risk is higher and extra care is required in optimizing the patient before surgery and while performing the operation. Alternatives to surgery should be considered in advanced cirrhosis, and alternative techniques should be used to reduce intra-operative bleeding, like **sub-total cholecystectomy** (see below). **Obviously, blood dyscrasias and anticoagulation may also increase the risk of bleeding**.

Anatomy

Variability of the biliary anatomy is said to be common, and is often cited as a risk factor for complications related to misidentification of biliary and vascular structures. So yes, you need to know that the **cystic duct** may be narrow or wide, short or long, enter the mid-CBD, or run down along it; course below, above or twist around the cystic artery — or even that there may be two cystic ducts as described nine times in the literature. You also have to know about the elusive and rare **accessory duct of Luschka**, draining the gallbladder directly into the liver, and often (wrongly) blamed for postoperative bile leaks. **You should also be aware that the right hepatic artery or one of its major branches (the same applies to anomalous branches of the right hepatic duct) can lie very superficially in the gallbladder bed and thus be injured during the dissection, after the cystic artery and duct have been adequately dealt with at the triangle of Calot.**

The key to dealing with all these variations is not to use them as excuses for mishaps. You should not even try to remember all the variations nicely illustrated in the textbooks. What you MUST do is be careful and meticulous with your dissection, and delineate the anatomy — whatever it is in the specific case — before clipping and cutting, even during the final step of separating the gallbladder from its bed! How you do that you'll read a little further below.

Pathology

$$A \times P = c$$

The Law of Anatomy and Pathology states that the product of anatomy and pathology equals a constant: the more pathology you have, the less anatomy you get.

Amram Ayalon

Different pathologies pose different specific difficulties when performing biliary surgery: inflammatory changes, gallstones, Mirizzi syndrome, cholecysto-biliary-enteric fistulas — see below.

Inflammatory changes

Inflammation is the most commonly encountered pathology that influences the difficulty of surgery, by causing adhesions to nearby structures, increasing vascularity, changing the quality of the tissues, and obscuring normal anatomy by edema and fibrosis. **Severity of inflammation, and timing along the inflammatory process, are factors that affect the operative difficulty and hence the risk of complications**. The decision whether to operate on a 'hot gallbladder' or wait for the inflammation to subside is multifactorial, **but if you decide to operate — take advantage of the edema of the early days and avoid the fibrosis that will follow shortly**.

Gallstones

Stones, the actual reason we remove most gallbladders (forget about biliary dyskinesia for a moment), come in a multitude of sizes and quantities (colour and shape don't really matter…), may affect the course of the operation and be associated with specific complications. A gallbladder packed with stones increases the risk of **stone spillage** (see below). **Small stones** are more likely to pass into the CBD, especially if the cystic duct is wide and valve-less. This may happen before surgery — presenting as jaundice or pancreatitis, or transient pain and elevation in liver enzymes, and be managed accordingly. But it may also occur during surgery, when you mobilize and manipulate the gallbladder. **Remember: pre-op jaundice or pancreatitis is the 'patient's responsibility', but postoperatively these are YOUR complications…** So please try to milk any offending stones out of the cystic duct before clipping it; it's the least you can do to reduce these annoying conditions — but this belongs to the next section…

Mirizzi syndrome

Mirizzi syndrome, described by the famous Argentinean surgeon in 1948, is a source of diagnostic uncertainty and operative difficulty. External compression of the CBD or common hepatic duct (CHD) by a stone located in the cystic duct, or Hartmann's pouch, leads to jaundice in the early stages, and actual bile duct erosion and fistula formation (between the gallbladder and the CBD/CHD) in more advanced stages. Apart from the jaundice, which can be alleviated by endoscopic retrograde cholangiopancreatography (ERCP) and stenting before surgery, the process is usually associated with severe fibrosis and distortion of the anatomy, and consequently the risk of bile duct injury is high. Proper pre-operative imaging, by magnetic resonance cholangiopancreatography (MRCP) and possibly by ERCP, is mandatory to get yourself ready for surgery. When erosion and fistulization ensue, bile duct repair or reconstruction has to be added to the cholecystectomy. **Failure to identify this pathology before the operation may result in a bile duct injury and bile leak**.

Cholecysto-biliary-enteric fistulas

These fistulas result from the combination of mechanical erosion of gallstones and chronic inflammatory reaction. Usually a big stone in Hartmann's pouch is the culprit, eroding its way to the nearby duodenum, or CBD, or even colon. The fistulous process is invariably embedded in fibrotic tissue with little remaining normal anatomy. Recognizing the presence of a fistula is the first step, and hints such as **air in the biliary tree** seen on plain X-ray should be pursued with further imaging. However, occasionally, the diagnosis is made only during surgery, when a contracted gallbladder is found stuck to an adjacent structure (or more than one), and whether an actual opening between the lumens exists or not may be impossible to tell. Taking down the fistula, not a simple task in itself, may leave a gaping hole in the target organ, which is not easy to fix (and, we hope, not missed!). **If severe adhesion without a clear fistula is encountered, it is better to leave a piece of gallbladder wall on the target structure than the other way round...** and if a fistula is diagnosed or highly likely, a GIA stapler may be used across it to separate the structure without leaving a hole.

The main question should actually be asked before surgery: if a fistula already exists — is the operation necessary? A cholecystocolonic fistula with resultant episodes of cholangitis must be fixed, but a cholecystoduodenal fistula, that lets the bile drain where it should arrive anyway may be left alone, especially when the patient is high risk and minimally symptomatic, avoiding a difficult and risky surgery. And if you happen to operate on a patient with **gallstone ileus** (if you are lucky you will encounter such a case once in a few years), do both yourself and the patient a favor and leave the gallbladder alone...

When to operate?

Biliary colic, the most common presentation of gallstones, poses no emergency and is usually solved by elective surgery whenever convenient. However, other complications of biliary stones such as acute cholecystitis or pancreatitis frequently provoke controversy as to the optimal timing of operation. Multiple factors influence this decision, including the specific pathology, condition of the patient, availability of the operating room and a competent surgeon. The risk of recurrent disease while awaiting surgery and the cost-effectiveness of early vs. late intervention should be also considered.

Acute biliary pancreatitis is usually treated non-operatively, and cholecystectomy is completed after the acute inflammation subsides. Operating too early on a patient with *severe pancreatitis* may cause secondary infection of the pancreatic process, especially if necrosis is present. On the other hand, waiting too long after the acute event may allow a repeated attack before the scheduled operation. **Operating on the same admission after resolution of symptoms, or within a week or two, is the common practice**, but in some environments OR availability may influence the timing of surgery. Whether to complete imaging of the ductal system before surgery (MRCP, endoscopic ultrasound — EUS), or during surgery (intra-operative cholangiography — IOC), or not at all (as most of the stones are small and pass spontaneously to the duodenum), is a debate that will not be settled here. If amylase or liver enzymes are not back to normal, the probability that a stone is still present in the CBD is higher and you better get some imaging of the ducts.

Acute cholecystitis has been shown in many studies to be better treated by an early operation, within the first few days after the onset of the disease (the 'golden 72 hours'). The edematous tissues, before fibrosis ensues, are easier to dissect, and overall recovery is quicker. While "operate as soon as possible" has become the prevalent practice in the USA, in other countries, 'cooling off' acute cholecystitis with antibiotics is widely practiced — being effective in most cases. Emergency operations for 'hot gallbladders' are generally associated with more complications than elective cholecystectomies on non-inflamed gallbladders; therefore, many surgeons still prefer to delay surgery despite the abundant literature supporting early surgery. Lack of immediate access to an operating room is another reason delayed surgery is practiced in some places. **Our recommendation: if you diagnose the acute gallbladder within 24-72 hours after the symptoms started, then go for it!** Of course, patients with multiple anesthetic risk factors, or on anticoagulants, should be 'cooled off' and postponed, to be operated under more controlled, elective conditions.

It is important to remember the alternatives when an urgent solution is needed for a septic patient, and LC is considered too difficult for the surgeon, or the patient, or both:

- Drainage of the gallbladder by **percutaneous cholecystostomy** usually solves the acute sepsis, allowing for an elective operation at a later date — the latter not being 'obligatory' in all such patients.

- **Open cholecystectomy!** Still a legitimate solution.
- **Referral** or getting help. Less surgical ego usually equals better patient outcome.

Choledocholithiasis

Stones passing from the gallbladder to the common bile duct (CBD) occur in about one tenth of patients — they can present with pain and elevated liver enzymes, acute pancreatitis, obstructive jaundice, ascending cholangitis or be asymptomatic. **It is highly recommended to diagnose and remove CBD stones** *before* **the operation, so that a simple laparoscopic cholecystectomy will follow**. CBD stones can be removed during the laparoscopic procedure, but in many (less experienced) hands, open CBD exploration surgery will be needed. A **missed or retained CBD stone** is an annoying complication that requires further intervention and disappoints the patient, who hoped that the cholecystectomy would permanently solve his problem. Missed CBD stones can contribute to postoperative complications, such as a cystic duct leak due to increased pressure in the CBD ('slipped clip'). Luckily, the need for repeat surgery is infrequent, thanks to our colleagues in endoscopy and invasive radiology.

When imaging of the CBD to rule out stones is indicated (e.g. jaundice, dilated CBD, elevated liver enzymes), non-invasive EUS or MRCP is usually preferred, and ERCP can be saved for obvious choledocholithiasis (e.g. persistent jaundice, stones seen by US).

Assimilation of new techniques

Since the advent of LC surgery has become much more technology-dependent, new techniques, instruments, devices and robotic machines appear in the market almost on a daily basis. The temptation to try new tricks, use new instruments and keep oneself in the forefront of surgery is combined with patients' demand (based on the internet and popular media) and pressure from the industry. *Single-incision laparoscopic surgery* (SILS), *natural orifice transluminal endoscopic surgery* (NOTES) and *robotic surgery* are the current hype, practiced widely without much evidence for a significant advantage over 'classic' laparoscopy. Adopting these new techniques is associated with a new learning curve for every single change, so new complications appear, some of them unique to specific techniques or devices. **No, we are not here to stop surgical progress, but to advise you not to lose your common sense in front of a dynamic and pushing surgical market** (see also ➲ Chapter 9).

Indications

> *When I was a resident all GBs with stones were chronic cholecystitis. In my early years all GBs without abnormal findings were normal (no surgeon ever liked this). In my mature years if I see two lymphocytes kissing its chronic cholecystitis! I don't know any surgeons who take out normal GBs unless it was just in the way.*
>
> **Miles J. Jones**

Most probably you are not one of those who believe that God has placed the gallbladder under the surface of the liver only so that it can be removed — preferably with the lap scope. However, looking around us we see not a few gallbladders removed unnecessarily and for dubious indications. The following are a few points which merit emphasis:

- **Asymptomatic gallstones** in the vast majority of cases do not indicate surgery. Exceptions are rare, for example: patients undergoing bariatric surgery and found to harbour gallstones which tend to become symptomatic after the weight loss, or patients living in countries where the incidence of gallbladder cancer is especially high. **Remember: asymptomatic patients cannot be improved!**
- **Non-specific symptoms**. The typical symptom of gallstones is pain in the right upper abdomen and/or the epigastrium. Attributing non-specific symptoms such as flatulence, dyspepsia, nausea, in the absence of pain, to the presence of gallstones only to justify LC usually **doesn't solve the patient's problems.**
- **Biliary dyskinesia**. In the USA, the laparoscopic era (or 'the easy GB' era), has seen a rising tide of cholecystectomies for the so called "biliary dyskinesia": where abdominal pain and diverse non-specific symptoms are attributed to dysmotility of the gallbladder, as documented by a radioisotope scan (HIDA) showing a decreased ejection fraction of the gallbladder (<35%). It has been estimated that at least **a third of the some ¾ million gallbladders removed each year in the USA do not contain stones and are labelled with this diagnosis. Perplexingly, in the rest of the world — not only in Europe, Australia, Asia and Africa but even in Canada — biliary dyskinesia is an unknown entity and the removal of stoneless gallbladders (acute acalculous cholecystitis excluded) is extremely rare**. We prefer to let others ponder or explain what makes the 'American gallbladder' so uniquely dysfunctional. But we do want you to remember this: **the lesser the indication — the greater the complication**.

Now go and proceed with an 'easy LC' for **biliary dyskinesia** in a morbidly obese patient (without gallstones) complaining about pain in the LEFT upper abdomen. What will you have to say if he sustains a CBD injury?

Intra-operative considerations

Beware of the easy-looking gallbladder and the overconfident surgeon.

During laparoscopic cholecystectomy (LC) you are only ever a 'clip away' from disaster — the following are a few tips on how to play it safe.

Critical view of safety (CVS)

Delineating the anatomy and correctly identifying the important structures is now considered the single most important factor in preventing significant complications, and especially bile duct injury, during LC. The concept of the **"critical view of safety"** popularized by Strasberg[1], involves complete dissection of the triangle of Calot, and identification of the cystic duct and artery as the only structures entering the gallbladder, before clipping or transecting any structure. This is accomplished by opening the peritoneum attaching the gallbladder to the liver, both anteriorly and posteriorly, thus mobilizing it away from its bed to create a large window (■ Figure 16.1). Documenting this view in the OR report, and preferably by a recorded image as well, is highly recommended, and could help in court if a complication occurs and is followed by a lawsuit. **The urge to identify and transect the cystic duct first should be wilfully suppressed, and**

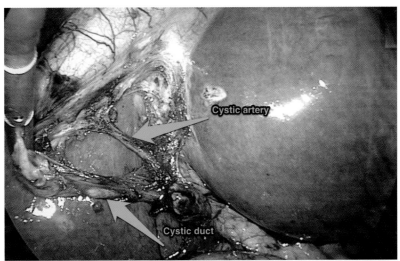

Cystic artery

Cystic duct

Figure 16.1. Critical view of safety — complete dissection of Calot's triangle with only the cystic duct and artery crossing the window.

---

1   Strasberg SM, Brunt LM. Rationale and use of the critical view of safety in laparoscopic cholecystectomy. *J Am Coll Surg* 2010; 211: 132-8.

postponed until the complete anatomy is clear, even in 'simple' cases. This is how 'classical' CBD injury occurs: what one is sure to be the cystic duct is actually the CBD. Even after the two desired structures are identified, it is recommended to clip/divide the rigid artery first, allowing the more elastic cystic duct to stretch a little more, away from the CBD. A caveat: having achieved the CVS doesn't give you the green light to rush and tear the gallbladder away from the liver while frying the latter. Instead, continue carefully and stay near the gallbladder avoiding the potential danger of an anomalous segmental right hepatic duct, coursing near the gallbladder bed on its way to the hilum.

Intra-operative cholangiography (IOC)

Intra-operative cholangiogram is a religion — not science.
Nathaniel J. Soper

Surgeons divide into mandatory and selective users of IOC — many of the self-declared 'selective' users rarely perform it at all. IOC is used to detect CBD stones and to delineate the biliary anatomy. Retained CBD stones may be visualized even in the absence of any pre-operative clinical or biochemical abnormalities, and some cite an incidence of 15% of 'silent stones' — but this is probably an overestimation and relevant mainly to the elderly population.

The advocates of **routine IOC** claim that most of these stones can be dealt with during LC (by flushing, using a choledochoscope or doing lap CBD exploration), thus preventing missed or retained stones in need of further postoperative treatments. According to the selective users, on the other hand, IOC should be offered only when choledocholithiasis is suspected on clinical, laboratory or imaging grounds (e.g. history of cholangitis, acute pancreatitis, jaundice, disturbed liver function tests, small stones and wide cystic duct, etc.), **but these are the exact patients in whom CBD stones can be detected and treated pre-operatively as discussed in the previous section**. Be it as it may, IOC will detect asymptomatic stones which we know will most likely pass spontaneously, thus leading to unnecessary escalation of the operation with its inherent morbidity.

The other theoretical (or alleged) rationale for performing routine IOC is to verify the anatomy and prevent, or immediately detect, bile duct injury. **However, careful dissection and an obsessive drive to obtain the CVS as described above should delineate the anatomy and prevent identification errors**. And in fact, insisting on a cholangiogram may actually lead to an injury if the cholangiogram catheter is inserted to the CBD instead of the cystic duct. (A needle cholangiogram through the gallbladder itself may be safer if the ductal structure is difficult to identify.)

By now you will understand why we belong among the many surgeons who use IOC selectively rather than dogmatically: we invite you to join us — the selective IOC users! However, there is one scenario which makes IOC mandatory: when you suspect a CBD injury! Therefore, you should be familiar with the technique if you perform gallbladder surgery, and if laparoscopic IOC is not possible then convert to complete it if needed! **The difference between immediate and late identification of CBD injury has a huge impact on early and late outcome!**

Tackling difficulties

We can only wish that all gallbladders would be simple, 'teaching' cases. But the great variability, both in anatomy and pathology of biliary diseases, means that the safe surgeon should have an armamentarium of tricks and maneuvers to tackle all the potential difficulties with minimal risk of complications. While experience and dexterity cannot be learned from books, some principles and guidelines are worth mentioning here.

Unclear anatomy

Inflammatory changes obliterate dissection planes; this is common in advanced acute cholecystitis but more so in chronic and fibrotic disease. But even a non-inflamed gallbladder can have a variant anatomy that is not easy to understand or dissect safely. The attempts to define the anatomy should never be abandoned, using the principles of a critical view of safety (with the aid of IOC if necessary) and using dissection tricks, some mentioned below, before any transection of structures is performed. It can never be said too many times: **conversion almost never will be considered a mistake — a failure to convert when necessary is always a mistake!**

Stone spillage

The combination of a delicate gallbladder wall and the presence of many small stones frequently results in a tear in the gallbladder during dissection and spillage of bile and stones. While bile can be aspirated (or irrigated, if you like to irrigate…), stones are more difficult to control. Finding and picking them up is annoying and time-consuming, and spillage may result in *lost stones* and late 'weird' infections due to stones serving as an infectious nidus. Rare complications such as bowel obstruction or erosion into structures like the urinary bladder have also been described. Thus, collect all spilled stones (especially the larger ones) and you better be ready for that by placing the collecting bag early during surgery, so the stones can be emptied from the gallbladder (if torn) directly into it or collected inside it before being lost. **Make an effort to leave the abdomen stone free…** it is rarely indicated to convert just to locate and collect lost stones, but invest time and effort to find them — that is if you failed to avoid this mess in the first place.

Wide cystic duct

Encountering a cystic duct which is wider than expected (some experience is needed here ☺) is a flag that should not be ignored. Sure, it may be a simple variant (commonly seen after a 'passage of stones'), but three things should worry you:

- **Is it really the cystic duct** and not the hepatic or the common bile duct? Make sure the anatomical identification is flawless.
- **Can I close it hermetically?** Clips may be short, or slip easily, and alternative closure techniques such as ligatures, or pre-tied loops, should be considered. Avoid the temptation to use a stapling device!! The non-absorbable staples can serve as a nidus for late stone formation.
- **Is the cystic duct so wide as to allow the passage of small stones?** 'Milk' the cystic duct backward to remove any stone that can later pass into the CBD. If you are an IOC aficionado — consider using it to rule out retained stones (if not — don't bother…).

Bleeding and hemostasis

The risk of bleeding during surgery is increased if the gallbladder is inflamed, the anatomy is obscured and in certain situations such as **cirrhosis** and **portal hypertension**. Avoiding operation in these situations is not always possible, and, therefore, familiarity with the various hemostatic techniques is mandatory. Clips, ligatures, sutures, electrocoagulation, argon beam coagulation — all may help but should be used wisely and cautiously. **It is a well-known fact that biliary duct injuries are associated with excessive bleeding and careless hemostatic maneuvers, and it is not uncommon to see many clips on X-rays in patients sustaining biliary injuries — a sign of frantic attempts at hemostasis**. If you encounter unusual bleeding, and find it difficult to control with simple measures, remember that natural coagulation may be better than what you can achieve by careless maneuvers. **Apply local pressure, preferably with small pieces of gauze, and wait a little**. Novices tend to forget that the camera magnifies the field — they may panic when pulsatile bleeding from a tiny branch of the cystic artery appears almost like an injured aorta ☺. **Pressure and patience (PP) are usually effective**, and harmless, and may give you time to think, recuperate, call for help or arrange for conversion. After a few minutes the flow of blood can change into a trickle, or the invisible pumper will suddenly come into sight, and if not — you have had the time to change strategy and have the team ready with you.

Exposure

Working through a 'keyhole' is not always easy. Obesity, hepatomegaly, adhesions and inflammatory changes may all interfere with your view of the surgical field and your ability to safely identify and dissect the necessary structures. **Open your mind to possible alteration of the standard technique, like variations in trocar placement (or number), and be familiar with other**

ways to expand the surgical field and enhance your view — adding a fifth (or even sixth) 5mm trocar will hardly interfere with cosmesis or the postoperative pain of an obese patient, but can significantly enhance retracting down the fat, or up a liver lobe, away from your view. **A suture passed through the abdominal wall can stabilize or pull away a structure that is in your way**. It can also be used to elevate the falciform ligament, and further expose the sub-hepatic space, especially when access to the CBD is required (as in CBD exploration). **And do not forget the availability of positional maneuvers of the operating table** — a steep anti-Trendelenburg position helps in bringing the 'deep' triangle of Calot, in a morbidly obese patient, into view!

Alternative dissection techniques

Two variants of dissection of the gallbladder are worth mentioning, as they are important in dealing with difficult scenarios:

- **Retrograde dissection**: although, according to the CVS principles, all LCs should start by dissecting the gallbladder from the liver ABOVE the area of the cystic duct and artery, sometimes it is not enough and identification of the anatomy is extremely difficult. This is more common with the chronically inflamed, contracted gallbladders, frequently described by the pathologist as *xanthogranulomatous*. Resorting to the equivalent of open surgery, and starting the dissection from the dome downward, may allow for gradual and safe separation of the gallbladder until it is 'hung' by the cystic duct. Remember that with these 'bad gallbladders' even starting above may quickly lead you to the hell down below, and ductal injury may still happen. You may need to combine this technique with the one mentioned in the next bullet. It was 'invented' by Max Thorek of Chicago some 100 years ago and has since been practiced by 'wise surgeons' (including us of course) — a technqiue which every surgeon has to master!
- **Subtotal cholecystectomy**: when anatomy is 'impossible', and the risk of CBD injury is high, it suffices to remove most of the gallbladder, leaving behind the most problematic part, namely a cuff of Hartmann's pouch connected to the cystic duct and artery. This is achieved by opening the gallbladder in a 'safe' place above the pouch of Hartmann, emptying the stones, and excising the upper part of the gallbladder. Usually it is possible to see the opening of the cystic duct 'from within'. The remaining (small) part of the gallbladder is closed by sutures (or tied with a loop, if possible), and a drain is left since a transient bile leakage can develop (albeit rarely). **Of course, if you are not familiar with endo-suturing, you will have to convert (see below) and accomplish the subtotal cholecystectomy — like in the good old days. Subtotal excision** is useful also when bleeding from the liver bed is expected, as in cirrhotic patients. Here, the 'posterior' wall of the gallbladder is left *in situ*, excising the rest of the gallbladder and destroying the remaining mucosa with the electrocautery.

Don't forget: call for help (that is if you have anyone to call) and consider converting. We hope, by now, that these last two options are already engraved in your mind...

Drains

The debate concerning the use of drains has been detailed in ⮎ Chapter 4. Luckily, in biliary surgery there is a wider agreement regarding the role of drains, as they have a specific purpose and rationale, namely **the diagnosis and treatment of postoperative bile leaks**. A properly placed drain may evacuate spilled bile, alert the surgeon to the presence of a leak and the possible need for further imaging or action, or prevent the need for additional interventions such as percutaneous drainage, ERCP or even reoperation. **A bile leak without a drain** *in situ* **leads to a** *spectrum* **of problems including sepsis, bile peritonitis, bile ascites or bilomas — but a drain usually saves the situation, converting the uncontrolled leak into a controlled bile fistula that is destined to close**. It follows, then, that a simple, straightforward cholecystectomy does not mandate leaving a drain, but when operating in 'bad conditions' like acute cholecystitis with an edematous cystic duct, or performing more complex biliary procedures like CBD exploration or hepaticojejunostomy, leaving a drain would be advisable. **Leaving a drain for 'bleeding' is more controversial; in general, meticulous hemostasis is the correct answer**. There are times, though, when surgical reality does not conform to absolute principles, and the gallbladder bed is 'wet' due to inflammation or coagulation disorders, and the surgeon feels he has reached the maximal hemostasis possible in these conditions — leaving a drain to monitor for possible rebleeding (beware the false sense of security it may provide, see ⮎ Chapter 3) or to prevent a local hematoma is certainly not a sin. And indeed, while we loathe the dogma implied in the term "routine drainage" we cannot criticise any surgeon who decides to leave a drain (we use a 7mm Jackson-Pratt®) in the subhepatic space after LC — provided the drain is removed promptly (within 24-48 hours) if not producing bile. **The truth is that we have never been sorry for leaving a drain after LC for it has saved our butts not a few times... and the reverse is true as well!**

Conversion

Mentioned several times already in this chapter, and many more times in other chapters, and other books, and M&M meetings, and court proceedings, etc., etc. — "when will they ever learn, when will they ever learn..." (do you remember the song?) — conversion seems to be the magic word in laparoscopy. And indeed, **what cannot be achieved safely by laparoscopy should generally be completed by opening the abdomen and in a timely manner — before further damage is done**. However, it must be remembered that conversion is not always magical, and may be associated with complications as well. Don't expect a difficult, fibrotic, contracted gallbladder with 'no anatomy' suddenly to change its nature when exposed to the open air. Don't lose your patience, don't rush, and remember that a fair amount of CBD injuries occur AFTER conversion. Call for help, before conversion if time permits (massive bleeding calls for immediate action), or after conversion (you may not be too familiar with open cholecystectomy these days...), as a new set of eyes and hands can make a lot of difference. **We never saw a patient dying *because* he was converted to open; we saw them dying or almost dying because they were not converted...**

> LC should take as long as it takes to do it safely and if it takes much too long it only means that it should have been converted earlier... **Moshe**

Postoperative considerations

The key to everything discussed below is this: LC is a day procedure. A few hours after the operation the patient should be able to walk to the bathroom and drink chai with milk or a cappuccino (a few of our patients ask permission to go out for a smoke...). His/her vital signs should be normal and the (incisional) pain controlled by basic analgesia. **Anything which deviates from the above — and by anything we mean anything and everything! — should warn you that not everything is *kosher*.** That the operation was straightforward does not mean that a disaster is not lurking inside (■ Figure 16.2).

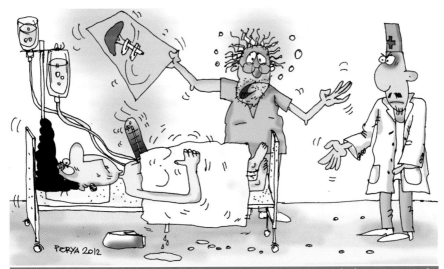

PERYA 2012

Figure 16.2. The surgeon telling his resident: "What an easy cholecystectomy it was!"

Bile leak

How do you feel when the 'prophylactic' drain you left after the LC is producing pure bile? Like s**t, eh? (But after saying the F word a few times do congratulate yourself for having left a drain!). Surely this complication is dreaded by any surgeon, as it may turn a simple, day-case operation, in which the surgeon is a hero (or even magician), into a complicated case full of shame, blame and loss of fame.

Bile leaks can be grouped into 'simple' and 'complicated', based on the specific anatomy, but even a **cystic duct leak**, which is considered simple and relatively easy to manage, can end with catastrophic consequences, probably due to infected bile. Rapid and severe SIRS can ensue, and is attributed to the elusive 'lethal bile' which can result in a rapidly progressing inflammatory response and may end with multi-organ failure. Strangely, at the other end of the spectrum, bile (probably non-infected) can gradually fill the abdominal cavity and be quiescent for several days — the patient presenting back with non-specific symptoms like malaise, abdominal swelling, ileus and mild jaundice.

The source of the bile can be:

- The **cystic duct** — common and 'easy' to manage.
- A **major bile duct injury (CBD, CHD)** — less common (we hope) and not so easy to deal with.
- The **injured liver parenchyma** in the gallbladder bed — a minor leak and self-limiting.
- **Accessory bile duct** (of Luschka), originating in the right hepatic lobe, and (originally) entering the gallbladder directly — rare, unpredictable and 'easy' to manage.
- **Anomalous bile duct**, draining a segment of the right lobe, joining the confluence of the main right and left bile ducts at the hilum — rare, unpredictable and 'difficult' to manage.

The following discussion will focus on the first two entities.

Cystic duct leaks

A **leaking cystic duct** can be the result of insecure closure of a wide or edematous duct, leading to slippage of the closing metal clips. A high-pressure system, caused by distal obstruction to flow as from a retained CBD stone, may also cause such a cystic duct blow-out. Attention to proper closure of the cystic duct before transection is of utmost importance, and can be achieved, if deemed necessary, by using sufficiently large clips, adding another 'safety' clip, or ligating the cystic duct. A simple, single-handed ligature technique has been popularized by the surgeon Serg Baido, and is described here[2]. You better get yourself familiar with this technique (http://www.youtube.com/watch?v=l9sKta2pZm4) — satisfaction guaranteed!

A leak from the cystic duct can develop immediately after the operation or be delayed for days. We have seen a leak developing already in the recovery room with the patient shouting with pain in his right shoulder (no, it is not always a 'gas pain'!); we have seen it presenting with bile in the drain in the morning after the operation — the patient completely well; and we have seen it presenting, out of the blue, 10 days after the operation — while the patient was almost forgotten…

What to do when a bile leak is diagnosed

What to do when a bile leak is diagnosed depends on the specific scenario, namely, is there a drain *in situ* which is draining bile, or isn't there one?

There is a drain which is draining bile

- Most importantly, do not get excited or hysterical — this is not the end of the world. Luckily, you have left a drain and now you have all the time in the world to decide what to do.
- **First assess the patient**: no signs of SIRS? Abdomen soft? White cell count normal? Biliribin and liver function normal? (Remember that even in the aftermath of uneventful LC, liver enzymes can be a little elevated and so too the leukocytes.) **If so, this means that the bile leak is well controlled through the drain.**
- **Now try and guess which of the sources mentioned above may be leaking**. Replay the operation in your mind: did you achieve the CVS? If so, it is extremely unlikely that one of the main bile ducts has been injured. Was the operation 'traumatic'? Did you have to 'dig' into the liver bed? The parenchyma may have been injured and hence the green output from the drain. How happy were you with the cystic duct closure; how many clips did you place? Was the cystic duct a little too wide for your clips? **But remember: shit happens and even a perfectly clipped cystic duct could leak!** It is comforting to blame the elusive accessory duct for the leak — but this is extremely rare.
- **So if the patient is 'well' do not rush with any further <u>invasive</u> steps** (i.e. ERCP). Just wait another day or two and monitor the patient (for SIRS, liver function) and watch what's coming out of the drain.

---

[2] Thanakumar J, John PH. One-handed knot tying technique in single-incision laparoscopic surgery. *J Minim Access Surg* 2011; 7: 112-5.

Meanwhile, to reassure yourself (and the vexed patient), you may want to obtain some non-invasive tests such as an ultrasound (to rule out a significant bile collection) or a HIDA scan (to document flow of bile into the duodenum) — and, if you really worry, an MRCP to show that the main bile ducts are intact. A bile leak from the liver surface in the gallbladder bed is likely to cease rapidly (unless it originates from an injured anomalous right segmental duct). Also, 'small leaks' from the cystic duct tend to cease spontaneously. A day later the drain may be dry! **But even if the bile leak persists beyond a few days there is no need to get panic-stricken**. (Lessons learned during the old days of open cholecystectomy and even the older days when ERCP was not available, taught us that the vast majority of well-drained bile leaks will dry up eventually — if there is no distal obstruction, e.g. CBD stones.) So often, when the clinical features and the non-invasive imaging show that the leak is well controlled and the CBD intact, one would discharge the patient home with the drain still in place, with daily follow-up in the clinic and/or by phone. That the patient drains 500cc of pure bile daily, a week after LC, should not elevate your blood pressure, because a day later it may suddenly drain only 50cc and a day later become dry! **In summary: a significant number of controlled bile leaks after LC can be managed with no more than reassurance and watching the patient and his drain**.

- Obviously, the patient should take part in the decision-making based on informed discussion. **He has to be informed about the other more aggressive option available, namely ERCP to delineate the anatomy (what exactly is leaking?) and leave a stent across the papilla** — to decrease ductal pressure and hasten closure of the leak. A reasonable approach would be to start with a 'wait and see approach' and if the leak persists beyond a week or so ('large' leaks from the cystic duct may take longer to heal...), resort to ERCP plus stenting. You have to reassure yourself and the patient that the expectant approach is safe. Trust us: it is!

- **Remember that ERCP and stenting, while safe and effective in most instances, are not free from complications** (e.g. pancreatitis, duodenal perforations, etc., and the stent will have to be removed endoscopically at some stage). In some places ERCP is not readily available or the local expertise is mediocre. So why rush into it frantically, when the chances of spontaneous closure of the leak — as long as the area is well drained and sepsis is controlled — are extremely high, and with patience and careful follow-up results are gratifying. Excavating our legal cases, we could find a case just like this: a few cc. of bile encountered in the drain immediately after an 'uneventful LC'; the patient rushed immediately for an ERCP (no evidence of leak!); the next day she is dying because of duodenal perforation. How futile and depressing!

- **Obviously, if the patient is not 'well', if you suspect that the leak is not well controlled through the drain** (this should be rare), **if you have reasons to worry about CBD injury... then proceed as outlined below**.

There is no drain and you suspect a bile leak

So your LC patient is not well, or not progressing as expected, as preached to you already *ad nauseum*. Now you suspect a bile leak but first you have to prove it:

- First curse yourself: "hell, why didn't I leave a drain!"
- No, the next step is *not* an ERCP; what you want to do is **actually diagnose the bile leak and exclude other serious complications**, such as visceral injury or pulmonary embolism (PE). Features suggesting a bile leak are SIRS associated with abdominal tenderness, distension and ileus. **Intraperitoneal bile is being reabsorbed into the 'system' resulting in a gradual but invariable elevation of the bilirubin**.
- **Abdominal imaging should be your next step**. Ultrasound and CT would document free intra-abdominal fluid but remember that the leak and accumulation of bile is rather slow and it would take more than 24 hours to have a significant amount of free fluid visualized. The advantage of CT scanning is that it helps to exclude other catastrophes such as duodenal injury. Starting the scan in the thorax excludes PE as well. Whether to start with ultrasound or CT depends on the clinical picture and institutional preferences.
- **To prove the actual leak we advocate the HIDA isotopic scan which is simple, non-invasive, highly diagnostic and widely available**. Within an hour or two after injection of the isotope you will see it accumulating under the liver; if the CBD is not transected or obstructed you will also see flow into the duodenum — which may make you less tachycardic ☺.

So you have diagnosed the bile leak. What now?

As always there are a few options to choose from the menu, depending on the patient, your own capabilities and those of your environment:

- If the leak is diagnosed immediately or very early (within 24 hours) after surgery — **relaparoscopy and reclosure** of the cystic duct is recommended by some surgeons, and has been practiced by us a few times. It must be remembered that it is not always that easy to accomplish this task laparoscopically, and if severe inflammation already exists — reclosure can end up with a releak, if not worse. **However, appropriate diagnosis, drainage and abdominal toilet are clear advantages of this approach**. In the worst case scenario you will end up with a leak controlled through the drain(s) — you know now how to proceed from here.

- If the patient is grossly septic due to bile peritonitis (the 'bad bile'), then **CT-guided percutaneous drainage** of bile or even a laparoscopy/laparotomy may be indicated.
- **In the majority of cases, however, the recommended *soup du jour* would be ERCP and stenting**. We need hardly add that all such patients should be placed on broad-spectrum antibiotics. **Usually the ERCP, with stenting, resolves the leak immediately without a need to evacuate the spilled bile**. If SIRS and abdominal symptoms continue, then re-imaging and percutaneous drainage of residual collections may be indicated.

If your postoperative assessment of a bile leak reveals a major duct injury then your heart sinks further. See the next section…

Major bile duct injury

If a postoperative biliary leak is dreaded by surgeons — a major bile duct injury is the materialization of a horrible nightmare (■ Figure 16.2). This problem may become manifest at various times and in several ways during and after LC, and for these reasons is discussed in this section of its own. The severity of this complication depends on the level and extent of injury, and the presence of associated (vascular) injuries. The time of diagnosis also has a major effect on outcome. It is useful to consider this topic under several headings: anatomy, general principles, mode of presentation.

Anatomy

An understanding of the anatomy of the catastrophe is crucial in any discussion of management. There are several **classification systems** to describe bile duct injuries. Although for practical purposes it is mostly sufficient to categorize them as 'partial' or 'complete', and 'high' or 'low', the more accurate classifications are important for planning the repair strategy by the hepatobiliary surgeon, who will eventually get involved in the case. The most popular classification has been offered in 1995 by Strasberg *et al* (■ Table 16.1) and considers the whole spectrum of such injuries, including the cystic duct and 'accessory' and aberrant-anomalous ducts discussed above. A recent classification which considers only **major duct injuries** has been offered by the European Association for Endoscopic Surgery (EAES). See below [3].

---

[3] Eikermann M, *et al*. Prevention and treatment of bile duct injuries during laparoscopic cholecystectomy: the clinical practice guidelines of the European Association for Endoscopic Surgery (EAES). *Surg Endosc* 2012; 26: 3003-39.

Table 16.1. Strasberg's classification of bile duct injuries [1].

- A. Leaks from the **cystic duct** or from the (accessory) duct of Luschka.
- B. Occlusion of an aberrant **right hepatic duct**.
- C. Transection without ligation of an aberrant **right** hepatic duct.
- D. Lateral injuries to a **major bile duct**.
- E. Transection or resection of a **major bile duct**.

  Grade E is subdivided into types 1-5 according to the level of injury as previously described by Henri Bismuth [2].

1. Strasberg SM, Hertl M, Soper NJ. An analysis of the problem of biliary injury during laparoscopic cholecystectomy. *J Am Coll Surg* 1995; 180: 101-25.
2. Bismuth H, Majno PE. Biliary strictures: classification based on the principles of surgical treatment. *World J Surg* 2001; 25: 1241-4.

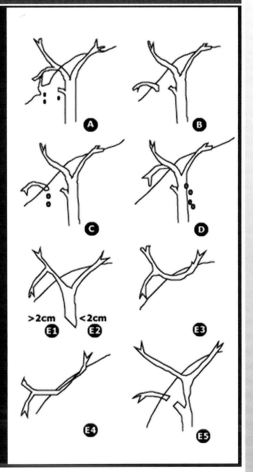

Naturally, **the higher the level of transection, and especially if part of the CBD is missing, the worse is the prognosis and the more difficult is the management and eventual reconstruction**. Unfortunately, the *classic* laparoscopic CBD injury, caused by misidentification of the CBD as the cystic duct, involves a 'high' injury and excision of a bile duct segment. Wrongful dissection of the CBD is commonly associated with excessive bleeding and sometimes chaotic hemostatic attempts by coagulation or clipping (if you find yourself in this situation it should cause you to pause and consider seriously if you are dissecting in the wrong place), and this is why CBD injury is often complicated by ischemia, which may cause failure of repair attempts, and lead to future stenosis.

General principles

This leads us to a discussion of the general principles of major bile duct injury. It is a serious injury with great implications for morbidity and mortality. For this reason, the early assistance, if available, of an **experienced hepatobiliary surgeon** is desirable. If the injury is recognized intra-operatively (less common), then ask for help immediately, otherwise ship the patient out to a liver center if the injury only becomes apparent postoperatively. The mode of injury of the duct is an important consideration in salvaging the situation. **If the injury is thermal,** or **complicated by ischemia** from excessive dissection, then a simple intra-operative repair is unlikely to be successful. On the other hand, a straightforward incisional injury, particularly if only partially circumferential, may be repaired over a T-tube. The last important consideration is if there has been **resection of a large portion of duct,** in which case expert help is essential.

Mode of presentation

Keeping in mind the above general principles it is practical to discuss diagnosis and management under *three* **different scenarios:**

- Intra-operative diagnosis.
- Postoperative jaundice.
- Postoperative bile leak.

Intra-operative diagnosis

This is rather rare, for what makes surgeons injure the duct — sloppy technique, impatience, arrogance, lack of attention to detail, inexperience — does not help them to realize the catastrophe they have just created. But what to do if one realizes that, "hell, this is not the cystic duct which I have just clipped and transected — this is the frickin' CBD!" **In general, early repair yields a better outcome, as long as it is performed by a competent surgeon.** So if you feel up to the job, if you have done a few enterobiliary anastomoses before, then go ahead: summon additional assistance — a second surgeon, even if not HPB trained, has the advantage of no emotional involvement with the mishap — convert (yes, WTF, convert!) and deal with it. Primary repair over a T-tube, especially for partial injuries (type D), is sometimes possible. For a 'clean' transection of the CBD without missing tissue, an end-to-end anastomosis over a tube is a viable option. However, for most significant type E injuries a Roux-en-Y hepaticojejunostomy is considered the chosen procedure, and despite the non-dilated duct is doable and has mostly a favorable outcome. Late stricture — often amenable to endoscopic treatments — is the most common long-term complication. But if you do not know how to tackle it, if no capable biliary surgeon is available to help, then your best option would be to terminate the LC, **place drains in the gallbladder bed and the proximal transected duct if possible,** wake up the patient and ship her to the nearby HPB referral center. **Remember Rod Stewart's song — *The first cut is the deepest?* Likewise here — the first attempt should be perfect**, as less than perfect reconstruction would render further attempts more complex and less successful.

Postoperative jaundice

The post-LC patient is doing well except that he develops jaundice. This occasionally happens in type E injuries after the surgeon has carefully clipped the CBD below, and hepatic duct above, before removing the intervening segment of duct — not realizing what he is actually doing. One should not get too excited if the bilirubin is a little elevated on the first postop day, but if it continues to climb (always along with elevated liver enzymes) you have to act. **Your hope is for retained CBD stones but dread ductal injury**. The next diagnostic step, whether to start with MRCP or ERCP, depends on local facilities and on how vexed you are. Treatment depends on the timing of diagnosis (early occlusion vs. late stricture), the extent of injury (a single occluding clip versus resection of the duct) and the condition of the duct (small vs. dilated). In selected cases endoscopic treatment with dilatation and stenting is possible. In most cases reconstructive surgery is indicated — get an HPB guru! — usually with an enterobiliary anastomosis. (For the management of postop jaundice due to stones see the next section.)

Postoperative bile leak

The duct is injured and leaks bile — into the drain or the abdomen. Here you have to proceed as described in the previous section on a leaking cystic duct: abdominal imaging, HIDA scan, ERCP. Rarely, under favorable conditions, early reoperation and reconstruction are possible. **However, in most instances, the diagnosis is delayed for a few days rendering attempts at reconstruction inadvisable because of systemic and local sepsis, thus mandating a staged approach — consisting of percutaneous drainage of collections, establishment of a controlled bile fistula, and, in selected patients (depending on the anatomy of injury), endoscopic stenting**. Late reconstruction, after sepsis is controlled and the patient is no longer catabolic, is usually by Roux-en-Y hepaticojejunostomy. By the time of surgery the bile duct is usually dilated, making anastomosis easier and less likely to stricture.

When a major bile duct injury occurs, it is a major blow to the surgeon's ego. Defence mechanisms like denial may cause further delay in diagnosis and management, and self-attempts to fix the injury may lead to further deterioration and worse outcome. This situation is one of the most difficult tests to the surgeon's integrity; calling for assistance, referral to a HBP surgeon or even transfer to another facility are probably the best modes of action. Full disclosure and honesty with the patient and family are mandatory, as they are the only possible ways to prevent a lawsuit. **Once submitted — it is almost always a lost case** (⟳ Chapter 10).

Retained stones and associated complications

The passage of stones from the gallbladder to the common bile ducts always escalates the level of complexity — both of the disease and its treatment. When pancreatitis or obstructive jaundice is diagnosed before surgery, diagnostic and therapeutic efforts will be made to confirm the presence of CBD stones, and remove them pre-operatively by ERCP. This is the most common approach, despite the availability of other options like laparoscopic CBD exploration. However, since CBD stones tend to pass spontaneously to the duodenum, many do not require any specific intervention — this is why, for example, so few patients with biliary pancreatitis have stones demonstrated on pre-op ERCP or intra-op cholangiogram.

It can happen, though, during the waiting time for the scheduled LC, or even during the operation itself, that another stone finds its way into the CBD. This is more common with the combination of a wide cystic duct and multiple small stones. Retained CBD stones can be found even after CBD exploration — the rationale behind leaving a T-tube, to allow postoperative cholangiography and confirm completeness of the clearance. Therefore, these stones are 'annoying' but less unexpected. On the other hand, retained stones after a cholecystectomy are a source of frustration: to the disappointed patient (presenting with symptoms "like before surgery") and to his surgeon.

Prevention, diagnosis and management

Although residual/retained CBD stones cannot be completely avoided, the incidence can be reduced by pre-operative and operative measures, as follows:

- **Pre-operative** investigation for CBD stones is recommended when there are clues to the passage of stones through the CBD, like elevated liver enzymes, or a history of pancreatitis or cholangitis. Complete resolution of symptoms and normalization of lab results may mean that the stone has passed — but not necessarily so. The availability and non-invasiveness of MRCP makes it a favorite diagnostic modality by many surgeons. **When a patient presents with elevated enzymes and bilirubin, it is wise, though, not to rush but follow the trend in the next few days. Investigation too early may show the stone that is destined to pass, and provoke unnecessary interventions**.
- **During surgery**, the presence of a wide cystic duct should alert the surgeon to the possibility of passing stones. 'Milking' of the cystic duct before clipping may return stones 'en passage' to their home-base. The application of a 'temporary' clip at the cystic duct junction with the

gallbladder early in the dissection may prevent migration of stones during the struggle to achieve the CVS. The question of routine cholangiography arises again — it is enough to say that most surgeons, including us, find it unnecessary.

- **After the operation**. When the patient presents, usually a few days to a week after surgery, with painful jaundice or pancreatitis, we should keep in mind that most cases are self-limiting, and represent 'the last stone in the system'. **Therefore, rushing to ERCP is usually unnecessary, and supportive care, repeated labs and a clear explanation to the patient are the mainstays of treatment**. Imaging should include ultrasound to rule out an obvious stone and significant bile duct dilatation, and MRCP if there is no quick resolution. ERCP should be reserved for cases when a stone is impacted, evident by no resolution of symptoms and labs, or by non-invasive imaging. In most cases ERCP and sphincterotomy will solve the problem, but rarely will fail, and repeat surgery will be needed, unfortunately.

Having read the above you understand that retained CBD stones are not really a 'complication' but rather a spectrum of the disease. Nevertheless, it is a source of anxiety to both patient and surgeon and must be managed and explained carefully.

Postoperative bleeding (see ⮌ Chapter 3)

Despite a meticulous technique and careful hemostasis, some patients will suffer from significant bleeding after cholecystectomy. The use of platelet inhibitors or anticoagulation, so common nowadays, increases the risk of postoperative bleeding, especially 'surface bleeding' like in the liver bed of the gallbladder. **Cirrhosis and portal hypertension** are obviously risk factors for excessive bleeding. "It was completely dry!" is the common reaction of the surgeon, and is usually the truth. But nevertheless, on-going ooze can result in significant blood loss. **Reoperation is sometimes necessary, as the accumulation of blood clots can result in the so-called "local DIC", and the bleeding will not cease without evacuation of the clots — even when no 'surgical' source of bleeding is found.** Leaving a drain in a 'less than dry' operation is condemned by some purist surgeons — but is not a sin as long as you don't rely on it instead of achieving appropriate hemostasis. **So our advice: leave in a drain when liver bed hemostasis is not perfect**; it will prevent the collection of a hematoma, allowing natural hemostasis to do its magic. **But remember**: a dry drain does not exclude a significant hemorrhage!

Significant blood loss with hemodynamic instability should warn the surgeon to the possibility of arterial bleeding. An injury to the right hepatic artery, sometimes running superficial near the gallbladder bed, may seem controlled during surgery due to vasospasm, only to resume bleeding after the operation. Attempts to control such an injury with clips and cautery, without accurate identification, may lead to the creation of a **pseudoaneurysm** that can bleed massively a few days after surgery. When the diagnosis is suspected and GI bleeding, due to **hemobilia**, should raise this possibility, angiography and embolization should be the preferred approach. **When reoperating for bleeding be careful with adjacent bile ducts — combined injuries of the two structures are oh so common**.

Visceral complications

When things go wrong after cholecystectomy, the mind is naturally directed to the biliary system. But, as in every laparoscopy (or surgery in general), complications can result from other systems and organs. We will not dwell here on general complications (pneumonia, etc...), but **injury to surrounding structures** has to be mentioned yet again (see also ➲ Chapters 6 and 9).

Duodenal injury is usually associated with a difficult operation when the first part of the duodenum is 'pulled up' by the inflammatory process onto the gallbladder, making its separation difficult. Rarely, a cholecystoduodenal fistula may exist and be unrecognized; its separation leaves behind an unsuspected duodenal hole. The **colon** may also be involved in an inflammatory conglomerate around the gallbladder — a potential source of postoperative infection if injured during dissection.

If detected during the operation, then repair, usually with drainage, is usually successful. **But unsuspected and undetected visceral injuries are horrendous disasters**. The spectrum of presentation ranges from a free duodenal leak, which if missed can kill within 24 hours, to a delayed presentation of colonic injury, with sepsis and peritonitis, sometimes a few days after surgery. Diagnosis is not always straightforward, delays are common, repeat surgery is usually required, and the overall prognosis from such missed injuries is bad, with high morbidity and mortality. **Thus, always suspect and be on the alert. Excessive pain after any LC should be promptly and carefully considered...**

'Post-cholecystectomy syndrome'

This somewhat historic diagnosis is worth mentioning as it is still occasionally used when no specific diagnosis can be reached. This condition is actually a basket full of different entities, most of which are well defined. The common denominator is that they appear after cholecystectomy, and have a similar presentation, mainly pain and dyspepsia. In some cases the symptoms are related to residual stones, as mentioned above. Peptic disease symptoms may be similar to biliary symptoms, and a missed diagnosis may have led to an unnecessary cholecystectomy. Some symptoms may be related to the cholecystectomy itself, such as diarrhea (explained by the continuous flow of bile to the intestine), and are expected to settle spontaneously within a few weeks, except in a minority of patients with stubborn symptoms. In elderly patients, persisting post-cholecystectomy syndrome may eventually prove to be caused by intra-abdominal cancer (e.g. gastric, colonic), the symptoms of which were wrongly attributed to gallstones.

Once residual stones are excluded, referral to a gastroenterologist is the best advice we can think of. **But essentially, the time to prevent post-cholecystectomy syndrome is 'pre-cholecystectomy' by proper evaluation and exclusion of other diagnoses mimicking gallbladder disease**.

Some late complications

Even long after successful biliary surgery, patients may sometimes haunt you (or other surgeons) with complications appearing months or even years later.

While most CBD stones originate from the gallbladder, true **primary CBD stones** can develop when CBD drainage is impaired. **Papillary stenosis**, more common in elderly people, may be related to past inflammation or passage of stones and resultant scarring. ERCP, sphincterotomy and stone extraction is the mainstay of treatment, but multiple stones and a very wide CBD may require surgical intervention, with CBD exploration and possible bilio-enteric diversion (e.g. choledochoduodenostomy).

Late cholangitis, even without the presence of stones, may result from an obstructed biliary flow due to a stricture. Partial CBD injury, or thermal injury, can lead to such a stricture presenting months after the original surgery. A bilio-enteric anastomosis can also result in late strictures. Don't forget the possibility that a stricture may be malignant, unrelated to the previous operation!

'Sump syndrome' is a specific complication seen after a side-to-side choledochoduodenal anastomosis, favored by some surgeons for CBD stones, with a wide duct, mainly in elderly patients. This operation, while being simple and relatively safe, and providing CBD drainage, leaves behind the distal part of the CBD, which may remain obstructed by residual or recurrent stones. Despite the alternative drainage route, this part can give rise to recurrent infections. ERCP and sphincterotomy should solve this condition, but reoperation and disconnection of the distal CBD, or even conversion to hepaticojejunostomy, may be needed.

Acalculous cholecystitis

Although not a complication of biliary surgery, we mention this entity as it is a biliary complication of other conditions. Usually (but not only) encountered in sick patients, in ICU settings, post-trauma or other operations, acalculous cholecystitis results from the combination of gallbladder distension (secondary to prolonged fasting) and a low-flow state (secondary to hemodynamic instability, pressor support or dehydration). The general condition of the patient usually prevents the possibility of heroic interventions and, if not quickly improved by antibiotics, percutaneous, transhepatic ultrasound-guided drainage is usually achieved. If not available — cholecystectomy may be required, as gangrenous cholecystitis may quickly ensue.

Summing up

After being familiar with the numerous possible complications listed above, you should be able to integrate the information and develop a coherent approach in a patient who is 'not well' after biliary surgery.

The recovery after LC should be 'easy and prompt'. Thus. a non-smooth postoperative course should alert us that something may not be as perfect as we think. **A difficult operation keeps us alert to postoperative problems; it's the 'easy' operation that can numb our surgical instincts and create a false sense of security**. Unexpected pain of unexpected severity, requiring repeated doses of narcotics; tachycardia; fever; abdominal tenderness; and, of course, signs of peritonitis or sepsis — these should all make you uncomfortable, and lead to some investigations — be it just an extra day of observation, or blood tests, or even imaging (ultrasound, CT, HIDA, MRCP) — according to the actual findings. Remember that bile in the peritoneal cavity may be 'silent', and be alert to the soft signs that may help you diagnose it earlier than on day five, when bile pours out of the umbilical wound.

You should by now appreciate the significant difference between **a drain and no-drain situation**. Although not recommended routinely after every cholecystectomy, placing a drain in a high-risk situation for a leak may save your butt, and may save the patient from another procedure. Difficult dissection, inflammatory conditions, edematous tissues, a very wide cystic duct or even if you assisted a junior resident and felt that not all his movements were as you like — a drain in these conditions, removed the next morning if all is well, is not a sin. In fact, it may be a *mitzvah!*

If you diagnose a problem, choosing the **correct route of action** is not always easy, and depends much on local practices, approaches and availability of imaging and interventional modalities. Non-operative management is possible in many situations, but it is mandatory to make the correct diagnosis. Start with the simple, cheap and less invasive tests — blood count and chemistry, ultrasound and a HIDA scan will together give you much of the information you need. CT, MRCP — will be added as needed, and ERCP can be both diagnostic and therapeutic, but is invasive and carries its own risks, so should be used wisely.

Early re-exploration may be suitable for some situations; it may give an early diagnosis and allow for early correction — or at least proper drainage if needed. It should, however, be used selectively, and not as a knee-jerk reaction to every post-op hiccup.

Be alert, attentive, and selective, don't hesitate but don't rush. If you know the potential biliary complications and think about them — in all likelihood you'll be able to prevent them, or treat them successfully. But never be ashamed to consult your local biliary guru.

Chapter 17

The appendix

Moshe Schein

> *Humans can survive easily without an appendix, but surgeons can do so only with difficulty.*
>
> **Rudolph Virchow**

> *It is not true that the appendix is worthless — it has put thousands of surgeons in expensive cars.*

> *If a patient has right lower quadrant pain and no appendectomy scar, put one there.*

Numerous wisecracks exist about the special love-hate relationships between surgeons and the appendix vermiformis so that I could fill the entire chapter with them. And indeed, acute appendicitis (AA) and appendectomies still are 'bread and butter' for us general surgeons. Appendectomy is considered a relatively minor procedure, commonly allocated to trainees and 'low-brow' surgeons — you will rarely find a distinguished 'Herr Professor' wasting his time on such a modest procedure. Also, laypersons do not seem to have too much respect for the humble appendectomy; true, the fear of the nasty *rupture* or *perforation* is deeply entrenched in their collective psyche, but in general they believe that appendectomy is not a 'big deal' and thus expect a smooth postoperative recovery — like after extraction of a non-molar tooth. This is even more so with the rapid ascent of laparoscopic appendectomy (LA), with its enhanced postoperative convalescence.

Table 17.1. Complications of appendectomy reported by members of SURGINET.

'Conventional' complications	Comments
Postoperative bleeding from appendicular artery/mesoappendix	Fatal cases described
Wound infections (superficial SSI)	Can develop also at a lap trocar site (usually the extraction trocar)
Prolonged ileus vs. early postop SBO	
Intra-abdominal or pelvic 'collections' or abscesses (organ/space SSI)	
Infected retrocecal hematoma	Hemostasis crucial!
Necrotizing fasciitis (deep SSI)	Can originate at the wound or trocar site
Cecal fistula	When the cecum is not adequately closed after perforation of the appendix at its base
Post-appendectomy phlegmon of the stump	
Bladder injury	Bladder should be empty before laparoscopic and even open appendectomy
Incisional hernia	More common after midline incision, rare after local RLQ incisions
'Typical' to laparoscopic appendectomy	
Incomplete appendectomy	Often causing recurrent appendicitis
Cecal injury by Endo GIA	
Delayed perforation of cecum	Difficult lap dissection of stump
Appendicular stump leak	This happens when you use clips
Inferior epigastric artery injured by trocar — abdominal wall hematoma	
Terminal ileum confused with appendix and cross-stapled	
Enterotomy	
Aortic injury in a child	Delayed recognition, paraplegia
Bleeding from Endo GIA stapler line	
SBO due to stray staples from a 3.5mm load of Endo GIA stapler	

Alas, life in general is not perfect and appendectomies are associated with a long list of potential complications, some 'minor', others potentially lethal. This is why we decided to dedicate an entire chapter to this little night crawler-like organ.

To start with, we obtained a **real-life perspective** from members of SURGINET (an international online forum of general surgeons), asking them which complications of appendectomy they had personally experienced, or observed over the shoulders of their colleagues. Their replies are summarized in ■ Table 17.1 and seem to encompass common and less common complications of LA and open appendectomy (OA). I will discuss all these complications — both prevention and management. I hope that after reading this chapter our young readers will realize what their older colleagues have learned from bitter experience — that appendectomy is not always a 'piece of cake'; and even if it appears to be so, the cake could fall apart quite easily. Thus, have respect for that rudimentary piece of tissue and acknowledge something which has been said by an unknown surgeon: **"There are two things in life that I will never understand: women and acute appendicitis."**

Pre-operative considerations

> *The proportion of perforated appendicitis is not a good measure of quality. The proportion of perforations may increase because you operate on fewer patients with non-perforated appendicitis. A high proportion of perforations may in fact be a good thing because it means you operate only on those patients who need surgical treatment.*
> **Roland Andersson**

> *As we achieve greater sensitivity in diagnosing appendicitis, we will likely increase the number of patients treated who might otherwise resolve spontaneously. These competing interests: improving diagnostic accuracy to reduce the number of unnecessary (and potentially harmful) operations and, simultaneously, not over-treating patients with appendicitis that may be self-limiting represent the newest challenges in the management of this disease.*
> **Frederick T. Drake and David R. Flum**

As this is not a *manual of surgical therapeutics* but a book on complications, we do not need to stress that optimal diagnosis, pre-op preparation and optimization (as discussed elsewhere in this book) lead to better outcomes. However, one issue has to be discussed in this section.

Is negative appendectomy a complication?

By 'negative' I mean that at operation the appendix is found to be 'white' — **normal**! Negative appendectomy can be further classified:

- Normal appendix with no other pathologies discovered — **unnecessary operation**!
- Normal appendix with another surgical pathology disclosed and treated (e.g. Meckel's diverticulitis) — **therapeutic operation**.
- Normal appendix with **another pathology disclosed and treated that could have been treated without an operation** (e.g. cecal diverticulitis, appendicitis epiploica) — **avoidable therapeutic operation**.

What is a 'normal' appendix? This issue is not always clear. There are various definitions of AA used by pathologists. Some even maintain that it is enough to rub the appendix with your finger, or torture it with your laparoscopic dissector, to produce the inflammatory changes that allow the pathologist to scribble the diagnosis of *early AA*. Some pathologists are loyal to their surgeons and always try to 'confirm' the pre-op diagnosis — have you ever seen a pathology report of a 'normal' gallbladder?

I know of a surgeon who did a 'negative' appendectomy on a patient who had his appendix already removed! **But by 'negative' or 'normal' I mean an absolutely normal appendix observed by you during the operation: not enlarged and not inflamed, not gangrenous, not perforated — nada! You know that it is normal and that the operation you are busy doing is unnecessary** and possibly dangerous. You do not need to wait for the pathology report, hoping the pathologist would comfort you with the words "early AA", so you can tell the family that "it could have ruptured..." **Stop cheating yourself and admit it: the appendix was 'negative' and the operation superfluous!**

Some 'old farts' (and young ones who impersonate the old) do not consider negative appendectomy a complication. In their old books they read that a 15% rate of negative appendectomies reflects cautious surgical judgment. A friend of mine during our training days in Johannesburg used to boast that half of his appendices were 'white'. We did not have any abdominal imaging in those days and he did not want to 'waste' his time by 'keeping and observing' the 'non-classical' cases. **But, fortunately, things have changed and today with the availability of modern abdominal imaging (US and CT), the various scoring systems of AA and, of course, the old understanding that it is safe to observe borderline cases, the rate of negative appendectomy should be well below 5%**. If yours is higher, then there must be something wrong with your practice, your system or perhaps you are simply an impatient 'surgical cowboy'!

Myself, now a lone surgeon serving an entire county, I have not removed a normal appendix during the last seven years. And no, I did not 'miss' or 'delay' any case *in need* of an appendectomy. For more details on our diagnostic approach to AA you can read elsewhere [1], but here I will mention only this: **in this day and age negative appendectomy should be considered as a complication!** It is associated with a non-negligible rate of morbidity and even mortality, and is easily avoided by careful clinical assessment supported by abdominal imaging. **Diagnostic laparoscopy**, popular among assertive surgical souls, is an invasive procedure under general anesthesia which, even if the appendix looks normal, ends usually with an appendectomy. **Yet another unnecessary operation — a complication!**

So now, when you are assured (almost beyond any doubt) that the patient suffers from acute appendicitis do you have to rush him immediately to the operating room? Not always!

Most *adult* patients with AA, unless appearing sick with advanced perforation, can wait until the morning and be operated under more favorable conditions. Appendectomy in the middle of the night, by a sleepy and tired (and non-optimal) surgical team, is increasingly considered an unnecessary ritual. So administer fluids and antibiotics and go back to bed!

What about non-operative management?

The prevailing attitude around the world is that a diseased appendix belongs in the formalin jar. Such a notion is buoyed by deeply entrenched dogmas: (unfounded) fear of progression of mild appendicitis to perforation; fear of litigation, surgeons perceiving that non-operative management is not the accepted standard of care in their communities; the perception that appendectomy (particularly laparoscopic) offers an instant remedy with minimal morbidity; reluctance to subject patients to an assumed prolonged hospitalization and antibiotic treatment, whereas following an uneventful appendectomy for mild AA they usually go home within 24 hours. And there are always the financial motives to consider. However, even strictly salaried surgeons often suffer from the syndrome of *funktionslust* isn't operating more fun than prescribing antibiotics?

---

[1] *Schein's Common Sense Emergency Abdominal Surgery,* 3rd Ed. Springer Verlag, © 2010: Chapter 28.

In reality however — based on solid evidence — a large percentage of AA cases can be treated successfully without an operation but with antibiotics (like acute diverticulitis). **This would be reasonable and reduce morbidity in the following categories of patients**:

- Patients with a prohibitive surgical-anesthetic risk (e.g. post-myocardial infarction) — those are the type of patients who decorate the mortality lists after appendectomy.
- Patients who refuse an operation.
- Patients in the middle of the Pacific Ocean, on a space ship or nuclear submarine, or in rural locations where a surgeon is not available.
- Patients who present with *resolving* symptoms, their assumed mild AA getting better when seen by the surgeon.
- Morbidly obese patients.
- Pregnant women (first trimester) with mild AA, where any operation may induce abortion.
- Patients with pure 'CT AA': an inflamed appendix visualized on CT but no clinical/laboratory evidence of systemic inflammation and minimal local signs.
- **Obviously, patients with an *appendiceal* mass or *phlegmon* should be managed non-operatively. This is accepted by most surgeons and is no longer controversial!**

Careful clinical assessment, augmented by imaging (or clinical scoring systems, if imaging is not available) should distinguish between the 'mild cases', which are mostly amenable to non-operative treatment (notably, many instances of mild appendicitis may resolve spontaneously without any treatment at all) and the gangrenous or perforated ones which are not likely to resolve and mandate an operation.

Last thing: when the decision to operate has been made, **do not forget to administer antibiotics**. During the operation you will decide whether the antibiotics will be considered *prophylactic* or *therapeutic* (see below and ➲ Chapters 4 and 5).

Intra-operative considerations

> *The appendix is generally attached to the cecum.*
> **Mark M. Ravitch**

I will postpone discussion of the intra-operative minutiae to the next section, where specific post-appendectomy complications will be listed and scrutinized. However, two 'operative' topics have to be mentioned here: the OA vs. LA controversy and the choice of incisions.

Lap versus open appendectomy

This is not controversial anymore. Numerous comparative studies, when taken together, reveal that LA achieves exactly the same outcomes as OA but is associated with reduced postoperative pain, earlier discharge (a few hours) and more rapid return to full activities (a few days); the rate of wound infections is also lower after LA. Some series claim that LA for **perforated appendicitis** is associated with an increased rate of intra-abdominal infections but other reports dispute this notion. It is no wonder then that LA has been enthusiastically adopted as the procedure of choice wherever surgeons have a video camera and lap instruments — from Boston to Bombay (sorry, Mumbai). Just look at YouTube — it seems that anyone who has a video camera is compelled to boast of his own dexterity with LA by posting a well-edited clip! (Can you find any clip posted by a surgeon who can remove an appendix with his fingers through a 3-6cm incision?).

I believe however that *overall*, **LA is more prone to serious complications — is more potentially dangerous than OA**. "This is not what the literature shows" you may claim but, as we all know, the **literature is biased**: randomized studies comparing LA to OA are not performed by laparoscopic *amateurs*, and surgeons are not keen to publish their disasters — would you write a case report describing how you damaged the aorta during LA? Would you post it on YouTube? ☺ So, in the 'real world', complications tend to go unreported or 'excluded' from the otherwise 'excellent results'. But looking around us, and reading between the lines, we perceive a long list of complications (some bizarre) which are more typical of LA, complications almost unseen in the good old days (see ■ Figure 17.1). I do not talk only about complications inherent to laparoscopy (e.g. trocar injury to the inferior epigastric vessel) but also about direct complications of the act of appendectomy. Can you recall a surgeon failing to remove the whole appendix during OA? Well, with LA, this has become not so uncommon. **This is not a tirade against LA: I do not claim that LA is an inferior procedure and that OA is preferable. I am just trying to warn you that LA is more prone to mishaps, especially if performed by a lone, inexperienced lap surgeon in the middle of the night; and the surgeon is reluctant to convert when facing difficulties**.

Talking about conversion to OA, it is my impression that the young generation of surgeons who are obsessed with laparoscopy have lost the skills of doing a difficult OA through a small RLQ incision. And this brings us to the next item: **the choice of incision(s)**.

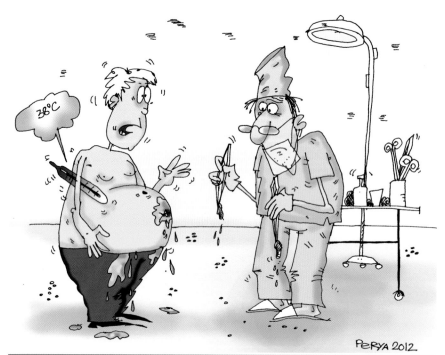

Figure 17.1. "Doc, you told me that laparoscopic appendectomy is safe."

Choice of incision for OA

There is no doubt that the classical RLQ muscle-splitting incision, centered on McBurney's point — you can incise the skin obliquely or transversely — is 'easier' on the patient and is associated with fewer early and late wound or abdominal wall complications than vertical incisions such as the midline or the paramedian.

I do not recall a single appendectomy which I could not successfully accomplish through a 'local' RLQ incision — including when the tip of the appendix lay near the gallbladder or when cecal resection proved to be necessary. When additional exposure is needed one has simply to extend the incision either medially or laterally, cutting the muscles if necessary. In my mind, a midline incision should be considered only when other pathologies, which cannot be accessed through the RLQ incision, are disclosed (e.g. perforated peptic ulcer, perforated sigmoid diverticulitis). **However, in this era of pre-operative imaging and/or laparoscopy, such surprise diagnoses should be rarities!**

So why do we still observe, hear and read about surgeons doing appendectomies through midline incisions?

One reason: when the surgeon decides to convert from LA to OA (usually for technical difficulties, often reflecting complicated AA) he intuitively does it by 'connecting' the infra-umbilical trocar site with the suprapubic one, thus creating a mega-midline laparotomy.

Second reason: the 'modern' laparoscopic surgeon is trained to 'see it all' — he needs to *see* any drop of pus in order to suck it out. The notion of converting to a limited RLQ incision to continue successfully the hitherto failed LA is counter-intuitive to him.

And thus the patient is punished with a long midline incision — more pain, longer recuperation, a higher incidence of SSI, dehiscence, and late hernia formation — while a smallish, local RLQ incision would suffice. **My advice to the young surgeon: learn to master difficult OAs. Mentors: from time to time, let your disciples start with OA rather than LA, especially when dealing with perforated AA**.

Postoperative considerations

In this section I will outline the complications listed in ■ Table 17.1 and discuss their prevention and management.

But first, **remember: always think outside the box!** One surgeon told us about a case he had: just before discharge, 24 hours following an 'easy' LA for simple AA, the young patient developed an acute abdomen with diffuse peritonitis. No, it was not leakage from a poorly occluded appendiceal stump but a perforated peptic ulcer. **After surgery, anything can happen!**

Before we start with infective complications, here are a few words about **postoperative antibiotics**. The *duration* of postoperative administration has been discussed in ⟳ Chapter 4. Here is a reminder:

- **'Negative' appendectomy or simple appendicitis** — no need for postop antibiotics. However, we won't condemn you for giving one or two postop doses.
- **Gangrenous appendicitis**. A day or two suffices.
- **Perforated appendicitis**. Rarely more than five days.

You could switch antibiotics from i.v. to oral as soon as the patient tolerates food and is ready to go home. In some countries (e.g. USA), you may decide to prolong the course in order to hinder potential litigators even if the evidence suggests that prolonged administration is unnecessary. This is the price we pay when forced to practice 'defensive medicine'…

Wound complications

- **Wound infections** (superficial SSI) are the most common complication of appendectomy. The more advanced the AA, the longer the incision, the fatter the patient (and so forth — see ⮫ Chapter 5) — the greater the chance of developing this complication. Logically, wound infections are less common after LA but can develop at any port site — especially the one used for extraction of the appendix (use an endobag!).
- **Deep SSI**: are rare but well described, including *necrotizing fasciitis* developing at a port site after LA for simple AA. Necrotizing fasciitis has been described originating even from an appendectomy wound which has been left open! **Never say never — always suspect and check everything**.

Details about prevention and management of wound infection please find in ⮫ Chapter 5. I suture ALL my post-appendectomy wounds; in 'dirty' cases I insert 'wicks' into the wounds for 2-3 days. Adhering to the principles outlined here and in ⮫ Chapters 4 and 5, the rate of wound infection in your patients should be negligible — as is mine ☺.

Intra-abdominal or pelvic 'collections' or abscesses (organ/space SSI)

This group of entities represents a *spectrum* which tends to be confused by clinicians and the literature — lumped together under the definition of "abscess". The spectrum ranges as follows:

- **Non-infected intraperitoneal fluid collections**. An example: a child underwent appendectomy for gangrenous AA. Four days later he is still spiking a temperature. Somebody ordered a CT which shows free fluid in the pelvis. Antibiotics are continued and the child recovers. The case is included in a published case series entitled: "Post-appendectomy pelvic abscess treated with antibiotics." Obviously, in such a case the fluid collection was not a walled-off abscess, and it may not have been 'infected' at all — the fever representing residual SIRS.
- **Infected intraperitoneal fluid collections**. Another example: a young adult with perforated AA and diffuse purulent peritonitis was treated

with LA. On postoperative day five there is still significant SIRS and ileus. CT shows a well-defined collection around the cecum. The patient continues to receive antibiotics: SIRS and ileus resolve within a few days. This fluid collection may have been infected (we will never know) but **not all infected fluid collections need to be drained — they commonly resolve thanks to the peritoneal defense mechanisms assisted by antibiotics**.

- **Intraperitoneal abscess**. Let us assume that the above mentioned patient does not improve on antibiotics. Three days later we repeat the CT, which now shows that the fluid collection has an 'enhancing rim' — an abscess. We proceed with CT-guided drainage, 25cc of pus is evacuated. SIRS resolves and ileus subsides.

- **Multiple intra-abdominal abscesses**. This is a consequence of advanced AA, associated with a prolonged and serious morbidity — requiring treatment with repeated percutaneous drainage or a reoperation.

For how to diagnose and treat intra-abdominal infection see ⟳ Chapter 4 or consult our other book [2]. Below is some advice about prevention specific to AA.

Both OA and LA should include the principles of 'source control' (appendectomy) and 'peritoneal toilet' (⟳ Chapter 4). **However, I believe that accomplishing these tasks laparoscopically is susceptible to more pitfalls and a higher rate of intra-abdominal infective complications** — as suggested by the literature and what we see in the 'real world'. *First*, during LA the appendix is more likely to be ruptured or macerated leading to contamination — the simple AA becoming 'perforated' by the surgeon. *Second*, the prevalent obsession of laparoscopists to 'irrigate/wash everything' is the cause of the postoperative fluid collections and abscesses! **Yes — the fluid collections represent the saline that you've instilled within the abdomen and didn't suck out completely.**

An old aphorism by Mark M. Ravitch is relevant even today: "The surgeon who can describe the extent of an appendiceal peritonitis has convicted himself of performing an improper operation." He implied (there was no laparoscopy at that time) that appendectomies are better done through a local RLQ incision, even when the peritonitis is diffuse. His point was that you don't need to actually see the pus in order to deal with it. You remove the appendix and insert the *Poole* sucker (gently!) and suck the right gutter, the pelvis, and all around. And then you mop everything with moist gauze pads. **You can**

---

[2] *Schein's Common Sense Emergency Abdominal Surgery*, 3rd Ed. Springer Verlag, © 2010: Chapters 49 and 52.

accomplish a **perfect peritoneal toilet through a 5cm McBurney incision**. If you *see* each drop of pus that you're sucking out, it means that you did too much — a midline incision, for example.

LA in cases of perforated AA when combined with generous peritoneal irrigation is 'too much' as well — and potentially harmful. **It spreads pus and bacteria from the RLQ, and the lower abdomen, all over the peritoneal cavity**. And then, if the surgeon does not suck out all fluid, collections and abscesses may develop. I do mostly OAs, only through a McBurney incision; I never irrigate or wash! Over the last 20 years I had a single patient who required percutaneous drainage of an intraperitoneal abscess in the aftermath of perforated AA. I never saw a 'collection'! **Dedicated laparoscopic surgeons who do not irrigate during LA share a similar experience — no collections, no abscesses!** Those who irrigate experience abscesses even after LA for simple AA. If you ask again: "where is the evidence? The literature does not talk about such things...", then you better not read this chapter, nor is this book for you.

Drains after OA or LA — do they prevent collections and abscesses? No, no, no! Please do not raise my blood pressure! Studies and experience taught us that they are useless. They prevent nothing, they only contribute to complications (⮕ Chapter 4).

Prolonged ileus vs. early postoperative small bowel obstruction

Between you and me, an ileus of 4-5 days after appendectomy for perforated AA cannot be considered a complication. But to the patient of the iPhone generation, who expects to be at home a day after the operation — sharing pizza with his girlfriend — but instead has to linger in the hospital with a nasogastric tube emerging from his left nostril, it represents a major complication.

The more advanced the AA, the more traumatic the procedure, the more prolonged the ileus may be. Occasionally, what initially appears to be an ileus actually is early postoperative small bowel obstruction (EPSBO). For a comprehensive discourse on this topic go to ⮕ Chapter 8.

Bleeding complications (see also ⮕ Chapter 3)

From my medical school days I remember a little boy who developed profound shock a day after OA. At reoperation his abdomen was full of blood. I was then so impressed by the attending surgeon's instant clinical diagnosis and the rush to the operating room that I decided to become a surgeon!

Luckily, since that day — more than 30 years ago — I have never experienced a post-appendectomy hemorrhage. But I have had a few 'near misses' and I am obsessed with meticulous hemostasis during appendectomy. I like to overrun the mesoappendix with a locking suture of 3-0 Vicryl®. But, of course, you can use whatever people are using these days: clips, Endo GIA™, Harmonic Scalpel®, LigaSure™ or even 'only' diathermy. **As you know — you can get away with anything — almost anything**…

The source of bleeding after appendectomy may be the appendicular artery, smaller vessels at the divided mesoappendix or abdominal wall vessels injured during insertion of laparoscopic trocars.

Deaths due to missed bleeding after appendectomy (more common after LA!) have been reported — oh what a prosaic and easily avoidable tragedy! **How to prevent it?**

Always, always after the completion of the appendectomy, after the cecum has been dropped down to its natural position, check yet again for hemostasis. The partial evisceration of the cecum and the appendix attached to it during OA, or its retraction forward and laterally during LA, places the blood supply on tension and may interrupt the blood flow, thus concealing bleeding. When the cecum is repositioned, its circulation recovers and bleeding from the divided artery or the meso may declare itself!

Therefore, I repeat, always, always recheck hemostasis *after* the cecum is back in place. At LA, suck again, look again: any bleeding? During OA, after the cecum has dropped back you cannot see it anymore. Before closing, suck again around the cecum with the Poole sucker, insert/remove a 4x4 gauze — look at its color. Do it again. If still RED, reinsert the retractors, re-expose the cecum and see what's bleeding. Usually it is a small 'pumper' (at LA it is often from the Endo GIA™ stapler line). A suture, a clip… makes it a 'near miss' — you have avoided embarrassment or disaster.

Now suck out the remaining blood. Old blood is an excellent culture medium for bacteria, becoming an infected hematoma or abscess. No, there is no need to *wash* out the old blood ☺.

Appendicular stump complications

Yes, that humble remnant of flimsy tissue which you have ligated, sutured, stapled, clipped, sealed, burned — however you have tortured it (my own practice is to transfix the stump at the level of the cecum with a 2-0 Vicryl® suture, taking a bite in the cecal wall as well) — can be the source of a range of complications.

Phlegmon of the stump

This can develop even in a 'perfect' stump abutting the cecum. Your patient had an uneventful appendectomy. Seven days later he returns with right lower quadrant pain and tenderness, a temperature and leukocytosis. The wound looks fine. This is a typical presentation of an appendix stump phlegmon. Nowadays the diagnosis is straightforward: a CT will demonstrate a *phlegmon* which involves the cecum — as opposed to a drainable abscess. A few days of antibiotic therapy will cure this relatively rare complication, which is not mentioned by standard texts.

The 'viral' spread of LA has increased the spectrum of stump complications: what previously had been the subject of esoteric case reports is being seen all over the place:

- **Stump leakage.** *Faulty closure of the stump* (studies in rats… and a few patients in India… 'proved' that clips or even thermal energy can adequately seal the stump… but this does not mean that you want to try it on your own patients!) leads to leak of appendicular contents resulting in an abscess or fecal fistula. Diagnosis is clinical assessment supplemented by CT; use your common sense for treatment decisions: percutaneous drainage and/or reoperation.
- **Stump appendicitis.** Patients can develop classical acute appendicitis at any time after appendectomy. Historically this rarely followed OA for complicated appendicitis, often by a relatively inexperienced family doctor/surgeon under adverse conditions. It has now become more common in the era of laparoscopic appendectomy, when during the procedure surgeons may misidentify the cecal base of the appendix and consequently leave a long appendiceal stump (partial or hemi-appendectomy). Patients and their physicians, and even emergency room docs, are not aware that AA can develop after the "appendix had been removed" and thus the diagnosis is often missed or delayed. A colleague told me about a patient who had undergone LA in another center (remember: complications always occur 'elsewhere' ☺). Subsequently, he presented to various doctors and centers with 13 (!) documented attacks of RLQ pain, tenderness, raised white cells and C-reactive protein. The patient had six (!) CTs before somebody (my colleague) diagnosed the stump appendicitis and treated it laparoscopically. Obviously, laparoscopic re-appendectomy may be difficult and result in **cecal complications** (see the next item).

The way to avoid stump complications during LA is to deal with the stump as accurately as is done during OA. The Endoloop® or the Endo GIA™ — whatever you use — has to be placed at the base of the appendix. **You have to visualize the appendix-cecal junction**. If you can't then convert! Leaving a long appendicular stump is *litigable*…

Cecal complications

In the days of OA, cecal complications occurred mainly in cases where the appendix had perforated just at its base — with the inflammation/perforation involving the cecal wall — leaving no proper stump for safe closure. Nowadays, laparoscopic dissection — especially in difficult/advanced cases, applying sources of energy near the cecal wall, or misfiring the Endo GIA™ — has increased the danger to the cecal wall. **The cecum can leak 'early' or even after five days (delayed thermal injury), presenting with a spectrum of sepsis, local phlegmon, abscess, peritonitis, and fecal fistula.**

Prevention: in general, **respect the cecum** — try not to brutalize it during OA or LA. When the appendix is perforated just at its junction with the cecum, fire a linear stapler across and *proximal* to its base, **including the cecum at the stapler line**. This can also be done laparoscopically. Take care not to harm or narrow the nearby ileocecal valve. If you do not have staplers, excise a disk of the cecum around the base of the appendix and close with sutures using your basic anastomotic technique.

What to do if you find the **appendix and cecum matted together within a gross inflammatory phlegmon?** The first thing you should do is to curse yourself and admit that you were stupid, for an appendiceal phlegmon/mass can and should be diagnosed before the operation and treated conservatively (as mentioned above). **Now you have two options**: to *abort*, close up and treat the patient with antibiotics or to *proceed* (I bet that your ego will drive you to take the second option). If appendectomy seems unsafe then a segmental cecectomy with ileocolic anastomosis is the obvious solution. Anyone who has a personal series of more than 2-3 cecectomies or right hemicolectomies for AA is much too aggressive.

Injury to adjacent organs

Such tragic (if not comic) mishaps are typically associated with the laparoscopic procedure and are addressed in ⊃ Chapter 9. Injuries to the small bowel, ureter, aorta and iliac vessels and of course the cecum have been described during (careless) LC. A few years ago I allowed a chief resident to take a junior resident through an OA. Half an hour into the procedure I was summoned from the tea room: "what should we do?" They were looking into the inside of the **urinary bladder! Always make sure that the patient has voided just before taking him to the OR!**

Mistaken diagnosis

Mistaken diagnoses were not uncommon in the pre-CT era. Those of us who do not use pre-op CT or use it sparingly will from time to time encounter not only a 'white' appendix but other pathologies responsible for the clinical presentation. Most such *mimicking* conditions could have been managed without an operation, but encountering them at surgery, while the patient is under general anesthesia, often goads the surgeon to *escalate* the procedure, to do more, with new potential complications. For example:

- **Perforated cecal diverticulitis**. Like sigmoid diverticulitis it can be managed conservatively. Confronting it at surgery usually prompts cecectomy.
- **Acute sigmoid diverticulitis**. Remember: the sigmoid can lie to the right of the midline. What would you do if you are surprised by the finding of non-perforated sigmoid diverticulitis during an appendectomy? Would you abort or escalate? You know the right answer!

The list continues: Meckel's diverticulitis, inflammatory pelvic disease, even ruptured ectopic pregnancy and so forth. This chapter is already too long and I have to stop. **The bottom line: having an accurate pre-operative diagnosis by obtaining an accurate road map (imaging!) is of great value. Why not use it?**

Legal considerations

Even the lowly appendix is a not uncommon source of malpractice litigation. The stated reasons for litigation in order of frequency are:

- Faulty technique (e.g. hemi-appendectomy, injury to adjacent structures).
- Misdiagnosis or delay in diagnosis.
- Operating room delays (e.g. your boss wants to finish his elective-private list…).
- Inadequate follow-up and failure to recognize/treat the complications.

I am hopeful, that after reading this chapter and ➲ Chapter 10, you will never have to defend an appendectomy case.

> "So I might have the immense privilege of relieving the pain, anguish, and threat to a wonderful small boy by making an incision in the right lower quadrant of his abdomen and taking out a pus-filled appendix skillfully and safely, my first operation… I felt that this was both a miracle and a privilege. I still do."
>
> Francis D. Moore

Chapter 18

The pancreas

Gregory Sergeant, Mickaël Lesurtel and Pierre-Alain Clavien

---

*God put the pancreas in the back because he did not want
surgeons messing with it.*

Ever since the first reports of pancreatic resection appeared, pancreatic
surgery has been considered an area of surgery that has to be kept well away
from residents in training. It is true that pancreatic surgery is associated with
a high rate of complications (i.e. most series report frequencies between 25
and 60%). However, the great majority of these complications can be
managed conservatively — without the need for reoperation. Nevertheless,
these complications impact profoundly on the length of hospital stay,
postoperative recovery and the general condition of the patient. In oncological
settings this often delays adjuvant chemotherapy or makes it impossible
altogether. The management of complications after pancreatic surgery
requires some expertise. **Indeed, it has been shown that there is a good
correlation between center volume and surgeon experience and
outcomes after surgery, and this is true especially with pancreatic
resection**. Clearly, experience and additional resources are needed to salvage
patients who develop septic and bleeding complications as a consequence of
pancreatic leaks and fistulas.

"Ductal adenocarcinoma of the pancreas is an incurable disease," said
Michael Trede, with some justification. And indeed, there are not a few
surgeons who adopt a *nihilistic* attitude concerning patients diagnosed with
this disease. On the other hand, there are the 'macho-type' surgeons who

believe that chopping out a pancreas after breakfast each morning is a mark of a great surgeon (■ Figure 18.1). But we do not want you to be nihilistic or macho — we want you to use your common sense.

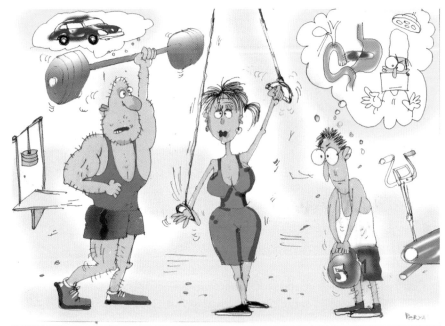

Figure 18.1. At the gym. Macho 1: "I drive a Porsche..." Macho 2: "I do a Whipple each morning!"

> Surgeons operating on pancreatic cancer today can be classified into three groups: the 'aggressive-radical' surgeon who will always attempt major extirpative procedures with resection of major vessels and vascular reconstruction; the 'nihilist-timid' surgeon who avoids getting involved in complex time-consuming risky procedures; and the 'rational' surgeon who will tailor the operation to the stage of the disease, and the patient's general condition and the ability to tolerate the operation.
>
> **Abdool R. Moosa**

Pre-operative considerations

> He who fails to plan is planning to fail.
>
> **Winston S. Churchill**

Resectability and operability

One of the most important ways to avoid complications after pancreatic surgery is to select those patients anatomically amenable to R0 resection (i.e. **resectable**) and who are not overly debilitated so they can tolerate such a major operation (i.e. **operable**).

Borderline resectability of pancreatic cancers may be classified according to the definition by Katz and colleagues at the MD Anderson Cancer Center [1]. **Borderline resectable tumors are those that abut the superior mesenteric artery (SMA), abut or encase the common hepatic artery over a short segment, or occlude the superior mesenteric vein (SMV)-portal vein (PV) axis with a suitable vein above and below such that a venous reconstruction is possible.** Some of these patients may actually profit from a neoadjuvant multimodal treatment strategy including systemic chemotherapy and perhaps loco-regional radiotherapy to downstage the tumor. It is notable that these therapies do not necessarily result in radiological downstaging, because of the difficulty in differentiating between tumor and fibrosis. For surgeons who are not familiar with vascular resection and reconstruction in pancreatic surgery, it is wise to refer these patients to expert centers that are familiar with this complex surgery.

In addition to this 'anatomical' group, two additional borderline resectable patient groups may be defined: those who have **questionable metastatic disease** and those patients with a **suboptimal performance status** or extensive medical comorbidity requiring prolonged work-up that precludes immediate major abdominal surgery. The latter considerations refer to the *operability* of the patient.

Patients with indeterminate or questionable metastatic disease may benefit from systemic chemotherapy first. This provides the opportunity to evaluate the natural history of the disease and avoids performing high-risk surgery in patients with systemic disease and an unfavorable prognosis. Similarly, for example, it is common for patients with pancreatic cancer to have a smoking history. These patients are therefore at increased risk of cardiovascular comorbidities that may need treatment first (e.g. coronary stenting). Another very common scenario is the *cachectic* patient who has recently been diagnosed with pancreatic head adenocarcinoma after a 15kg weight loss over three months. **These severely malnourished patients have a high incidence of postoperative complications and it seems logical that every effort be made to improve their nutritional and immunological status prior to pancreatic surgery, with the aim of avoiding a great amount of peri-operative morbidity.**

---

[1]   Katz MH, *et al*. Borderline resectable pancreatic cancer: the importance of this emerging stage of disease. *J Am Coll Surg* 2008; 206: 833-48.

Exploratory laparoscopy

> Back in 2004, I was fortunate to spend a few weeks at the Johns Hopkins, known as the Mecca of pancreatic surgery. I was delighted to see the great John Cameron at work. I remember he was starting a case in a patient with an adenocarcinoma of the head of the pancreas and performing a large midline laparotomy to realize a fraction later that even the 'greatest' surgeon may be confronted with peritoneal carcinomatosis. **GS**

In spite of all the studies around, we still proclaim a pragmatic approach regarding diagnostic laparoscopy in pancreatic surgery. For proven adenocarcinoma (especially in borderline resectable cases) or high suspicion thereof (e.g. a large mucinous cystadenoma), in the absence of jaundice (or if the patient already has a biliary stent in place), we recommend starting any planned pancreatectomy with a **diagnostic laparoscopy. These patients will be spared an unnecessary laparotomy if peritoneal carcinomatosis or previously undetected liver metastases are revealed**. In patients with obstructive jaundice, failed ERCP and stenting, and those with gastric outlet obstruction, we do not start with diagnostic laparoscopy, **because in these patients we would consider doing a palliative bypass anyway**. The assessment of local resectability is difficult during diagnostic laparoscopy; however, if the *ligament of Treitz* or the *mesenteric root* seems to be involved, the likelihood of mesenteric artery abutment, encasement or invasion is very high. In any event this information is usually known from pre-operative imaging.

Jaundice

New evidence refutes the classic dogma that operating on jaundiced patients results in more complications. **There is generally no need for pre-operative ERCP and stenting in obstructive jaundice unless the patient presents with cholangitis, intense pruritus or organ failure (often renal failure) necessitating treatment and resulting in a delay to surgery. Indeed, pre-operative stenting is associated with more infectious complications peri-operatively, often because of contamination of the biliary tract**. Nevertheless, the experienced surgeon knows that surgery in severely jaundiced patients is often more difficult and is associated with more diffuse oozing of blood, especially when dissecting the hepatoduodenal ligament. In addition, such patients are often referred to you with a stent already in place — surgeons like to operate, gastroenterologists like to insert stents...

Chronic pancreatitis

Surgery for chronic pancreatitis is in a league of its own. **The chronic inflammation may lead to profound scarring and obliteration of all common anatomical planes, including the bursa omentalis (lesser sac), the retropancreatic tunnel in contact with the SMV and the hepatoduodenal ligament**. Furthermore, it is not rare that these patients suffer from **segmental portal hypertension** because of splenic vein thrombosis or portal vein stenosis, which increases the risk of intra-operative bleeding. Therefore, we believe that if a surgeon does not do a lot of pancreatic surgery, he should stay far away from chronic pancreatitis. Although the intra-operative course is often complicated with increased blood loss, the postoperative course generally goes well.

Recent acute pancreatitis

I tell patients that the pancreas is like somebody's wife: she doesn't need a reason to be pissed off and, once she is, you had better just lay low and not touch her until she feels like being in a better mood.

Karen Draper

Acute pancreatitis may complicate ERCP with papillotomy for bile duct drainage, and less frequently after tumor biopsy. Earlier in the chapter we summarized our very selective indications for ERCP. **Also, we do not generally recommend performing biopsies or fine-needle aspiration of pancreatic lesions unless they are cystic**. With modern imaging (e.g. triple-phase contrast computed tomography, contrast-enhanced MRI and DOTATATE-PET [2] scans), it has become easier to correctly differentiate lesions in the pancreas without the need for invasive endoscopic procedures or biopsies. **A recent acute pancreatitis may render a surgeon's life miserable during the resection. In the event of an acute pancreatitis after ERCP or biopsy, we recommend delaying the scheduled pancreatectomy for a few weeks**. In some severe cases, it may preclude future resection and even lead to premature death of the patient. Management of the complications of acute pancreatitis (such as infected pancreatic necrosis) is beyond the scope of this chapter.

---

[2] Ga-68 DOTATATE-PET — a new somatostatin analog.

Portal vein stenosis or occlusion

Be prepared for considerable blood loss.

Portal vein stenosis or occlusion is usually caused by tumor encasement, true tumoral invasion (rather rare) or post-radiotherapy fibrosis. However, this does not automatically preclude resection if the segment to be resected is not too long (ideally less than 3cm) and if the proximal segment of the SMV is still open. More important is whether the outflow distal to this stenosis or occlusion is preserved. If the outflow (e.g. cavernous transformation of the hilar part of the portal vein) is not preserved, the risk of postoperative mesenteric vein thrombosis is dramatically increased.

Another problem associated with severe stenosis or occlusion is the generation of a venous collateral circulation (segmental portal hypertension), leading to increased intra-operative blood loss.

Intra-operative considerations

Intra-operative bleeding

If it were not for the frightful hemorrhage which so frequently attends them, operations would be robbed of nearly all their terror, and few men would shrink from their performance.
Samuel Gross

When working in close proximity to large vascular structures it is not unimaginable to end up, once in a while, with sudden massive bleeding from one of these sources: the hepatic artery, portal vein, superior mesenteric vein and superior mesenteric artery with its branches to the uncinate process and jejunum. **The bleeding most frequently originates from a tear in the portal or mesenteric vein either during retropancreatic tunneling or during dissection of the uncinate process from the portal vein**. Our advice: don't panic! Control the bleeding by compression of the vessel proximally and distally with a sponge stick by your assistant. Next, fix the source of bleeding under vision — give it one try! **If you fail, call a more experienced colleague to help you** (now you understand the advantage of doing such cases in a dedicated center!). Don't start blindly placing sutures, clips or vascular clamps…

The soft pancreas

I'm tired of all this nonsense about beauty being skin deep. That's deep enough. What do you want, an adorable pancreas?

J. Kerr

A normal and soft pancreas remains the pancreatic surgeon's greatest enemy. It is far from adorable. The good thing is that the attentive surgeon can almost always predict from pre-operative imaging when the pancreatic texture will be soft with a small pancreatic duct. In duodenal, neuroendocrine or small distal bile duct tumors, the pancreatic duct remains small and the pancreas usually keeps its soft texture. In such cases, when suturing the **pancreatic anastomosis**, you should be at your gentlest, taking care not to readjust your needle when it's in the pancreas and not tearing your suture through the tissue when tying. **We believe that a duct-to-mucosa pancreaticojejunostomy is the best anastomotic technique in a soft pancreas**; however, if you don't do pancreatic surgery often, it might be better to stick to the technique that you're most comfortable with. Indeed, the diversity of reported techniques used is endless and none has repeatedly been shown to be superior to the others. **In patients with a soft pancreas, we recommend draining the pancreatico-enterostomy because of the high risk of postoperative pancreatic fistula (10-30%).**

Extended vs. locoregional lymphadenectomy

Whether to perform an extended or a locoregional lymphadenectomy is an old discussion. Extended lymphadenectomy is not associated with improved survival, but it is associated with increased postoperative morbidity and may therefore delay initiation of adjuvant chemotherapy. Of course, you may resect enlarged or PET-positive lymph nodes outside the locoregional field. But you should bear in mind that positive inter-aortocaval lymph nodes from cancer of the head and positive celiac trunk lymph nodes from tumors of the body and tail are actually considered to be M1 disease with a poor prognosis. **Therefore, don't be excessive in the extent of your lymphadenectomy.** Remember: the patient does not benefit from the massive chylous ascites or therapy-resistant diarrhea which may result from extensive celiac dissection.

Portal vein resection

Before engaging in portal vein resection and reconstruction, we like to control all the afferent and efferent venous branches. It is equally important to mobilize the mesenteric root in order to avoid traction when performing an end-to-end anastomosis. If a long segment (>3cm) is resected or, despite mesenteric mobilization, excessive tension at the anastomosis still exists, it's wise to use an *interposition graft*. We prefer to use an autologous (e.g. external iliac vein, left renal vein) or homologous venous graft over a synthetic prosthesis. Whether or not the splenic vein should be routinely reimplanted after resection of the portosplenic junction is unclear. To forgo reimplantation of the splenic vein may decrease portal venous flow, possibly contributing to an increased risk of postoperative thrombosis. Another risk of splenic vein ligation is the development of gastric varices and a 30% chance of UGI bleeding if the patient survives for long.

To drain or not to drain?

The evidence is limited in spite of what your 'experienced' colleagues may claim. Most centers routinely leave one or two *low-suction* drains in the vicinity of the pancreatic and bile duct anastomoses. Others have shown comparable or even reduced postoperative pancreatic fistula rates with the use of *passive drainage* or no drain at all. **However, when we lie in bed at night (yes, even HPB surgeons have to sleep sometimes), we have never regretted leaving in a drain**.

We usually place one or two BLAKE® radiopaque silicone drains, unless the pancreas is hard and atrophic, and the pancreatic duct is large. In those patients we do not leave in a drain and, as previously mentioned, in this situation the leakage rate should be lower than 5%. Another reason to leave a drain (albeit an academic one, despite this being a pragmatic book), is that the International Study Group of Pancreatic Fistula (ISGPF) has defined postoperative pancreatic fistulas based on the drain/plasma amylase ratio >3 on postoperative day three. This is until now the most commonly used classification system.

Postoperative considerations

> *Know your enemy and know yourself and you can fight a hundred battles without disaster.*
>
> **Sun Tzu, The Art of War**

Pancreatic fistula

You've performed a Whipple three days ago in an obese 65-year-old patient with an ampullary carcinoma. The amylase level in the drain is 200U/L, while it is 70 in the blood. You want to take the drain out; however, your senior resident reminds you that the pancreas was soft. Indeed, you commented after the procedure that you had just made an anastomosis in 'butter' and you pulled out two sutures while tying the posterior wall of the pancreaticojejunostomy. You're the boss so you decide to take the drain out anyway. At five days postoperatively, your patient develops a low-grade fever and vomits three times. You start a gastroprokinetic agent and i.v. antibiotics. His fever resolves. The evening before discharge he develops sudden abdominal pain, hematemesis and hypovolemic shock. You call your interventional radiologist. Twenty minutes later (already in the arteriography suite), the patient has no palpable pulse.

The most feared complication after pancreatectomy is pancreatic fistula. Not just because of the prolonged postoperative course it is associated with, but rather **because it can be the cause of uncontrolled abdominal sepsis and acute postoperative hemorrhage** — the latter being the most frequent cause of postoperative mortality after any type of pancreatectomy (that is independent of underlying comorbidities!).

The difficulty in managing pancreatic fistula often lies in its timely diagnosis. When patients have drains, increased amylase levels provide sufficient proof. However, in some cases, patients may develop postoperative septic signs (e.g. fever >38°C and tachycardia), gastroparesis and abdominal discomfort. One strategy could be to just start antibiotics empirically, add some prokinetics and remain in denial of a potential severe complication. **A safer strategy would be to stick to the principle of SOURCE CONTROL and perform an abdominal CT scan to look for undrained collections, take blood and urine cultures, check lines... early on.** Indeed, undrained collections are a major risk factor for acute bleeding due to erosion of the gastroduodenal artery stump, hepatic artery or splenic artery stump (the latter in the case of distal pancreatectomy). **Therefore, these collections should be drained as soon as possible by the interventional radiologist.** Due to the frequent dorsal location of these undrained collections, this may be difficult or impossible, requiring **surgical drainage**. Obviously, only fools would be tempted to try and redo the pancreatic anastomosis!

However, most of the time, if you are careful and you keep the intra-operatively placed drains *in situ* (because the amylase levels in the drain were high at postoperative day three and five), these well-contained pancreatic fistulas can generally be managed conservatively. **In fact, amylase-rich drain fluid is usually clear during the first postoperative day and becomes greenish (little enteric backflow) or grayish (peri-anastomotic necrosis) at postoperative day four or five.** If the fistula is well drained, your patient may stay asymptomatic, eat and even go home with his drain. In the case of a *pancreaticogastrostomy*, a Salem nasogastric tube (connected to wall suction) to keep the stomach empty may reduce the fistula output. In both situations you will then progressively shorten the drain until the fistula dries up (this may take a few weeks). **Conservative management may suffice in 80% of pancreatic fistulas.**

Occasionally, in cases where the leak is associated with an abscess or collection which is not reachable by a percutaneous route, a relaparotomy is necessary. Although advocated by some, we are very reluctant to perform *completion pancreatectomy* as the mortality rate of this procedure in this particular setting is extremely high. **We prefer to drain extensively, striving for improved control of the fistula.**

Pancreatic fistula after distal pancreatectomy is usually more frequent although less problematic, since there is no pancreatico-enterostomy (and pancreatic juice remains unactivated), as long as it is well drained. When a fistula persists, papillotomy and *pancreatic duct stenting* may be useful to improve drainage of the pancreatic juice into the duodenum and reduce the fistula output.

Postoperative hemorrhage

Down the slippery slope...

Acute postoperative hemorrhage may lead to the death of your patient within a few minutes. **Remember: early postoperative bleeding after pancreatectomy is usually due to failure to achieve secure hemostasis** before closure (often related to transection of the small bowel mesentery close to the ligament of Treitz), or is secondary to **coagulopathy. Late postoperative hemorrhage** on the other hand is **highly suggestive of bleeding from erosion of a pseudoaneurysm of a major artery.** A leaking pancreaticojejunostomy or hepaticojejunostomy may liberate corrosive pancreatic or biliary juices that may digest the susceptible adjacent arteries. The typical bleeder is the stump of the gastroduodenal (GDA) artery (■ Figure 18.2). **In other words, until proven otherwise, delayed major hemorrhage**

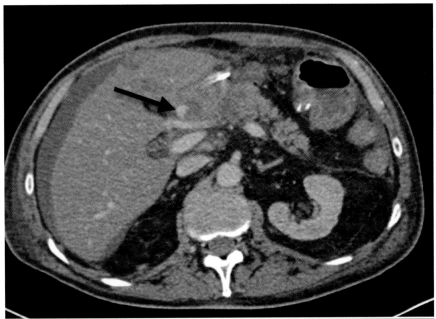

Figure 18.2. CT angiogram after a pancreaticoduodenectomy with presence of a perihepatic hematoma and contrast blush (arrow) at the hepatic artery.

after pancreatic surgery must be attributed to a bleeding arterial pseudoaneurysm. And pancreatic fistula is associated with this life-threatening complication in 75% of cases. Patients with known pancreatic fistulas must therefore be carefully followed in order to diagnose any pseudoaneurysm.

In half of the cases, repetitive small amounts of blood in drains or in the gastrointestinal tract (nasogastric tube, hematemesis or bloody stools) — so called *sentinel bleeds* — can herald massive hemorrhage. Given the potentially fatal outcome of major visceral arterial bleeding, any episode of sentinel bleeding must prompt immediate investigation and treatment. In this case (in a stable patient), your reflex must be to immediately obtain a good quality **contrast-enhanced CT scan** with an arterial phase to localize any pseudoaneurysm and/or a contrast extravasation. **The treatment of choice is angiographic embolization by your interventional radiologist**, because surgical management of the bleeding source is often a messy nightmare, commonly ending up with a hazardous completion pancreatectomy and prohibitive mortality rates. Instead, the help of your experienced interventional radiologist may save your patient's life in more than 80% of cases (to say nothing of your coronaries). During angiography, the treatment consists either of selective embolization of the pseudoaneurysm with coils or the insertion of a covered stent graft in the hepatic artery to occlude the bleeding stump of the GDA, while preserving vascular patency (■ Figure 18.3). When you are sure that your patient does not bleed anymore, you may think about a delayed relaparotomy to evacuate any intra-abdominal hematoma or to optimize drainage of the pancreatic fistula if necessary.

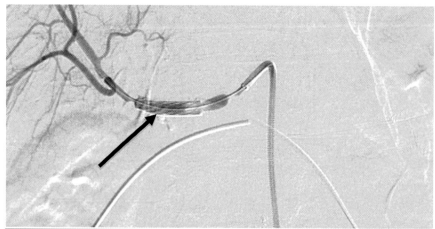

Figure 18.3. Covered stent (arrow) grafting of the stump of the GDA identified as the bleeding source.

Ischemic complications

The typical scenario is the fellow who jumps into a duodenopancreatectomy case without carefully looking at the pre-operative CT scan. He missed the replaced right hepatic artery. Because of vascular spasm during dissection of the hepatoduodenal ligament, this artery is difficult to visualize. While transecting the bile duct, the replaced artery is cut. Ischemia of the right lobe of the liver associated with a hepaticojejunostomy will lead to right liver abscesses.

Most of the ischemic complications after pancreatic surgery are due to anomalies of the celiac axis or the SMA. **These anomalies should be recognized and anticipated with a contrast-enhanced CT scan including arterial and portal phases**.

One such anomaly is a **replaced right hepatic artery**. It usually arises from the SMA, runs behind the 'pancreaticoduodenal block' and posterior to the common hepatic duct towards the right liver, forming its primary blood supply. Thus, it has to be preserved unless it is involved with the tumor. It should be routinely recognized on a pre-operative enhanced CT and sought during dissection of the hepatoduodenal ligament. If injured, revascularization might be attempted but is usually not feasible either because of the small size of the artery or the tissue defect. Revascularization with a synthetic graft should be avoided because of the risk of infection. If no revascularization is possible or the injury has been missed, you may count on, or hope for, collateral arteries from the left hepatic artery, the diaphragm and the retroperitoneum, to nourish the right lobe. But if the collateral blood supply is not sufficient, be prepared for the development of right liver abscesses due to superinfection of infarcted liver areas, via the hepaticojejunostomy.

Another potential cause of postoperative liver ischemia is **stenosis of the celiac axis**, due to extrinsic compression (by the median arcuate ligament syndrome [MALS]) or atherosclerosis. In such cases, retrograde blood supply to the liver comes from the SMA through the pancreaticoduodenal arcades and the GDA. **Since the GDA is divided during pancreaticoduodenectomy, the liver blood supply may become compromised**. If suspected on pre-operative imaging or noted during surgery, reduced flow in the common hepatic artery must be tested by an **intra-operative GDA clamping test** — the surgeon assessing the strength of the pulsating blood flow in the hepatic artery before and after clamping of the GDA. When in doubt, assessment of hepatic artery flow by Doppler is necessary. **When there is a hemodynamically relevant stenosis, the GDA should not be divided since vascularization of the foregut (liver, pancreas and stomach) depends on the SMA**. In such cases, either the median arcuate ligament must be exposed and divided or the celiac trunk needs to be revascularized if there is severe atherosclerosis. **When a stenosis (often large calcified atheromatous plaques seen on CT) is recognized pre-operatively, endovascular dilatation and stent grafting may prevent the need for intra-operative reconstruction**.

Postoperative thrombosis of the SMA and hepatic artery is extremely rare. Its cause is probably multifactorial including extensive fibrosis (e.g. post-radiotherapy) or inflammation, pre-existing vasculopathy and missed intra-operative intimal dissection.

In conclusion, ischemic complications usually lead to (irreversible) liver ischemia resulting in major hepatic cytolysis and liver necrosis. Most patients develop superinfection of the infarcted areas of liver, probably due to biliary tree contamination through the hepaticojejunostomy. This accounts for significant mortality and morbidity after pancreatectomy and justifies particular attention.

Delayed gastric emptying

Delayed gastric emptying (*gastroparesis*) is a frequent problem after pancreaticoduodenectomy. In many cases, the gastroparesis is *idiopathic* with no apparent underlying cause. Thus, in some centers (not ours), erythromycin is routinely used to decrease the incidence of this complication. However, before using the term "idiopathic" one has to rule out an underlying problem such as obstruction of the gastrojejunostomy (usually due to edema and therefore self-limiting) or a retrogastric collection. When the latter is suspected, you better perform a CT scan and treat the cause. Symptomatic treatment combines decompression of the stomach with a nasogastric tube and intravenous gastric prokinetics (e.g. erythromycin). Obviously, nutrition should be maintained, preferably by the enteral route. **Remember: before blaming the gastrojejunostomy or 'nature', do exclude a pancreatic leak!**

Chylous ascites

This very rare complication develops more frequently after **extended lymphadenectomy**. It declares itself with a change in the drain's output from a serous to a milky character. The presence of triglycerides, chylomicrons and lymphocytes in the fluid can help to confirm the diagnosis. Most patients should respond to conservative treatment which consists of a low-fat diet (using medium chain triglycerides). Some patients benefit from bowel rest and parenteral nutrition. Peritoneal paracentesis is often required and octreotide has been shown to be effective on account of its ability to inhibit lymphatic flow. In cases resistant to the above modalities and maneuvers, lymphoscintigraphy-guided surgical intervention may become necessary to interrupt the leaking lymphatic vessel.

Portal vein and superior mesenteric vein thrombosis

Portal vein thrombosis (PVT) is a relatively uncommon finding (<5%) after pancreatic resection without portal vein resection. Nevertheless, early PVT or SMV thrombosis is associated with an increased postoperative mortality. The initial symptoms are generally non-specific; however, high postoperative transaminases and sepsis because of ischemic bowel should alert the surgeon. A duplex ultrasound of the portal vein or an abdominal enhanced CT scan quickly tells us whether portal vein flow is preserved.

When there is poor tolerance of the PVT with signs of liver failure or bowel ischemia, we would proceed with a relaparotomy. A thrombectomy of the portal vein is performed both proximally to the SMV as well as towards both the right and left portal vein. Acute PVT may, however, be well tolerated. Indeed, in such patients, pre-operative tumoral occlusion of the portal vein induces development of venous collaterals that minimize the consequences of postoperative PVT. Then, anticoagulation with heparin may be sufficient to avoid extension of the thrombus to the SMV.

As usual the best way is to avoid such a situation. In portal vein reconstruction it is paramount to avoid tension because this generally narrows the anastomosis. Distances up to 3cm are easily bridged with a primary anastomosis if the whole mesenteric root is completely mobilized. During a primary end-to-end portal vein anastomosis a *'growth factor'* may be used to prevent stenosis and to allow the anastomosis to expand following reperfusion: after performing the anterior and posterior wall anastomosis with two running sutures (we use Prolene®), the knot is deliberately placed away from the vessel wall at a distance of about 1cm — leaving the suture intentionally slack. When the clamp is released the portal flow fills the anastomosis nicely, it dilates and there is no narrowing or leaks. When longer distances have to be bridged both autologous or homologous vein grafts (as mentioned above) or synthetic grafts (certainly not our first choice) may be used.

Postoperative diarrhea

Postoperative diarrhea is a relatively common problem; in most cases it is readily treated but may be extremely resistant to therapy. We empirically classify postoperative diarrhea into one of three categories:

- **Malabsorptive**: a consequence of exocrine pancreatic insufficiency. Treatment with pancreatic enzymes should solve the problem.
- **Neuropathic**: a consequence of injury to the neural plexus surrounding the celiac trunk or SMA. This entity is the most difficult to treat and may need long-term treatment with loperamide and opium tincture.
- **Iatrogenic**: a consequence of the intake of gastroprokinetic drugs or secondary to antibiotics (e.g. *C. diff.* colitis).

In conclusion, in pancreatic surgery (maybe more than in any other surgical field), it is not just the technique, but also the anticipation and management of postoperative complications that are crucial for a favorable outcome. These factors contribute to the difference between specialized and non-specialized surgical teams and the **improved ability of the former to salvage the complicated patient**.

Chapter 19

The liver

Erik Schadde and Pierre-Alain Clavien

For a long time the liver has been the general surgeon's Pandora's Box. Cutting into the liver opens the door to bleeding, bile leaks and other complications with potentially dire consequences for the patient and endless travails for the surgeon. **The reasons for the special status of the liver in abdominal surgery are obvious**: it weighs about three pounds, has double inflow — arterial and portal venous, with the portal vein carrying about one-sixth of the cardiac output — all connecting to a sponge of capillary vessels that are hidden within glistening brown liver tissue. The blood drains into three major veins the size of fingers that flow into the vena cava about 1cm below the right heart. Throughout the organ there is an intricate capillary network of bile ducts.

Since the vascular and biliary structures are not visible from the outside, operating on the liver is like flying at night or during bad weather: you have to rely on auxiliary modes of navigation and most of the time the forces of nature will be up against you. Given that the umbilical fissure divides the organ into two lobes visible from the outside, most elective liver surgery prior to the 1950s transected the liver along this plane. In 1952, the French surgeon, Lortat-Jacob, was the first to describe an anatomical right liver lobe resection and from there techniques were developed that make liver surgery as safe as surgery on other parts of the human body. Let's now look at the main issues that have advanced liver surgery to where it now stands: surgery that may be performed routinely and safely. This of course depends on many factors...

Pre-operative considerations

Functional compromise of the liver tissue

Many primary liver tumors arise in livers damaged by viral hepatitis, fibrosis or even cirrhosis. This functional compromise may lead to **postoperative liver failure** and, frequently, death. General surgeons have long known that patients with cirrhosis carry a higher risk of mortality even for procedures unrelated to the liver. Resecting part of the dysfunctional parenchyma of a diseased liver is an even greater challenge. C. G. Child from the University of Michigan developed the well-known "Child" scoring system to assess the mortality risk prior to shunt surgery in patients with cirrhosis and portal hypertension. When the classification was used for liver resections, it became clear that only patients with "Child A cirrhosis" may undergo liver resections with expectations of a reasonable outcome. **But even in patients with Child A cirrhosis, there are those who are at increased risk of mortality and severe complications**. These patients may be identified by more specific testing such as the *indocyanine green (ICG)* test or other metabolic liver function tests. The well-established group from

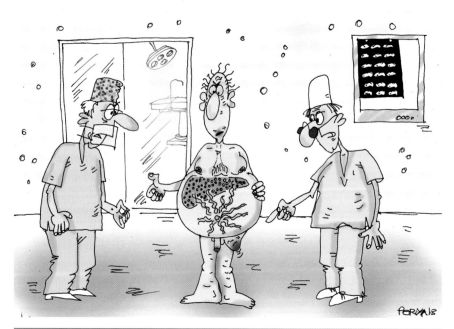

Figure 19.1. Surgeon to internist: "Sir, but he is Child C..." Internist: "I don't care who your Child C is, but this chap needs his hernia fixed!"

the Barcelona Clinic has proposed measurement of portal pressure using the **transjugular hepatic vein wedge pressure. As a rule of thumb, any pressure gradient >12mmHg between the portal vein and vena cava, or any plasma retention of ICG greater than 15-20% after 15 minutes, precludes performing a** *major liver resection* **in cirrhotic patients.** Whether *minor resections* are safe depends on the judgment and experience of the surgeon. **Be aware that in the presence of portal hypertension even minor resections may lead to unstoppable bleeding and decompensation of liver function.**

Among patients referred to you for liver surgery identify those with potential parenchymal compromise and test their functional capacity to undergo a major resection.

But then you have to familiarize yourself with the Child's scoring system and its offspring, the "Child-Pugh classification" (■ Figure 19.1). Google it up!

The size of the liver remnant

> *It's not the size of the dog in the fight, it's the size of the fight in the dog.*
>
> **Mark Twain**

The main consideration in avoiding liver failure and death after resections is **how much liver you may remove with impunity.** Lortat-Jacob described a 60% liver resection in 1952 in a patient who survived without functional compromise and fully recovered. Tom Starzl described a 90% liver resection in 1975 in an otherwise healthy 19-year-old woman, who became critically ill but ultimately recovered normal liver function.

There is almost unanimous consensus that 30% of the liver should be preserved given normal baseline liver function and that at least 40-50% of the liver should be preserved in cases of functional compromise due to underlying parenchymal disease.

Whom should you definitely refer to a liver center?

The pioneering days in liver surgery lasted until the 1970s when major liver resections were commonly associated with a mortality of up to 20%. Since then a large volume of water has flowed down the Limmat River (do you know where it is?) and liver surgery has undergone progressive standardization and specialization. **There is now general consensus that the mortality at experienced centers for major liver resections should be below 5%, and close to 0% for minor resections**. Evidence from most areas of highly specialized fields in surgery indicates that both center, as well as individual surgeon's experience counts in preventing complications and mortality. The bottom line is this: you should not get involved in doing elective liver surgery unless you or your partners do a fair volume of it. What constitutes a fair number is the subject of debate, but let's pick a number: **you should perform at least 30 cases a year to perform elective liver surgery at all!**

Now given these challenges, should one as a general surgeon touch the liver at all unless one has no choice, like in trauma surgery? There is no doubt that some experience in liver surgery should belong to any general surgeon's portfolio. **The best preparation to be comfortable with liver trauma is elective liver surgery**. On the other hand, the key to preventing complications after liver surgery is to know when to refer cases for elective tumor resections to experienced centers. To perform an uncomplicated resection for benign and malignant liver tumors, not much is needed than appropriate experience, solid training (optimally, a formal fellowship), knowledge of the anatomy, a single shot of antibiotics, an adequate subcostal retractor, intra-operative ultrasound, the ability of your anesthetist to provide you with a low peri-operative central venous pressure (CVP) and familiarity with a parenchymal transection method of your choice. **However, if you are dealing with** *patients*...

- Older than 70 years.
- With viral hepatitis, non-alcoholic steatohepatitis (NASH), fibrosis or cirrhosis, obstructive cholestasis or extensive pre-operative chemotherapy.
- With tumors in a difficult location close to the three hepatic veins or vena cava as well as perihilar tumors, large or multiple tumors that frequently require extended resections.
- Who will not tolerate a low CVP or in whom a low CVP will be difficult or impossible (e.g. those with pulmonary hypertension or congestive heart failure).
- Who are at higher risk for peri-operative bleeding (e.g. anticoagulation, anti-aggregants, thrombocytopenia).

Then — to prevent excessive M&M — you better refer them to a specialized liver center, like ours, for example ☺.

Intra-operative considerations

The problem of exposure

Firstly, there is the problem of exposure and access to the liver. Differently from the way the liver is depicted in the textbooks, it is a curved organ: the right lobe dives deep into the depths of the right sub-diaphragmatic space. To the operating surgeon's hands (as opposed to the anatomist's eyes) the right posterior segments truly lie posterior to the anterior segments. Ease of exposure was the reason why left liver resections were initially preferred. When Lortat-Jacob described the first anatomical right hepatectomy he chose a thoraco-abdominal incision to adequately expose the vena cava, the right hepatic vein and the small draining veins of the right lobe. Since then, sophisticated **subcostal retractors** like the *Fowler* or *Thompson* retractor have been developed and they make a thoracic incision almost obsolete. Transverse subcostal incisions (*Chevron* or *rooftop*) are used by most surgeons today with a few variations on the theme. These incisions transect the rectus muscle and cause a fair amount of postoperative pain, but the fascial borders of the abdominal muscles close well in two layers, the closure has ample blood supply, and eviscerations and hernias are rare. Sometimes a midline extension of the bilateral subcostal incision (named after the famous *Mercedes* logo) is helpful to get at the hepaticocaval junction. If you find yourself in a situation of having to do a liver case without subcostal retractors in a smaller hospital (or the 'developing world'), a *Balfour* retractor can be used as a subcostal retractor — one side is placed in a subcostal position and the retractor is extended.

Fully movable operating room tables have made it easier to operate on the liver as well. Experienced liver surgeons will frequently tilt the table to the right and the left to let gravity help with retraction.

In general though, have subcostal retractors available and know how to use them when you perform liver surgery.

The problem of bleeding

Bleeding is the major problem to be overcome during liver surgery. The control of bleeding from major vessels has been the daily bread (with or without butter) for general surgeons since Ambroise Paré ligated a carotid artery in a battlefield hospital in 1637. The bleeding encountered from liver tissue, however, has a different quality — **it is the seeping, non-stoppable**

bleeding from parenchyma that does not only originate from identifiable blood vessels but also from an abundantly perfused parenchyma. A clear source frequently cannot be identified and only compression with the surgeon's fingers or sponges or packs stuffed into the abdominal cavity can ultimately stop it — that is if the coagulation system is intact. A tear in the liver from trauma results in bleeding, clot formation or — if not treated appropriately — exsanguination. Early liver surgeons soon realized that bleeding would not always stop by compression only. Multiple attempts to suture liver tears were described but suturing liver tissue is like suturing soft cheese — like French *Camembert* rather than our own cherished *Emmenthaler*. Therefore, *bolstering techniques* were described to anchor sutures.

A major step forward in the management of liver hemorrhage was the introduction of the *Pringle maneuver*. In 1908, J. Hogarth Pringle published a description of en-masse clamping of the entire hepatic inflow pedicle including the hepatic artery and portal vein to control bleeding encountered during liver trauma. **This maneuver is now electively used in modern liver surgery to reduce blood loss during parenchymal transection**: the lesser omentum is opened and a right-angle clamp passed behind-around the hepatoduodenal ligament through the foramen of Winslow to encircle all hepatic inflow structures and clamp them either with a tourniquet or a soft vascular clamp.

Besides compression and the use of the Pringle maneuver for parenchymal transection, it was felt that ligation of individual parenchymal vessels could further reduce blood loss. To free the vessels from the liver parenchyma, a 'finger fracture technique' (aka *digitoclasia*) was developed: the vessels, identified as a 'resistance' between the palpating thumb and the index finger, are freed and ligated with individual ligatures. Today, liver surgeons use a variety of techniques for parenchymal transections: the curved Kelly clamps (clamp crush technique), ultrasound dissection devices (e.g. CUSA® — Cavitron Ultrasonic Surgical Aspirator®), pressured water dissection (with the Waterjet® device) or sealing devices (e.g. LigaSure™, Enseal®). **There is no evidence to date that any of these new techniques is superior to 'clamp crush' — probably still the most widely used technique today.**

The most intractable bleeding that really compromises visibility of the operative site comes from the hepatic veins. A particular problem is that side branches of hepatic veins tend to tear off from the main hepatic veins during dissection. A good technique is to just keep up hand pressure for a while — most bleeding from veins stops this way. Sometimes careful stitches with 6-0 monofilament sutures are necessary.

Bleeding from liver parenchyma does not depend only on inflow but also on venous outflow. Pressure in the hepatic veins corresponds well with

CVP. The anesthetist should monitor and reduce CVP by using reverse Trendelenburg positioning (head up!), vasodilatory drugs and diuretics. **Randomized studies have demonstrated that keeping the CVP low (<5mmHg) during the operation decreases blood loss during hepatectomies by a factor of three**. Despite all of this the transfusion rate in major liver surgery is still around 20%.

If the CVP is too high and cannot be lowered quickly, **packing and waiting** is the good-old and well-proved strategy. Don't push your head through the wall during an excessively bloody parenchymal transection because there will be 1.5L of blood in your suction canisters faster than you think. Tell the anesthetist kindly that part of the team will take a coffee break while **he should further lower the CVP** (of course, we would leave the most junior member of the surgical team to watch the abdomen… and the anesthetist). You will return relaxed, refreshed and find a completely different situation after 30 minutes or longer if necessary.

Remember: if you want to perform liver surgery without losing too much blood (the less blood you lose the lower the M&M!), be comfortable with a parenchymal transection method, selectively use the (intermittent) Pringle maneuver (cycle of 15-minute Pringle followed by 5-minute reperfusion) and have a skilled anesthetist (every hospital has to have at least one of them ☺), who keeps the CVP under 5mmHg.

The problem of hidden anatomy

Navigating through the inner liver anatomy remains a challenge. In 1897, the Scottish surgeon, James Cantlie, realized during an autopsy that the true anatomical midplane of the liver runs along the gallbladder fossa and not the umbilical ligament. The supply of the eight liver segments through a complex branching pattern of the Glissonian triad was not clear until the French anatomist Couinaud published his observations in the 1950s; not incidentally at the same time the first anatomical resections were performed. **The theoretical advantage of anatomic resections is the relative paucity of bile ducts and blood vessels in the watershed area between liver segments**. To aid in directing the parenchymal transection plane, some surgeons swear by intra-operative ultrasound, whilst others consider 3-D reconstruction of dynamic CT images helpful. In Japan, it is still quite popular to inject blue dye into segmental portal vein branches to delineate segmental borders on the liver surface. The natural variation of the standard liver anatomy gives theoretical support for the use of this exercise in high-risk procedures (e.g. live donors in liver transplantation). To become competent you should transect the liver a few times with somebody experienced by your side. **In liver surgery, knowing how to follow a map is not enough**.

> **Remember:** do not engage in elective major liver surgery without feeling comfortable with its inner anatomy and being able to use intra-operative liver ultrasound.

Intra-operative disasters in liver surgery

Liver surgery (like trauma, vascular, thoracic and heart surgery) harbors a true potential to lose a patient on the table from torrential hemorrhage. Intra-operative death may occur even in experienced and busy centers although it should be an exceedingly rare event. **It is important to review the area of highest risk during any major liver surgery, to choose each step carefully and to avoid performing risky maneuvers without a security rope**.

Bleeding from the vena cava and the hepatocaval junction

Bleeding from the vena cava and major hepatic veins needs to be anticipated when tumor masses abut these structures or the patient has been operated in this area before and is now undergoing a repeat resection. **Bleeding from the cava-hepatic vein junction and vena cava due to avulsed draining veins, a dissecting right angle or simply because of too much pulling (e.g. on the right lobe) may be stemmed by just holding pressure for 2-3 minutes or can develop into a real problem that cannot be managed without total vascular exclusion. Therefore, it might be wise to prepare a *Pringle tourniquet* around the porta hepatis, a tourniquet around the infrahepatic vena cava and one around the suprahepatic vena cava as a security rope before your fall.** You should have sent cases that involve the vena cava and major hepatic veins to a high-volume center, but in case you find yourself in a difficult situation like this, it is essential to know how to perform total vascular exclusion and to limit its time appropriately.

Bleeding from the **anterior face of the vena cava** is usually only a problem if the caudate lobe has already been detached by transecting and ligating the small draining veins. If the bleeding occurs while the caudate lobe is still attached to the vena cava — like while passing a right-angle or stiff plastic tube for a 'hanging maneuver'[1] — it is always self-limiting since the caudate lobe tamponades the bleeding.

Injury during dissection of the portal triad

Bleeding from the portal vein may be one of the most treacherous problems because this vein is occasionally thin, sutures less well than the cava and tends to stenose when it is repaired, unless an appropriate 'growth factor' is allowed by leaving the suture loose (see ⟳ Chapter 18, page 375). Injury may occur during dissection of the porta hepatis especially if a digit is used behind the porta to push up the portal structures, thus collapsing the vein which is then not recognized properly as the finger-thick 'blue' vein. Draining veins from the pancreas into the portal vein need to be carefully tied off with 4-0 ties to avoid tears of the portal vein. Tears in a retropancreatic location and those beyond the primary bifurcation of the portal vein in the liver hilum may be particularly difficult to manage. **Tumor involvement of the portal vein** should be addressed by placing clamps proximally and distally, excising the affected segment as in the surgical management of cholangiocarcinoma. However — sorry for stressing this yet again — these tumors should be referred to an experienced center.

Very rarely, dissection of the extrahepatic hilar structures for a hepatectomy may lead to an injury of the **common hepatic artery** or the contralateral (right or left) hepatic artery. **A future liver remnant after hepatic resection cannot live on the portal vein alone**. Integrity of arterial flow needs to be preserved and a patch repair or repair with an interposition graft has to be attempted at all costs by recruiting the help of a vascular or transplant surgeon (a solid liver surgeon has to possess all such skills!).

Postoperative considerations

Bile leaks

> *Only a sailor, not a clerk, should be running the ship.*
> **Ivor Lewis**

The most common complication after liver resection is a bile leak.

---

1   Liddo G, *et al.* The liver hanging manoeuvre. *HPB* 2009; 11(4): 296-305.

You performed a wonderful left lobe resection ("a walk in the park", you mentioned to one of your partners) with only 300ml blood loss in a young non-cirrhotic patient with a giant hepatocellular carcinoma. Because you are not a 'drain surgeon', you did not insert a closed suction drain after the surgery, and the patient did well for the first four days. Laboratory values were perfectly fine after surgery. On the day of discharge the patient has a low-grade temperature at 38.3, but you blew it off because the patient feels well and wants to go home badly. From the corner of your eye, however, you saw your chief resident shrug his shoulders signaling his internal disagreement. Five days later he will admit the patient with a high fever and abdominal pain. A CT scan shows a large fluid collection at the cut surface of the liver. You convince the interventional radiologist to tap the collection and insert a drain. The intern on duty calls you and declares that pus came out and that it is *just* a 'deep surgical space' infection and no bile is seen in the drain. On Monday, the drainage fluid has turned bilious and you switch the antibiotics to a brand that costs a small fortune per week. The drain now puts out about 800cc a day, but the bilirubin level is only 2.1mg/dL. You know that when there is a large volume of ascites, the bilirubin may very well be diluted and you trust your gut feeling that this is a bile leak. A small leak from the transection surface can occur even after the nicest liver resection and you explain that to your patient. He is in pain with the pigtail right under his costal margin and has developed an ileus with vomiting. He hasn't really eaten well since the surgery and now a nasogastric tube puts out 2L of bilious succus a day. Your chief resident wants to do an ERCP every day but you calm him down pointing out that ERCPs are not without risk of pancreatitis, etc., which is the last thing one needs in this situation. By the end of the week your nutritionist calls you and asks whether you would mind starting the patient on TPN. You don't disagree but silently hope that the problem is just going to resolve over the weekend. On Saturday you watch finals of the World Cup and shortly after the kick-off you receive a call that your patient is tachypneic and hypotensive on the ward despite prophylactic heparin. The patient gets intubated and a chest X-ray shows a large pulmonary effusion on the left and a chest tube is inserted. A CT of the abdomen shows a large fluid collection. Your intensivist, who obviously does not appreciate soccer, calls you and suggests to take the patient back to the operating room "because something is not right". You drive in to talk to the family and make a plan. You decide that the abdominal fluid collection should be drained with a second drain and an ERCP performed on Monday. Since there is no leak visible on ERCP your hypothesis is that the biliary leak is occurring from an 'excluded' liver segment of the right lobe. On Wednesday, you indeed take the patient back to the operating room where you have to dig yourself through a horror show of green adhesions — a bile leak cannot be found on the liver surface very easily — while your chief resident talks about presenting this 'interesting case' in the next M&M conference. **Your initial "walk in the park" has transformed into a nightmare**.

This case exemplifies the potential of bile leaks to cause a spiral of problems that may seriously endanger your patient's life. Most bile leaks are minor — from small bile radicals on the surface of the liver — and are self-limiting with appropriate drainage. However, bile leaks may also originate from major intrahepatic bile ducts and from injuries to the main duct near the hilum requiring early ERCP and stenting. **In the presence of a bile leak with a 'blank ERCP', one should think of excluded ducts (disconnected from the main bile duct system), often requiring surgical revision**.

The mortality of patients with bile leaks is about three times higher than those without a bile leak. No systematic review and no randomized trial will provide the answer to how to prevent and how to manage these leaks. Every liver surgeon has bile leaks but it is one thing to have a complication and another one to manage it well and anticipate potential pitfalls.

Our 'take' on these matters is as follows:

- **There is no clear evidence that the routine leaving of drains behind improves the detection and management of bile leaks as long as you have a good interventional radiology service to drain postoperative fluid collections**. Many bile leaks remain undetected (some are even asymptomatic and clinically insignificant) or show up late after removal of drains. However, if you happen to perform a liver resection in an African district hospital without a CT scanner and interventional radiology suite, we recommend the placement of a closed suction drain at the end of the operation... and wish you much luck ☺!
- **Be aware that left hepatectomies, central resections of segments 4, 5 and 8, and biliodigestive anastomoses will have a higher risk of bile leak**, while the method of pedicle division (intra- or extrahepatic), parenchymal transection (fancy dissection devices versus clamp crush) or laparoscopic versus open liver resection have no obvious impact on the incidence of bile leaks. Whether anatomic resections are less prone to cause bile leaks than non-anatomic is (despite the theoretical benefits of the former) a matter for debate.
- **If there is no reduction of bile output over the first 4-5 days after drainage, consider an ERCP with sphincterotomy and stent placement to detect** and treat major bile leaks and allow early re-exploration for leaks from excluded segments of the liver.

- After secondary interventional placement of drains repeat a CT to confirm resolution of the abscess or fluid collection, even if the drain is drying up — don't just trust your drainage tube.
- Be your own *surgical microbiologist* when you treat leaks and abscesses. Consider the possibility of resistant organisms; start with empiric broad-spectrum antibiotics, narrowing their spectrum based on sensitivity of appropriately collected specimens taken *during* source control. **Don't culture inlaying drains** since they will always be colonized with every organism which lives in the hospital and you will have to cover *everything* — the common advice one gets from the so called 'infectious disease experts'.
- **Anticipate problems** of anorexia, ileus (and the risk of aspiration especially in elderly patients) and pleural effusion. Watch for dehydration and electrolyte imbalances due to the large volume of bile output from the drain, which could result in renal failure. Expect complications related to the procedures needed to fix these problems, such as the use of chest tubes, intubations and endoscopies. Residents frequently tend to run behind the cascade of problems arising from a simple complication: **somebody needs to steer the boat and anticipate the next disaster**.
- **Fixing the leak from an excluded bile segment in the above described case is not an easy task**. Elective resection of the excluded segment and even ethanol ablations or portal vein embolization to atrophy the respective segments have been proposed in the literature. If possible, we would go for resection — of course, such reoperations can be like climbing the north face of the Eiger and should be performed in an experienced liver center.

Post-resection liver failure

The second most common complication and the main cause of death after liver resection is postoperative liver failure.

This **perfect storm scenario** (see facing page) serves to illustrate the causative factors of postoperative liver failure, which depends on many factors:

- **The function of the liver parenchyma**, which may be compromised by hepatitis, steatosis, chemotherapy-induced toxicities or fibrosis, each of which could be present to a mild degree, but not declaring

A 76-year-old diabetic patient is referred to you with three large liver metastases from colorectal cancer. You performed a colectomy on this patient two years ago for a T4 N2 tumor and you remember him well since he developed an anastomotic leak, spent several weeks in the ICU, and required a diverting ileostomy and a subsequent ileostomy takedown. Now he is found to have liver metastases on CT, and has received another few cycles of chemotherapy, together with Avastin®. The 'mets' are in the right lobe extending beyond the middle hepatic vein to segment 4. Your radiologist predicts that after the planned resection about 26% of the liver will remain. Platelet levels and liver function tests are all normal and the liver has a normal appearance on CT and ultrasound. You decide to proceed with an extended right hepatectomy.

You encounter extensive adhesions and you lose a fair amount of time and blood to even visualize the liver. You take down the liver's diaphragmatic attachments on the right and left to be able to rotate it well. During mobilization of the right lobe and the small draining veins into the vena cava, you injure the vena cava. You lose about 200cc of blood within a few seconds and your chief resident has to pull over the liver while you are trying to get control. You have to increase the skin incision and it takes more than a few minutes until the bleeding has stopped. The first-year anesthesia resident, who had told you at the beginning of the case how excited he is about this being his "first liver resection case", has trouble keeping down the CVP because, as he says, "the patient's blood pressure doesn't tolerate the rotation of the liver around the axis of the vena cava very well". You ask him to elevate the patient's head, and his attending finally arrives after what appears like an eternity, but finally you are happy when things proceed: you prepare the inflow vessels by transecting the right hepatic artery and portal vein, place a tourniquet to be ready for a Pringle maneuver in case you need to, and proceed along a resection plane slightly to the right of the umbilical fissure. During the parenchymal transection using the 'clamp-crush technique', there is again extensive bleeding from a few openings of large veins, while the CVP is still too high. You decide to 'Pringle' the liver on three occasions, for 15 minutes, to be able to see the intrahepatic structures you need to ligate and cut. The patient becomes unstable and the anesthetists have to use high doses of 'pressors' to keep the blood pressure up but, at last, you manage to complete the resection. After six hours, way longer than you felt was necessary, you eventually bring the patient out to the ICU extubated. Four units of blood had to be transfused.

The level of transaminases is now measured in multiple thousands, platelets are falling and the INR is rising to 2.3. Your patient requires several liters of volume resuscitation because he is oliguric on the first postoperative night and requires noradrenaline. Despite this his blood pressure runs low, although he suffered from arterial hypertension pre-operatively. Veno-venous hemofiltration is started because of the rising potassium levels. Because both the INR and bilirubin continue to rise for the next several days you perform a Doppler ultrasound to document normal hepatic arterial inflow. The patient turns gradually yellow and on day five after the surgery, his bilirubin is 10mg/dL, and his INR is 2.8. You know that his chance of survival is 'fifty-fifty'...

themselves with a decreased platelet count or signs of elevated portal pressure. These changes are not easy to detect unless you perform a pre-operative liver biopsy. It is also difficult to predict the eventual impact of these changes if you are already planning to have a small liver remnant.

- **The parenchyma can be further damaged during the surgery**: lack of portal venous and arterial *inflow* due to Pringle maneuvers with a total occlusion time of more than 45 minutes and *outflow* congestion due to partial occlusion of the left hepatic vein (which drains the liver remnant) because of prolonged torqueing of the liver around the fixed axis of the vena cava. While intermittent inflow occlusion with 10-15-minute occlusion intervals and 5-minute recovery has been associated with less blood loss and cytoprotection, **more than 45-60 minutes of total Pringle time might cause ischemic damage**. The diseased liver likely tolerates much less.

- **The ischemic liver parenchyma releases factors that contribute to low blood pressure and cause intra- and postoperative renal dysfunction**. Overzealous administration of fluids might contribute to swelling of the parenchyma and outflow congestion, further compromising hepatic cell function. Overzealous use of 'pressors' causes arterial vasoconstriction and further diminishes hepatic flow.

- There seems to be a minimum amount of liver cells that need to be left behind after resection to avoid a syndrome that has been named **"small-for-size"**, since the amount of liver cells required for appropriate metabolic function depends on the weight of the patient. Depending on different studies and schools of liver surgery, **the appropriate amount of liver in the liver remnant should be anywhere between 20-30% of the total liver volume**. With 26% in this case, it seems that you have been too aggressive — not knowing exactly how good the metabolic function of the liver parenchyma is, given the pre-operative chemotherapy and variable amounts of damage inflicted during the surgery.

Liver cell dysfunction expresses itself with progressive coagulopathy (rise in INR) and intrahepatic cholestasis (rise in bilirubin) that have been shown to be reliable prognostic factors for outcome. Among the many definitions for postoperative liver failure there is one thing you need to know: **the prognosis is guarded if the INR and bilirubin are still rising five days after surgery — unless manageable factors such as biliary obstruction or infection exist**. Infection, in most cases resulting from bile leaks, aggravates the picture in postoperative liver failure.

How to deal with postoperative liver failure is a difficult question: the mortality is around 50%, yet some livers recover. Ventilation, dialysis, optimizing nutritional status, treatment of infections and careful monitoring of vascular flow (duplex ultrasound) and liver function are the mainstay of treatment. We definitely recommend transferring patients who develop this problem to a high-volume center without any delay.

Remember: if you would like to perform elective liver surgery, get the appropriate training and stay busy to keep your experience up. If you wish to avoid complications follow our advice (■ Table 19.1).

Table 19.1. Avoiding complications in liver surgery.

Pre-operatively

- Know how to assess diseased parenchyma.
- Have the ability to perform liver volumetry based on CT and MRI.
- Know which patients to refer to high-volume centers.

Intra-operatively

- Master a parenchymal transection method.
- Have a good subcostal retractor in your armamentarium.
- Know how to use intra-operative ultrasound for resection.
- Be aware of the main steps that can get you into trouble during the resection.

Postoperatively

- Be proactive in the management of complications.
- Be knowledgeable about bile leaks and postoperative liver failure.

"A bad liver is to a Frenchman what a nervous breakdown is to an American. Everyone has had one and everyone wants to talk about it."

Art Buchwald

Chapter 20

The breast

Danny Rosin

> *Asya brought it (her breast) close to his face and held it for him. "Kiss it! Kiss it!" she demanded… he nuzzled it with his lips like a suckling pig, gratefully, admiringly… its beauty flooded him…Today it was a marvel. Tomorrow it would be in the trash bin.*
>
> **Cancer Ward, Alexander Solzhenitsyn**

Breast surgery is conceived as 'simple'. There is not much to prepare pre-op (just diagnose and localize the tumor), and there's no complex intra-op maneuvers (chop it out and close nicely), so obviously not many complications are expected… And that's also the reason we skipped the regular chapter format of pre-, intra- and postop considerations. BUT — as you'll soon find out — things are more complicated than one thinks, and complications are more common than one is willing to admit… So please read on!

Breast surgery used to be simple. The surgeon's role was to achieve the removal of some fatty tissue, even the whole breast, maybe fiddle around with the axilla — not a major technical challenge. Traditionally, lumpectomy was considered a first-year resident case. It all seemed so simple, so what complications could we expect apart from some minor wound infections and the occasional seroma or hematoma?

Well, it seems that this is not the case anymore, as breast surgery has become almost a subspecialty. Dedicated breast surgeons have evolved, who not only master the surgical technique but are involved in decision-making and need to know much about oncology, genetics, and plastic surgery — in order to provide the patient with answers, and a treatment plan, and be part of the multidisciplinary team.

In light of this evolution, complications in breast surgery can be divided into:

- **'Regular'**, local postoperative problems of the surgical field.
- **Long-term** complications related to the breast and the axilla.
- Complications associated with the **oncologic treatment** (mainly radiation) and the **plastic-reconstructive** procedures.
- Issues that are not complications per se but pose difficulty in management, both during surgery and after it, and are related to the **breast pathology** itself.

'Regular' postoperative complications

Wound infection (see ⊃ Chapter 5)

Luckily for breast surgeons (and patients), breast surgery belongs to the group of 'clean operations' and hence wound infections are quite uncommon. However, wound healing problems in this sensitive and 'sensual' organ, although considered 'minor' by most surgeons, may seem disastrous for the patient, causing significant despair and cosmetic disruption.

Prevention
While the debate on whether prophylactic antibiotics are universally indicated for clean operations is not over yet, **there are high-risk situations in which prophylaxis should be given**. These include patient factors such as obesity, diabetes, steroid use, immunosuppression, and local factors such as irradiated tissue, a high risk for fluid collections and drain usage, or the presence of a localizing wire. Other technical factors may help in decreasing the chance of infection, as is true in surgery in general: avoiding dead spaces, avoiding excessive tissue burning, meticulous hemostasis, gentle tissue handling and perfect closure of wounds. **Do your patients a favor — avoid skin staples on the breast!**

Treatment
Techniques for overcoming established infection can range from simple antibiotic treatment (covering Gram-positive cocci as the most common etiology), through needle aspiration, to opening the wound for drainage and debridement. In some cases wound disruption has already happened, and open wound management waiting for secondary healing (or at least delayed primary closure) is mandatory.

Hematoma (see ⮕ Chapter 3)

With no major named blood vessels in the breast tissue, hematomas should be uncommon. Perforators arising from the pectoralis muscle may bleed and retract, but usually can be controlled during surgery. Surgeons always claim that "it was dry when we closed". But still, bleeding after conclusion of the operation can occur, resulting in painful hematomas, which only rarely have hemodynamic significance, but may lead to disfigurement and further wound healing problems.

Prevention

Prevention of bleeding complications during surgery has been outlined in ⮕ Chapter 3.

Treatment

Checking the coagulation profile is mandatory (after unexpected bleeding has occurred). Blood transfusions are rarely needed. The main question is whether local pressure is enough to control the bleeding and limit the resultant hematoma size, or is reoperation needed to stop the bleeding and evacuate the hematoma. A large retained hematoma may take a long time to disappear, often leading to pain, fever, secondary infection and spontaneous drainage which can be messy and frightening for the patient. **Despite the natural reluctance to reoperate, early hematoma evacuation and hemostasis is a worthwhile exercise, shortening the recovery period and ultimately leading to a better cosmetic outcome**. Having said this I have to stress that reoperation for bleeding after breast surgery is rare — almost anecdotal! So be careful that you won't be forced to do it.

Skin flap ischemia after mastectomy

The main task in achieving a 'perfect' mastectomy is separating the skin from the breast tissue in the correct plane. Leaving thick and 'healthy' skin flaps may threaten the patient with retained breast tissue and possibly residual cancer cells (or a future risk of cancer, if prophylactic mastectomy is the procedure), while very thin flaps jeopardize the skin blood supply with resultant ischemia and necrosis. This struggle is more evident when immediate reconstruction is planned, as the added stretch on the skin from the silicone implant may further impair skin perfusion. This will result in the plastic surgeon's frequent cries to the surgeon: "you are ruining my flaps!" Large flaps, often the result of skin-sparing surgery with large breasts, are more at risk of inadequate perfusion, especially at the flaps' edges, away from their blood supply. Increased tension at closure, usually the result of large tumors needing wider excision, is a well-known factor in the genesis of skin ischemia.

Skin ischemia may present as minor discoloration, which often improves spontaneously, but sometimes results in wound disruption, wound (or graft) infection, and frank necrosis, requiring reoperation for debridement and secondary closure.

Prevention and management

Keeping the flaps healthy and well perfused, in their optimal thickness, is one of the 'secrets of the trade', learned over time. There are different techniques to raise the flaps, including traction and diathermy dissection, sharp knife or scissors dissection, and closed dissection, sometimes with the aid of subcutaneous infiltration with saline. **While surgeons will often swear by their grandmother's breast that their technique is superior, it is probably experience and dedication that results in creating the perfect flap**.

Avoiding closure under tension is important, and can be achieved by careful planning of the incision, sometimes in non-conventional directions. Raising the flaps further away from the breast tissue margins, above and below, may recruit more skin for a tension-free closure. In extreme cases, coverage by mobilization of distant flaps or even by skin grafts should be considered, with the aid of a plastic surgeon.

When ischemia does occur, close observation is essential, to determine whether and when reintervention is needed. Debridement of necrotic skin to healthy and bleeding edges and achieving tension-free closure are the keys to management of this frustrating complication. In cases of immediate reconstruction, prosthesis removal, or replacement of a permanent prosthesis with a temporary expander, should be considered.

Seroma

Fluid collections are common after operations involving wide dissection and resultant large dead spaces (like mastectomy) or where cavities are left behind (like lumpectomy). **The question whether to leave a cavity behind or close it splits the breast surgery community, but currently, with the increasing popularity of *oncoplastic* surgery, mobilizing breast tissue in order to close cavities and reshape the breast is becoming the favored approach**.

Prevention and treatment

As mentioned, some breast surgeons prefer leaving behind a cavity, to be filled with seroma which will keep the breast contour intact. Unfortunately, this effect is short-lived, and the end result may be less cosmetically appealing (see below). Closing cavities by mobilizing tissue from around the lumpectomy site may reduce seroma formation, and result in a small but acceptable deformation, which tends to be stable despite scar maturation and post-radiation changes. **When large collections are expected, due to wide dissection (mastectomy) or lymphatic channel disruption (axillary dissection — see below), prophylactic drainage (always use suction-closed drainage systems!) is recommended, until the output decreases**. Timing of drain removal is not written in stone, and depends on the surgeon's notion of how long is 'too long' and how much output is 'low enough'. Even after drain removal, fluid reaccumulation is not uncommon, and frequently requires further maneuvers, such as repeated needle aspiration (do it under sterile conditions!) and compression dressings.

Persistent seroma after mastectomy

Fluid collections under the skin flaps after mastectomy occur almost invariably, as a consequence of the wide dissection and resulting dead space. Hematomas are also frequent, and even if minor they may contribute to the accumulation of fluid. Drainage is therefore considered mandatory, and usually results in a decreasing amount of secretion over a week or so, depending on local factors. In some cases, fluid secretion and accumulation persists, sometimes in the presence of foreign bodies like a silicone graft, especially with the addition of covering material like a collagen sheet (AlloDerm®), now commonly used. A large hematoma can become 'organized', resulting in a longstanding, encapsulated collection.

While most such collections will disappear over time, it may take weeks or months in some cases, during which time the patient suffers inconvenience, pain, disability, and the need for repeated visits and possibly repeated needle aspirations. Secondary infection is not uncommon.

Long-term drainage, either by the original drain, or more commonly through a secondary drain inserted percutaneously, may eventually lead to resolution. **Rare cases will not be solved without surgical intervention, in which the fibrotic capsule of the seroma is treated, by partial or complete excision, or sometimes by cauterization of its discharging walls**.

Wound disruption

Almost 100 years ago, William Halsted, the father of modern breast surgery, said: "The surgeon who removes a breast with a malignant tumor should be the mortal enemy of the one who will be closing the wound." But fortunately, these days we are not as surgically aggressive as Halsted wanted us to be; while in his time giant, gaping chest wall wounds were the rule, today we see this only after the rare 'toilet mastectomy' (please use the politically correct modern term — *palliative mastectomy*) for neglected-advanced breast cancer. However, wound infection, hematoma or seroma can all lead to disruption of the wound closure, resulting in a productive, painful wound and agony for the patient.

Prevention

Current breast closure techniques are mainly adopted from plastic surgery, frequently using delicate, intradermal absorbable sutures. Closing the skin only, especially over a retained cavity, may result in a weak closure with a relatively high risk of dehiscence. **Layered closure, partially moving the wound tension into deeper subcutaneous tissue, should lower this incidence**.

Treatment

When wound dehiscence happens, the main question is immediate closure vs. delayed closure vs. non-closure. In a clean wound, disrupted due to an expanding seroma, immediate closure under local anesthesia is possible and hastens recovery. Antibiotic coverage may reduce the risk of secondary infection. If a large hematoma is the culprit, evacuation and closure may be better performed under the controlled and convenient environment of the operating room and under anesthesia. In cases of wound infection leading to disruption, treating the draining open wound is safer, leading to either secondary closure, or delayed approximation when infection is controlled (see ⟳ Chapter 5).

Cosmetic issues

> *The female psychologically identifies with the breast, which represents her narcissistic and sexual reality and also her relationship with others and with culture.*
>
> **Dominique Gross**

While the main outcome measures of breast surgery are oncologic, cosmetic aspects are also at the core of this discipline. The importance of the breast as a feminine organ led to the revolutionary shift from mastectomy to breast-conserving surgery (BCS) as the mainstay of breast surgery. Often, however, the struggle to keep the breast 'intact' leads to major disfigurements, questioning the value of breast preservation (■ Figure 20.1).

Deformation

Removing a significant amount of breast tissue, as required in removing a breast tumor, always results in a reduced breast volume. While initially this lost volume may go almost unnoticed, especially if a fluid-filled cavity replaces the

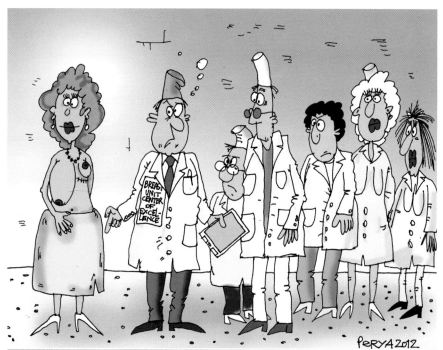

Figure 20.1. Surgeon to residents: "This is an example of superb cosmetic outcome after breast-conserving surgery..."

missing tissue, the final cosmetic outcome may be evident only months later, after scar maturation and contraction, and secondary radiation changes. Dimpling, skin retraction, cavitation, nipple deviation and complete breast disfigurement are different levels of breast deformation commonly seen after breast-conserving surgery — lumpectomy.

Prevention

Modern oncoplastic techniques, involving cavity closure, tissue mobilization, nipple repositioning and careful scar planning, are intended to reduce breast deformation, and are beyond the scope of this text. Avoiding cavities and collections often results in a stable outcome, that will change only minimally with scar maturation or radiation effects.

Treatment

When deformation is significant, plastic surgery may offer some solutions, ranging from filling defects with autologous fat injections, through local repair by tissue flaps, to completion mastectomy and reconstruction, in extreme cases. Most women will 'get used' to the end result and elect to avoid further surgery, and therefore the importance of prevention and careful planning cannot be over-emphasized.

Asymmetry

Asymmetry is expected when one breast is severed. While contour can be kept relatively intact, breast volume is sometimes significantly reduced, and further contraction is expected by the radiation effect, especially in large breasts. Oncoplastic techniques can be used to combine tumor removal with breast reduction surgery, sometimes combining contralateral reduction for immediate symmetry. Some surgeons prefer a late adaptation of the second breast, as the final breast size only becomes apparent at the end of all oncologic treatment.

Scarring

Scarring depends in large part on skin attributes, and any tendency for hypertrophic scar and keloid formation is mostly outside the control of the surgeon. There are, however, techniques that can be used to reduce unsightly scars. Using natural skin lines, such as creases, peri-areolar lines or Langer's lines (mainly circular in the breast) may result in more delicate scars. **Supporting the scar with the underlying tissue by using layered closure prevents scar widening**.

Pathology-related complications

Failure to detect the lesion ("It was palpable")

While a large percentage of lesions are nowadays detected by breast imaging and are too small to be palpated, breast surgery — especially in lesions clinically assessed as benign (e.g. fibroadenoma) — is often based on palpating the lesion and planning the operation accordingly. Occasionally, the surgeon may be surprised at surgery by not feeling the lesion which was so clearly felt at the clinic. **Large, dense or nodular breasts may be responsible for such confusion and injecting local anesthesia may cause palpable lesions to 'disappear' within the infiltrated tissue**. Also, a hematoma related to the previously performed needle biopsy could be mistaken for a mass, which is absorbed before surgery.

Another reason for failure to detect the lesion is a '**dislodged wire**'. Poorly anchored localizing wires, marking the lesion to be removed, can be dislodged during removal of covering dressings or while moving and positioning the patient.

Missing the correct lesion is another potential problem. The surgeon must be sure that the lesion he palpates is indeed the lesion which has been described by the imaging studies and sampled by the biopsy. Attention to detail here is crucial, as a benign palpable mass can easily distract the surgeon leading to removal of the wrong lesion.

Prevention and management

Pre-operative needle localization is better performed in cases where the mass is not prominent, even if the surgeon thinks he can palpate it. In the case where the surgeon is no longer sure where the mass is, **aborting the operation** and getting proper localization is preferred. If ultrasound is available, and can detect the lesion, on-table localization may be possible and the procedure can continue as planned. In the case of a dislodged wire, unless the surgeon is sure of the correct direction and depth of the lesion, guesswork is not recommended. Postponing the procedure is preferred, rather than facing the patient after surgery and admitting that another 'proper' operation is required

No lesion found by the pathologist

Rather than happily announcing to the patient that "there is no cancer", the surgeon should worry that the lesion has been missed. In some cases the lesion could have been completely removed already at the biopsy procedure, especially when vacuum-assisted biopsy (Mammotome®) was performed. **All cases of needle-localization surgery should have a specimen-radiography confirmation**. If, nevertheless, no lesion is found at pathology, repeat breast imaging is required to confirm the absence of the original lesion. Misidentification of the patient or the specimen should be suspected and actively excluded.

Positive surgical margins

While operating on a discrete palpable lesion makes it easier to keep the surgical margins away from the tumor, **the presence of intraductal pathology (e.g. DCIS) around a well-defined invasive mass is not uncommon, resulting in pathology in a wider area than expected, with a high risk of positive surgical margins and the need for repeat surgery**. In cases of surgery after previous ('neo-adjuvant') oncologic treatment, definition of the residual tumor margins may be tricky.

Better defining the tumor margins pre-operatively is sometimes possible with advanced imaging techniques, including MRI, especially in cases prone to difficulty in obtaining clear margins, including post-chemotherapy surgery and invasive lobular cancers. Multiple wires for defining resection margins may be used. Excising additional margins around the lumpectomy specimen may confirm that margins are indeed clear, and avoid the confusion associated with 'close' margins (the controversy surrounding what exactly is a close margin is beyond the scope of this chapter). **Anyway, positive or close margins are so common (up to a third of patients) that we wonder whether this should be described as a complication. All patients undergoing partial mastectomy should be warned about this potential problem and the possible need for a reoperation.**

Positive sentinel lymph node only at paraffin sections

The approach to axillary nodes has dramatically changed over recent years, and the true significance and implications of involved lymph nodes is no clearer today than it was in the past. Evidence is accumulating that with modern oncologic treatment surgical axillary 'clearance' is probably unnecessary and does not affect the outcome in most cases. **Therefore, the practice of getting a frozen section of a sentinel lymph node to decide whether completion of axillary lymph node dissection is needed is becoming outdated.** (If you will wait long enough, everything will become outdated, including yourself...). However, in cases where a frozen section is performed and found negative for cancer cells, a certain percentage of these nodes will prove eventually to harbour tumor cell on further pathologic analysis. While this false negative result cannot exactly be considered as a complication, it may be perceived as such, and therefore requires a thorough discussion, with the patient as well as with the oncologist, on the necessary further action — if at all needed.

The problem of re-lumpectomy

The battle is between margins and cosmesis and we must think like the 'oncoplastic' surgeon.

Marvin J. Silverstein

The desire for breast conservation can be overwhelming, and may lead one to wonder where the limits are. **Of course, the woman's preference must be considered, but the surgeon also has an obligation to influence the course of events.** Unfortunately, re-lumpectomy rates are rather high, up to 30% in some situations. Re-lumpectomy is associated with an increased chance of breast deformity. In some cases clear margins are not achieved even after repeat surgery, usually due to widespread intraductal carcinoma. **One has to avoid the mentality of 'one more try', or 'salami slicing', before the decision to complete a mastectomy is taken.** Reducing the rate of positive surgical margins was discussed above. Further imaging before deciding on the extent of further surgery is important, and MRI has a significant role in defining multifocality and multicentricity. Frank discussion with the patient regarding the surgical options, including mastectomy and reconstruction, is important, and may reduce suffering and disappointment... and the risk of litigation.

Axilla-related complications

A significant number of breast surgery complications are related to the axillary part of the operation. While before surgery most women are mainly concerned about the breast part of their intended surgery, it seems that the axillary part dominates their postoperative suffering. **Fortunately, the extent of axillary intervention has markedly decreased over the last decade. The assimilation of the technique of sentinel lymph node biopsy, and the changing concepts regarding the significance of axillary metastases, and the effect of axillary surgery on outcome, have led — and it is a continuing trend — to a reduced frequency of axillary clearance operations.** Nevertheless, many patients still suffer from postoperative axillary complications, both in the short-term recovery period and, more significantly, in the long term, with disabling problems that are often difficult to manage.

Lymph collections

Disruption of the lymphatic channels leads to free flow of lymph into the operated axilla. **Several factors affect the volume of lymph output, including the extent of dissection, and the amount of fat and lymph nodes within the axilla.** Axillary drains are almost invariably used after axillary dissection, and usually removed after 5-7 days when the amount of discharge is decreasing, but repeated collections are not uncommon and may require needle aspiration if symptomatic. Rarely, with persistent drainage, leaving the original drain for a longer period or reinsertion of a drain is needed, at the increased risk of infection. Attempts have been made to reduce the amount of lymph leakage, and even avoid the need for drainage altogether, by using lymphatic-sealing dissection with devices such as the Harmonic Scalpel®, but this is not yet accepted as a standard of care. **Replacing cutting, tearing and blunt dissection with meticulous tissue dissection and lymphatic sealing (sutures, clips) is probably advantageous, and in some studies has been shown to reduce drain output and facilitate its earlier removal.**

Pain

Perhaps the commonest symptom after axillary dissection, which, unfortunately tends to be a longstanding one, is pain. The combination of sensory nerve damage (it is not easy to preserve the intercosto-brachial nerves crossing the axilla), scarring and the added tissue damage of radiation therapy, often leads to chronic disability, combining hypo- and hypersensitivity, with pain radiating along the arm and forearm, and pain on movement of the arm and shoulder. While postoperative pain may be relatively mild and short-lasting, this neuralgic-type pain can appear later, weeks or months after surgery (not uncommonly following radiotherapy), and may last for years.

In patients who undergo only sentinel lymph node biopsy, the risk of chronic pain is much reduced, but not completely eliminated. This may be related to the amount of dissection needed to identify the sentinel node, and the possibility of nerve injury still exists.

Prevention and management

While preservation of the motor nerves in the axilla is considered mandatory (see below), sensory nerves are commonly sacrificed for the sake of lymph node retrieval. Trying to avoid injury to the axillary sensory nerves is recommended, but even meticulous preservation of the nerves cannot completely prevent neuropraxia and the resultant neuralgia. The **additive damage of axillary dissection and axillary radiation** markedly increases that risk for chronic pain. **Combining these two treatment modalities should be done only after serious multidisciplinary discussion, as axillary dissection may not have a clear survival benefit.**

Treatment of chronic pain is difficult and frustrating, and combining physical therapy with referral to a pain specialist is recommended. Explaining to the patient why now, six months after surgery, she has more pain than a week after surgery, is not a simple task.

Lymphedema

Disrupting the lymphatic flow through the axilla may lead to stasis and consequent swelling of the involved arm. As is true for other types of tissue damage, radiation therapy aggravates the problem by scarring and blocking even more lymphatics. The resultant lymphedema may vary from minor, mild, intermittent distal swelling to a severe permanent swelling of the whole extremity. Skin changes and ulceration, pain, and limitation of movement may render the limb non-functional in extreme cases. **Lymphangiosarcoma** of the upper extremity can develop in longstanding, neglected cases of severe lymphedema.

Fortunately, we rarely see these cases of severe lymphedema nowadays. Performing only a sentinel lymph node biopsy or avoiding axillary surgery altogether has contributed to this decrease in incidence, and even if axillary dissection is carried out, its extent is usually less than in the past, avoiding complete clearance of all lymphatic structures up to the apex of the axilla.

Prevention and management

Limiting the extent of axillary dissection, only to what is really necessary for the oncologic outcome, is the key to further reducing the incidence of this disabling complication. Thus, when axillary dissection is indicated, preserving part of the lymphatics draining the arm (sparing level 3 nodes) is currently the recommended practice. Further damage to the remaining lymphatics should be prevented, and any advantage of adding radiation treatment should be well considered. **Inflammatory processes may cause reactive lymphadenopathy that may further disturb the remaining lymphatic flow, leading to lymphedema even years after surgery. For this reason, injuries and infections of the limb should be prevented as much as possible**. The treatment of established lymphedema is difficult and only partially successful. Physical therapy and lymphatic massage may reduce the degree of swelling, and a compression sleeve may be necessary for continuing control.

Motor nerve injury

There are two motor nerves which cross the axilla and are at risk of injury during surgery:

- The **long thoracic nerve**, running down the chest wall, supplies the serratus anterior muscle. Nerve damage may lead to pain, weakness and limitation of shoulder movement, but the hallmark of this injury is *winging of the scapula*.
- The **thoracodorsal nerve** runs along the subscapular artery at the posterior wall of the axilla, to supply the latissimus dorsi muscle. Injury will lead to dysfunction in shoulder movement.

Identification and preservation of these nerves is essential as permanent injury (transection) may lead to significant disability. **Avoiding the use of muscle relaxants during axillary dissection will help the surgeon to identify the nerves, as mechanical (pinch it with your dissecting forceps!) or electrical stimulation will lead to a warning muscle contraction.**

Frozen shoulder

A frozen shoulder, which causes limitation of shoulder movements due to pain and stiffness, may be the severe end result of the various complications mentioned above. Avoidance of shoulder activity will lead to an ongoing decrease of range-of-motion, stiffness, pain, and eventual contractures and calcifications of the joint. To avoid losing shoulder functionality, awareness and early interventions are important. Physical therapy, including passive and active movements, should prevent further deterioration and regain shoulder function.

Post-reconstruction complications

Fluid collections and high drain output

As described above, the presence of large flaps and dead space, combined with the presence of foreign bodies, may lead to persistent fluid accumulation. The increased risk of secondary infection is especially significant in the presence of a graft, and long-term drainage, until the drain is 'completely dry', is often practiced (at the price of infection secondary to the presence of the drain itself). The swelling may also be perceived by the patient as a cosmetic failure, despite being reversible and self-limiting. While a surgeon may easily accept an output of 50cc per day as low enough to allow drain removal, the plastic surgeon will often insist on 10-20cc only...

Dehiscence and graft infection

Wound problems in the presence of a silicone graft may have many possible end results, ranging from a minor dehiscence requiring local treatment or simple reclosure, to complete disruption with graft exposure, infection, and inevitable removal. While never a lethal complication, **the agony associated with the failure of breast reconstruction is major, as it is usually based on high expectations, i.e. to leave the hospital with an attractive pair of boobs despite entering it in order to have one removed**.

Meticulous surgical technique, aimed at achieving well-perfused skin and durable closure, assisted by antibiotic prophylaxis, decreases the incidence but does not completely eliminate the occurrence of reconstruction failure related to wound healing problems.

Ischemia and necrosis of the breast reconstruction site

Tissue-based breast reconstruction, using pedicled or free grafts, allows for the most natural replacement of the removed breast, in terms of both consistency and appearance. The price, however, is a long and complicated operation, often with the use of microsurgery techniques for delicate vascular anastomoses. Not surprisingly, partial or complete ischemia of the mobilized tissue is not uncommon. Minor slough of skin edges, and relative ischemia of the fatty tissue at the periphery of the graft, far away from the feeding vessel, are to be expected, and usually heal spontaneously. **'Fat necrosis' lumps may appear, even months after surgery, and need to be differentiated from real masses and recurrent malignant disease. This often requires a needle biopsy for confirmation.**

Complete graft failure, with vascular thrombosis and tissue necrosis, is a major complication that mandates reoperation and graft removal. The incidence of this may be reduced by proper patient selection, avoiding high-risk conditions like vasculopathy, thrombophilia and even smoking. Treatment may be difficult, as the wide tissue defect that remains is difficult to close. It may not even allow a temporary synthetic reconstruction, and the whole episode leads to great disappointment.

Donor site issues

Even with successful tissue reconstruction of the breast, the donor site, usually the abdominal wall, may suffer short- and long-term complications. The specific type of reconstruction determines the type of associated complications.

With the now less-favored transverse rectus abdominis myocutaneous (TRAM) flaps, the resultant defect in the abdominal wall, even with mesh-based closure, often leads to abdominal wall weakness, bulging, asymmetry and even hernias. The deep inferior epigastric perforators (DIEP) flap uses skin and subcutaneous tissue only, leaving the muscle in place and keeps the integrity of the abdominal wall (often combined with abdominoplasty) intact. However, wound healing problems of the abdominal wall, with infection and dehiscence, are sometimes seen. These problems, despite being remote from the breast, may affect oncologic care by delaying necessary adjuvant treatment until healing occurs.

Luckily, all these post-reconstruction issues give more headaches to the plastic surgeon than to you ☺. **Your (the general surgeon's) job is to serve as the patient's advocate: to find her the best plastic surgeon you know or — in some cases — to deter high-risk and old women from resorting to complex post-mastectomy reconstruction.** A padded bra is not the end of the world in an aging woman. The majority of husbands would agree; use them to persuade their wives that reconstruction may not be a good idea!

Post-radiation complications

Although these complications are related to oncologic treatment carried out after surgery is 'complete' (therefore no surgical 'guilt'), and may even be considered as expected side effects — we should, nevertheless, be familiar with them, as the patient will continue to come under your follow-up, and be concerned, and sometimes even complain... So, a brief description is warranted:

- **Short-term skin changes**. Ranging from mild, sun-burn-like redness, to severe second-degree burns with blisters and skin peeling, these changes are usually self-limiting, and need local care like any other burn, including pain control and local agents. The occurrence depends on the amount of radiation and its delivery technique. Severe cases are now infrequently seen with modern radiation planning and techniques.

- **Pain**. Chronic pain has been discussed above, and is partly related to chronic tissue damage inflicted by the ionizing radiation. Edema, fibrosis and microvascular changes may lead to chronic pain in the irradiated breast and axilla, and extra tenderness around the scars. Secondary inflammatory changes, including redness and skin edema, may be painful (mainly a burning sensation), and are often difficult to differentiate rom inflammatory carcinoma, sometimes requiring biopsies to rue out this possibility.

- **Breast deformation**. While the primary injury to the breast contour is done by the surgeon, further deformity may evolve over months following surgery, due to the progress of the scar contraction. Added tissue damage, from radiation treatment, contributes further to the resultant deformity by causing tissue edema and then fibrosis. While the cosmetic effects of the radiation are difficult to predict, less scarring may lead to less eventual disfigurement. As mentioned above, avoiding seroma-filled cavities may reduce eventual scar tissue formation and contraction, and result in a reduction of late effects of radiation upon the final cosmetic outcome.

- **Adjacent organ injury**. Directing the ionizing radiation to where it should do its magic is a complicated task, dependent upon clever physicists and wise radiation oncologists. Modern radiotherapy is based on careful planning, with the use of 3D CT imaging and multi-directional beams, all aiming to minimize collateral damage. **Nevertheless, nearby organs are still occasionally harmed by stray photons, finding their way to the heart or lungs**. Early radiation pneumonitis, late radiation fibrosis, and chronic cough with deteriorating pulmonary function tests still affect breast cancer survivors.

- Left-sided radiation therapy with a significantly high dose **reaching the heart** may damage all its components, including the pericardium, the myocardium, the valves, the coronary arteries and the conduction system. Pericarditis is the typical manifestation of acute radiation injury, and follow-up years or decades later may reveal chronic pericarditis, cardiomyopathy, coronary disease, valvular damage and conduction disorders.

- **Prevention** is in the hands of the radiation oncologists, and treatment is in the hands of the pulmonologists and cardiologists. Surgeons are exempted on this one. However, discuss these potentially serious delayed effects of radiotherapy during your routine pre-operative 'lecture' on BCS vs. mastectomy — the latter option obviously obviates (in most cases) the need for radiotherapy. **Patients should know that BCS is not always a panacea. Years ahead they may pay the price for choosing to retain a few grams of fatty tissue.**

Recurrent local disease

The delicate line between what can be considered a complication and what results from the natural course of an aggressive disease is often difficult to define. But in general, surgeons, especially the soft-hearted ones, may feel responsible, or even guilty, when a patient returns, months or even years later, with a recurrent tumor at or near the previous surgical scar. While distant metastatic disease is perceived as an inevitable outcome of both tumor biology and the stage at presentation, local recurrence may indeed be related to the surgical technique.

The debate regarding what is considered to be acceptable surgical margins is clearly beyond the scope of this book. Keeping to good old practices of: staying away from a palpable tumor, removing 'extra margins', adopting oncoplastic techniques for wide resection, getting specimen mammography for wire-localized non-palpable lesions, and making accurate and clear markings for the pathologist, all help in reaching the goal of complete surgical excision. **Involved and close margins should be appropriately addressed, better after a multidisciplinary discussion about the best course of action (re-excision now? chemotherapy first? radiation boost only? completion mastectomy?) and proper imaging.**

Legal complications

'Failure to diagnose breast cancer' is one of the most common reasons for physicians to be sued in US. One must remain suspicious, but still use some common sense. Sometimes you can't do both.

John Kennedy

Women tend to be emotionally attached to their breasts, more than they are to other parts of their bodies. The diagnosis of breast cancer represents a huge stress to the woman and her family, and against such a background even relativity minor complications are commonly amplified. That a wound complication may delay the scheduled adjuvant radio/chemotherapy for a week or so is not clinically significant but to the breast cancer patient it could seem a tragedy.

It is no wonder then that in a society in which breast cancer has become a profitable industry, surrounded by hype, breast surgery-related litigation for alleged and true malpractice is so common. With improving standards of care, litigation concerning 'wrong side surgery' (yes, the normal breast chopped off, the cancerous left *in situ*) or unnecessary mastectomy (this was common in the old days when surgeons would proceed immediately with mastectomy based on misinterpretation of frozen section results) has declined drastically. However, litigation concerning a 'missed diagnosis' or 'delayed diagnosis' of breast cancer is common. **In fact, studies show that malignant neoplasm of the female breast continues to be the most prevalent and the second most expensive condition resulting in malpractice claims lodged against all physicians, and that radiologists are the most frequently sued specialty.** While the last part of the latter sentence sounds comforting to our surgical ears, we surgeons — who commonly are dominant in the overall care of breast cancer patients — are often being sued as well.

There is good evidence to show that a delay of up to three months in diagnosis does not adversely affect the patient's treatment or prognosis. But often the 'evidence' has little impact on the decision of the jury: multi-million dollar awards have been decided for the patient even for a delay of diagnosis as short as six weeks. Usually, the longer the delay the higher the average award.

Mishaps, real or perceived, of reconstructive breast surgery are commonly litigated as well. As we doubt whether a reconstructive-plastic surgeon would ever bother to open this book (you do not get paid for reading books!) we won't dwell further on this topic.

Remember: in dealing with the breast you have to be extra careful, super considerate and immensely tender — not only to the patient but also to her breast. You cannot take any chances with the diagnosis of cancer. "Beware a lumpy area that does not feel right and images as normal", "A typical breast cancer is easy to diagnose — it is the atypical one in a young patient that causes diagnostic problems" [both quotations by Michael Dixon].

And try to keep up to date despite the fact that "the medical profession can invent tests for breast disease faster than they are found out to be useless." [David Dent].

Let me conclude with another quotation from Professor David Dent of Cape Town.

"Actually, one's mind is amazing at rationalization. I thought our mastectomy complication rate was about zero. Certainly mine was. That is until we went into an international multicenter prospective trial of prophylactic antibiotics, with a full-time data handler, who visited each patient and the intern daily. Our complication rate was about 25%, with seromas, wound infections (Isn't the edge just a little red? No its infected!), hematomas and partial dehiscences. Mostly very small stuff, but there. Complications are in the eye of the beholder."

David Dent

Chapter 21

The thyroid, parathyroid and adrenal glands

Saba Balasubramanian

> **This chapter has been subdivided into the following four sections:**
>
> 1. Basic considerations.
> 2. Thyroidectomy.
> 3. Parathyroidectomy.
> 4. Adrenalectomy.

1   Basic considerations

Many of you may find texts about endocrine surgery boring — endless series of lab tests; long lists of drugs some of which are difficult to spell; convoluted illustrations of hormonal feedback mechanisms; a limited menu of uninspiring excisional procedures and a depressing number of potential complications with life-long consequences. So let me try and bring before you a simplified and more inspiring version.

Background and pre-operative considerations

Endocrine surgery is performed by surgeons from a variety of backgrounds such as general surgery, head and neck/ENT and yes — even urology. The relatively low prevalence of surgical endocrine disease and the distribution of cases across several specialties and surgeons make accumulation of volume and experience difficult. Procedures in endocrine surgery are **purely excisional** (almost the only specialty without any element of reconstruction — if we exclude parathyroid autotransplantation of course!). This can lead to the perception that complications are easy to avoid. In addition, **postoperative hormonal problems** (such as hypocalcemia and adrenal insufficiency) are sometimes not considered 'surgical problems' and some patients are referred to physicians or endocrinologists for management. Although good collaboration and multidisciplinary input is critical to the treatment of complex endocrine disease, an in-depth understanding of acute postoperative hormonal derangements by the surgeon facilitates early recognition of the problem and appropriate treatment.

As with any surgical procedure, the need for surgery should be carefully considered. Is the surgery to:

- treat suspected or confirmed **cancer**?
- treat **hormonal over-activity** and thereby specific symptoms or associated diseases?
- treat **compressive symptoms** (as in a goiter)?
- prevent *future* problems such as airway compression with large goiters, osteoporosis, renal impairment or vascular complications in primary hyperparathyroidism?
- improve cosmesis/aesthesis (in patients with a large goiter)?

The **extent of surgery** — as always, the more you do, the higher is the potential for complications — is dependent on the pathology and sometimes (oddly enough), the environment in which you work in. The various procedures relating to the thyroid, parathyroid and adrenals are:

- **Thyroid**: total thyroidectomy; subtotal thyroidectomy; Dunhill's (total on one side and subtotal on the other) procedure; hemi-thyroidectomy and isthmectomy. Prophylactic or therapeutic lymph node dissections may be required alongside thyroidectomy in some patients with thyroid cancer.
- **Parathyroid**: focused/targeted parathyroidectomy; unilateral exploration and bilateral exploration with excision of one/more glands (sometimes subtotal resection or total resection with auto-transplant is required). A thymectomy is recommended in MEN1 syndrome and renal hyperparathyroidism.
- **Adrenal**: unilateral or bilateral adrenalectomy. A partial adrenalectomy is occasionally performed in certain situations such as bilateral phaeochromocytoma to reduce steroid dependence. Occasionally,

radical resection of adjacent organs such as the kidney may be required in large adrenal cancers with local invasion.

Although operative findings may often dictate the extent of surgery, the **pre-operative plan and the underlying rationale should be discussed with the patient.** This is important as it influences patient expectations of outcomes including the need for postoperative hormone replacement and the potential need for further surgery. In certain instances, the extent of surgery may be tailored to local circumstances. **A subtotal resection may be preferred to total thyroidectomy in Graves' disease or multinodular goiter in situations where compliance with lifelong thyroxine replacement may be difficult to ensure. Life-threatening hypothyroidism may be a greater risk than the recurrence of disease and the risks of re-do surgery.**

Surgeons should also ensure that patients understand the risk of potential complications. Table ■ 21.1 provides a fairly comprehensive list of complications specific to endocrine surgery.

The need for detailed explanation of the potential risks should be balanced against the risk of inducing unnecessary anxiety over very uncommon complications. This could be considered paternalistic by some surgeons and patients' advocates; however, surgeons have to be able to draw a line somewhere along the slippery slope of rare complications and their even

Table 21.1. Specific complications related to thyroid, parathyroid and adrenal surgery.

Type of complications	Thyroidectomy	Parathyroidectomy	Adrenalectomy
Endocrine-specific	Hypocalcemia Recurrent disease	Persistent/recurrent hypercalcemia Hypocalcemia	Adrenal insufficiency Persistent/recurrent disease
Access-specific	Hypertrophic scar/keloid	Hypertrophic scar/keloid	Port site or incisional hernia
Adjacent structural damage	Airway compromise Voice change (RLN damage)	Voice change (RLN damage)	Liver/major vascular injury (right side) Spleen/pancreas/major vascular injury (left side)

rarer consequences. For example, I do not counsel patients about the potential need for a tracheostomy during routine, first-time thyroid and parathyroid surgery, as I consider this complication to be extremely rare. Elaborating on such complications risks needless and undue anxiety and may result in patients deciding against surgery that would clearly be in their best interests.

Further in this chapter, I will attempt to explain not just the preventative and management aspects of complications, but also the pathophysiology underlying these problems. **General complications** such as infection and bleeding, access-related complications such as hypertrophic scarring, keloid formation and wound dehiscence/hernia are not discussed here. Also not discussed are the management and complications relating to lateral compartment neck dissections occasionally needed in the treatment of thyroid cancer.

2 Thyroidectomy

The extirpation of the thyroid gland for goiter typifies, perhaps better than any operation, the triumph of the surgeon's art....

William Stewart Halsted

Pre-operative considerations

Ensuring an euthyroid status before thyroid surgery is essential to prevent peri-operative *thyroid storms*, which are fortunately extremely rare now. In patients who are hyperthyroid, antithyroid drugs (+/- beta-blockers) can often help restore euthyroid status in a few weeks. Occasionally, patients may present with a **thyrotoxic crisis** — very unwell with tachycardia, other tachyarrhythmias and heart failure — and will require rapid correction of their thyroid status before surgery. We treat these patients with a combination of medications including antithyroid drugs (carbimazole or propylthiouracil), Lugol's iodine (iodine in high doses paradoxically suppresses thyroid hormone synthesis and release in the short term — the Wolff-Chaikoff effect), cholestyramine (interrupts the enterohepatic circulation and increases removal of thyroid hormones from the circulation), beta-blockers (antagonizes the effects of thyroid hormones and reduces peripheral T4-T3 conversion) and, rarely, steroids.

A pre-operative **vocal cord check** is indicated in patients with voice change, but not mandatory in all cases. However, it is routinely performed in most centers (you can call it "defensive management"...). Abnormalities are rarely detected (one in several hundred asymptomatic patients), but if found do have the potential to change the need for or the extent of surgery required.

A baseline **calcium and vitamin D estimation** may help detect and treat patients with hypocalcemia and/or vitamin D deficiency, thereby reducing the risk of transient **postoperative hypocalcemia**, especially before total thyroidectomy.

Patients with a pre-operative diagnosis of **medullary thyroid carcinoma** (MTC) should have a diagnosis of phaeochromocytoma excluded by biochemical testing. If a phaeochromocytoma is detected, adrenal surgery should take precedence over thyroid surgery to reduce the real danger of a hypertensive crisis during thyroidectomy.

Lastly, think about whether the patient has a **retrosternal goiter**. Most retrosternal goiters can be delivered through the neck. However, in cases where the extension reaches the carina or beyond, it would be sensible to be prepared for a *sternotomy* or have someone to help you out, if the need arises!

Intra-operative considerations

Looking for the recurrent laryngeal nerve after previous thyroidectomy needs all the sensitivity of detecting a landmine in Angola.

David Dent

The **recurrent laryngeal nerve** is the most important structure to be identified and preserved in thyroid surgery. The thyroid lobe needs to be mobilized and retracted medially to see the nerve in the tracheo-esophageal groove as a glistening white, cord-like structure with a tiny vessel running on its surface. On the right side, the nerve often has an oblique course and does not run in the tracheo-esophageal groove. The very uncommon scenario of a **non-recurrent nerve** should also be borne in mind on the right side. Sometimes, in very large goiters, significant dissection and mobilization may need to be done to reach the plane of the nerve. In these instances, care should be taken to recognize the nerve if it aberrantly lies *on* the lobes instead of *beneath* it. One way to avoid nerve damage in this situation would be to dissect on or just beneath the thyroid capsule. **Ideally, the nerve should be tracked up to its entry into the larynx as injuries to the nerve often occur at this point**. In some situations, however, (when it is clear that the thyroid lobe has been dissected away from the plane of the nerve), it may be considered unwise to dissect all along the length of the nerve as this may injure the blood supply to the parathyroid glands. Occasionally, if the nerve cannot be identified clearly and the thyroid lobe has been devascularized and almost completely mobilized, it may be considered judicious not to further explore the area to avoid inadvertent injury to the nerve or the parathyroid glands. If a surgeon finds himself/herself to be in this situation more often than the occasional instance, I would suggest further mentorship and guidance by an experienced endocrine surgeon. The issue of routine identification of the recurrent nerve during a subtotal resection is debatable. I have rarely had the need to do a subtotal resection and hence would not consider myself competent to answer this. However, a good understanding of the course of the nerve (especially at its entry into the larynx) would help avoid injury during a subtotal resection; even if the nerve is not identified near the laryngeal entry.

Intra-operative nerve monitoring is increasingly being used during routine thyroid surgery. There is little evidence to suggest that this reduces the risk of nerve injury. However, if there is loss of signal on one side indicating nerve damage, surgery on the other side may be limited or delayed or avoided thus minimizing the chances of bilateral cord paresis.

An alternative technique is not to expose the nerve but to use, in benign disease at least, stay sutures placed in the lobe and use them to lift the lobe while gently peeling out the thin layers off the gland, thus staying very close to the thyroid capsule avoiding the area where the nerve is. Finally, a tiny segment of the posterior thyroid capsule might be left on purpose on top of Berry's ligament to avoid the nerve at its entrance to the larynx. **Ari**

I do not recommend that the **external branch of the superior laryngeal nerve** should be identified in all cases; knowledge of the variations of its course along with careful dissection close to the thyroid capsule should prevent injury in most cases.

A detailed awareness of the anatomy of the **parathyroid glands** and their relationship to the thyroid, inferior thyroid artery and recurrent laryngeal nerve enables the preservation of viable parathyroid glands. Postoperative **hypoparathyroidism** is often due to devascularization of the parathyroid glands and uncommonly due to inadvertent parathyroidectomy. Visualization of all parathyroid glands is not essential during a thyroidectomy. However, if they can be seen early in the dissection, care can be taken to avoid damage to them and the vasculature that often runs on the thyroid capsule. If not seen, capsular dissection is crucial to their preservation. Obviously, ligating the branches of the inferior thyroid artery ('on the gland') rather than the main artery reduces the chances of parathyroid ischemia. If at the end of the procedure, a parathyroid gland appears ischemic (pale, not black which simply implies venous congestion), it could be excised, minced and implanted in a well-vascularized muscle bed (e.g. in the sternomastoid). Care should be taken to avoid oozing in the bed.

Changing course and limiting the extent of surgery based on intra-operative findings is the hallmark of an experienced and wise surgeon. If surgery on one side of the thyroid has been difficult and there are concerns about nerve integrity, careful consideration needs to be given to continuing surgery on the other side. If surgery is for a benign multinodular goiter, lobectomy on the other side can be abandoned, and revisited at a later date if really necessary. Similarly, resorting to near total or very occasionally subtotal resection (on one side) may be necessary to avoid damage to the nerve and/or parathyroid glands. This may also be true for thyroid cancer as delayed completion of thyroidectomy has little impact (if any) on prognosis. **A patient with an intact thyroid lobe and no airway compromise is in a much better situation than a patient who has undergone total thyroidectomy but ends up with a tracheostomy** (because of bilateral recurrent nerve palsy).

Given the extremely good prognosis of thyroid cancer in general, the emphasis is on keeping the morbidity of surgery to a minimum. In patients undergoing central node dissection, the extent of dissection can also be modified (at least on the contralateral side) depending on the risk of postoperative hypoparathyroidism and nerve injury.

The shape of the patient's neck often influences how elegant a thyroidectomy will be. In this respect, I would much rather operate on a giraffe than a hippo!

What about drains? I do not use drains routinely, but would not say "never" either! I drain after procedures that include a central neck dissection and occasionally following re-do surgery. I believe that drains do not reduce reoperation rates for bleeding, but do add to postoperative morbidity and lengthen hospital stay. I am, however, not too excited by this debate and am happy to accept the opinion of people who feel otherwise. If you do choose to leave a drain, remember to remove it the next morning, after the dreaded bleeding failed to materialize.

Postoperative considerations

Acute airway compromise

Although rare, the most worrying short-term complication following thyroid surgery is acute airway compromise — it is the fear of this problem that limits the more general adoption of thyroidectomy as a day-case procedure. The reasons are often multifactorial: hematoma and airway edema are common predisposing factors. Bilateral nerve palsy is rare and rarer still (in the developed world) is *tracheomalacia*. **Post-thyroidectomy tracheomalacia** is reported mainly from developing countries and is likely to be related to very large, longstanding goiters resulting in weakening of the tracheal cartilages; this is often compounded by coexisting malnutrition. Significant bleeding usually occurs in the first six hours of the procedure, but it may present in a delayed manner up to 48 hours later. I suspect that the increasing use of modern vessel-sealing technology and clips (as opposed to ties) has slightly increased the risk of bleeding; however, overall rates should still be low (around 1%).

Early identification of airway compromise and rapid assessment are crucial to optimal management. **A patient with significant respiratory distress following a thyroidectomy needs the following measures instituted rapidly**:

- Sit the patient upright and start oxygen.
- Assess the wound and evacuate any hematoma (often at the bedside by removing the skin or subcuticular stitches). **Yes, immediately ripping the wound may be lifesaving!**
- A single dose of intravenous steroids may help reduce airway edema.
- Urgent intubation and reoperation under anesthesia to stop the bleeding.

Voice changes

> *Unilateral recurrent laryngeal nerve damage produces voice changes, but not choking: they graduate in the choir from singing "Ave Maria" to "Old Man River".*
>
> **David Dent**

Voice change such as hoarseness or weakness following thyroid surgery is common and does not necessarily reflect significant or lasting nerve damage. The vast majority of such change settles spontaneously and pre-operative counseling has immense value in reassurance. Some centers offer **routine postoperative laryngoscopy** to all patients; the optimum timing of which is debatable as very early examinations pick up a greater number of patients with transient cord paresis, the majority of which settle spontaneously. **Speech therapy** is effective but in some cases further intervention such as vocal cord injection or medialization of the cords may be needed. Some patients experience change in voice quality despite no evidence of damage on laryngoscopy. In some instances, this can be due to damage to the external branch of the **superior**

laryngeal nerve, the effects of which may not be obvious at laryngoscopy. Be that as it may, unless your patient is an opera mezzo-soprano, the vast majority of such cases end with... happy endings ☺ (■ Figure 21.1).

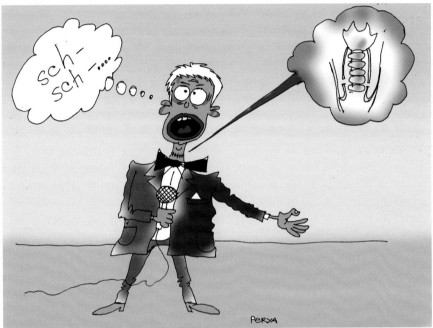

Figure 21.1. Opera singer trying to sing after a thyroidectomy and injury to the recurrent nerves on both sides... [1].

Hypocalcemia

It seems hardly credible that the loss of bodies so tiny as the parathyroids should be followed by a result so disastrous.
William Stewart Halsted

Post-thyroidectomy hypocalcemia is a consequence of hypoparathyroidism in the vast majority of patients. Hypoparathyroidism may be due to direct parathyroid damage, gland devascularization and/or inadvertent parathyroidectomy. *Transient* hypoparathyroidism is much more common. It may be asymptomatic or may manifest as tingling, numbness and paresthesia in the extremities and peri-oral region — do you still remember what the *Trousseau* and *Chvostek* signs are? Occasionally, symptoms may be non-specific and include nausea, lethargy and a feeling of being unwell.

---

[1] This is only a caricature. In real life a patient with bilateral nerve injury will end up with a tracheostomy more often than not...

A clearly defined protocol should be in place to detect and treat hypocalcemia appropriately. Postoperative hypocalcemia can sometimes manifest as late as 72 hours after surgery. Several centers make use of a low parathyroid hormone (PTH) level in the early postoperative period as a marker of postoperative hypocalcemia and treat patients with calcium/vitamin D supplements even if asymptomatic. A low serum calcium level along with a low PTH level clinches the diagnosis. Occasionally, a low postoperative serum calcium level is not due to hypoparathyroidism but due to **hungry bone syndrome**. Increased bone turnover is a hallmark of severe *hyperthyroidism* and in these patients there is a significant calcium shift from the circulation to the bones following surgery. This is typically associated with a *high PTH level* (that is secondary to the hypocalcemia). **It is important to differentiate between the hypocalcemia of hypoparathyroidism and the hypocalcemia of hungry bone syndrome** as there is a subtle but significant difference in how these two kinds of hypocalcemia are treated. In the former, calcium is given along with activated vitamin D such as alfacalcidol or calcitriol (as there is little PTH available to activate vitamin D in the 1-alpha position) and in the latter, calcium supplements alone are all that is needed for a short period of time. Inactive vitamin D may sometimes be needed if there is associated vitamin D deficiency. Patients started on alfacalcidol or calcitriol should be monitored carefully as there is a distinct risk of developing hypercalcemia in the weeks to months following surgery. Most patients can be weaned off their supplements within 3-12 months after surgery. Some, however, require longer-term supplementation and in these patients the treatment should aim to keep the serum calcium in the low normal range as aiming for higher levels will increase the risk of hypercalciuria and its attendant complications. In the long term, hypocalcemia due to hypoparathyroidism may be associated with an increased risk of renal impairment and bone disease.

Are you asleep yet?

3 Parathyroidectomy

Has the patient renal stones
Painful, brittle, broken bones
Complaints of thirst and constipation
Next to peptic ulceration
And you doubt his mental state
Determine calcium and phosphate
Sure the underlying mechanism
Might be hyperparathyroidism.

Hajo A. Bruining

There are several issues in parathyroid surgery that are in common with thyroid surgery. These include complications related to the laryngeal nerves and airway problems, which have already been covered and will not be repeated here. **Parathyroid surgery should only be done by surgeons who do it frequently.** Although an 'adequate volume' has not been universally agreed, my view is that this should only be done by surgeons who do at least one case a month.

Pre-operative considerations

The key to an adequate outcome is a clear diagnosis. With increasing earlier diagnosis and the recognition of entities such as *normocalcemic hyperparathyroidism* and *hypercalcemia with normal but non-suppressed parathyroid hormone (PTH)*, it is important to ensure that the biochemical diagnosis is correct. The primary objective of surgery (i.e. correction of hypercalcemia) should be clearly explained. This will reduce the risk of continuing end-organ damage — bone and kidney. **However, clinical effects such as broken bones, further renal calculi, worsening renal function and pancreatitis may still occur in patients following successful surgery.** Patients with symptoms 'attributable' to primary hyperparathyroidism (such as tiredness, bone and joint pains, mood changes, irritability, headaches and forgetfulness) should be counseled that symptom relief is only a secondary goal and may not always be achieved. Coexisting vitamin D deficiency should be identified and if present, postoperative hypocalcemia should be anticipated. Treatment of vitamin D deficiency could be started pre-operatively if the serum calcium is not very high; if too high, then correction could be done following surgery.

Several **pre-operative imaging techniques** (ultrasound, Sestamibi scan, CT scan, MRI, selective venous sampling) and **intra-operative modalities** (ultrasound, intravenous methylene blue, frozen section, intra-operative PTH assay, radioguided techniques) are available and different protocols are used in different centers to reduce the risk of failure. Although the use of pre-operative imaging has not been convincingly demonstrated to improve success rates in parathyroid surgery, it has now become the norm. **Failure to localize abnormal parathyroids on pre-operative imaging should raise the suspicion of multi-gland disease or a small, single adenoma, occasionally in the intrathyroidal position.** The **surgical approach** (targeted/focused surgery, unilateral exploration and bilateral exploration) depends on the results of pre-operative imaging techniques. **Our practice is to obtain an ultrasound and MIBI scan and offer targeted/focused parathyroidectomy only in patients with concordant results on dual imaging.** Centers that use intra-operative PTH (IOPTH) assay may be more liberal in the use of focused/unilateral approaches.

Any combination of localization techniques and surgical approaches is acceptable as long as the success of first-time surgery is constantly audited and maintained at around 95%. It is not acceptable to perform focused/targeted surgery with the view that bilateral exploration can be performed if the initial operation fails. The second operation often involves a return to the same side of the initial operation to look for the other gland on that side! Most patients prefer a single successful operation to a 'small incision' operation with a higher chance of failure. I often explain to patients that the morbidity (pain and scar length) of a bilateral exploration is only marginally higher than a focused operation. Paradoxically, the only cases of nerve injury following first-time parathyroidectomy I have seen and heard have occurred following a focused operation!

In patients with serum calcium >3.0mmol/L (>12mg/dL), intravenous hydration is a reasonable precaution before surgery. For those with higher levels, calcium levels should be lowered over a period of days before surgery with a combination of sodium-containing intravenous fluids, loop diuretics and occasionally intravenous bisphosphonates.

Intra-operative considerations

The principles underlying nerve identification and preservation have already been covered. The approach to identification of the parathyroid glands should be systematic and sequential.

During a targeted parathyroidectomy for single-gland disease, the enlarged gland identified on pre-operative imaging can usually be identified with little difficulty. However, as the incision is small and exposure is often limited, there is potential to damage a closely situated recurrent nerve.

During a bilateral neck exploration, the **identification of abnormal glands** should be possible with careful dissection and exploration. If the glands are not identified in their usual locations, other sites such as the para/retroesophageal space and thymus should be explored. Very rarely, ectopic glands have been found very high near the skull base or in the carotid sheath. Very occasionally, if three normal glands have been identified and the search is on for the fourth gland, consideration should be given to the possibility of a near normal size parathyroid adenoma in the subcapsular or intrathyroidal location.

Postoperative considerations

Many of the complications have already been dealt with in the section on thyroid surgery. **Hypocalcemia** after parathyroid surgery is more commonly seen in populations where presentation is delayed and is due to severe *hungry bone syndrome*. This can result in patients needing several grams of oral (+/- intravenous) calcium a day for days to weeks. In the developed world where the disease is much milder and detected early, hypocalcemia is uncommon except in the following three scenarios:

- **MEN1 syndrome** — where the aim of the operation is to remove all except a small remnant of one parathyroid gland (i.e. subtotal parathyroidectomy). The alternative is a total parathyroidectomy and autotransplantation.
- **Renal (secondary) hyperparathyroidism** — as in MEN1 syndrome.
- **Re-do parathyroid surgery** — where residual normal parathyroid tissue may be minimal or absent.

The treatment follows the principles already discussed and as emphasized earlier, a distinction needs to be made between hypocalcemia of hypoparathyroidism and that due to increased bone turnover. This is to decide on whether active vitamin D (alfacalcidol or calcitriol) is required for the treatment of hypocalcemia.

Failure to cure hypercalcemia is the complication dreaded by parathyroid surgeons! Contrary to popular opinion, it does not always reflect inexperience or technical incompetence. Reasons for failure have been explored at length in various textbooks and reviews, but in brief they can be summarized as follows:

- Failure to recognize and/or inadequate treatment of multi-gland disease.
- Small adenoma in the usual location (but unidentified by the surgeon).
- Adenoma in an ectopic location in the neck or mediastinum.

How should patients with persistent hypercalcemia be managed?
Several factors need to be considered before a decision to reoperate is made:

- Has the calcium level improved or is it as high as before the operation? The former is seen in patients with multi-gland disease where one or more glands have been removed. The latter is seen in situations where an ectopic adenoma has not been identified.
- Why has the operation failed? Is it due to multi-gland disease that was not recognized at first surgery or is it because an adenoma (single-gland disease) was not identified?

- How strong are the indications for surgery in the first place? Is it for severe hypercalcemia, marked osteoporosis or renal impairment or is it for minimally symptomatic disease with borderline hypercalcemia? **The latter could be managed conservatively**.

If re-do surgery is indicated, most surgeons would agree that it should be done by an experienced parathyroid surgeon (i.e. usually somebody more experienced than you!). A full review of the factors discussed above and discussion of intra-operative findings with the original surgeon are essential. I would strongly recommend further localization tests unless it is clear that the reason for failure was multi-gland disease and the location of the remaining glands has been clearly documented at the first surgery.

4 Adrenalectomy

General considerations

The best outcomes following adrenal surgery are seen in units where there is a close collaboration between the endocrinologists, anesthetists and the surgeons. The importance of patient selection, careful biochemical diagnosis and appropriate peri-operative management cannot be over-emphasized. As with other procedures in endocrine surgery, the biochemical diagnosis (be it functioning or non-functioning) is important for appropriate counseling, management of expectations and pre-operative preparation. The **minimum biochemical work-up** includes steroid biochemistry and urine or plasma levels of catecholamines and their metabolites. Renin/aldosterone levels should be estimated in patients with hypertension and/or hypokalemia. The results should be carefully considered in the context of current medications which may interfere with the estimation of the levels of several hormones. If in doubt, consult a friendly endocrinologist or biochemist!

Biopsy of adrenal lesions is rarely indicated. Even if required in instances of suspected adrenal metastases or lymphoma, **it is vital to ensure that a phaeochromocytoma has been ruled out by biochemical testing**. Failure to observe these basic principles can have catastrophic consequences. Most endocrine surgeons have heard of instances where biopsy or similar intervention in an adrenal mass without a biochemical diagnosis has resulted in a myocardial infarction as a result of an undiagnosed phaeochromocytoma. **It is for this reason that retroperitoneal masses discovered at an emergency laparotomy done for unrelated causes should not be biopsied or explored**.

The **surgical approach** to the adrenal lump should be dictated by the surgeon's experience, size of tumor and the risk of adrenal cancer. **In general, most authors would avoid a laparoscopic approach in large tumors (>10cm) suspected to be adrenal cancers due to the risks of capsular rupture and the potential increased risk of local recurrence**. Capsular rupture should be avoided in both adrenal cancers and phaeochromocytoma as they are prone to 'seeding' and result in locally recurrent disease. Both open and laparoscopic techniques can be performed via the anterior, lateral and posterior approaches. Further details are beyond the scope of this chapter. The specific peri-operative issues relating to different syndromes in which an adrenalectomy is considered are outlined below.

Phaeochromocytoma — pre-operative considerations

Blood pressure should be adequately controlled with maximally tolerated alpha-blockade. Different regimens are in use to achieve this objective. Our practice is to start patients on phenoxybenzamine (an irreversible alpha-blocker) at a dose of 10mg twice a day. In the ten days leading to surgery, this dose is gradually escalated by 10mg every 48 hours to maximally tolerated levels. Patients often report nasal stuffiness (due to the vasodilatory effects of the drug on the nasal mucosa) and symptoms of postural hypotension and tachycardia. They are usually encouraged to increase oral fluid intake in an attempt to 'fill the vasodilated' circulation. **A well-filled circulation is thought to ameliorate the fall in blood pressure that often occurs immediately after tumor excision**. In patients in whom severe tachycardia is troublesome, beta-blockers may be used. **It is important to stress that beta-blockers should not be used until alpha-blockade has been achieved as this may precipitate a hypertensive crisis due to unopposed alpha-agonist action**.

Phaeochromocytoma — intra-operative considerations

Phaeochromocytomas tend to be more vascular than other adrenal tumors. These tumors tend to draw arterial supply not only from the known sources (the aorta, renal artery and the inferior phrenic artery) but also from the surrounding retroperitoneal and lumbar vessels. The intra-operative cardiovascular hemodynamic changes are best managed by an experienced senior anesthetist who closely monitors the patient throughout surgery using arterial and central venous catheters and is well equipped with a variety of intravenous vasoconstrictor and vasodilatory drugs. Good communication between the surgeon and the anesthetist facilitates a smoother course during surgery. For example, it is advisable to warn the anesthetist before the main adrenal vein is divided, so he/she is prepared to deal with the inevitable drop in blood pressure.

It is important to perform meticulous surgical control with clips or sutures, etc., of all the small arteries — about 40 of them — going to the gland, when the dissection progresses. They might not bleed now, but can bleed later. **Ari**

One may save the need for the Finnish meticulousness by using one of the common vessel-sealing devices like the Harmonic Scalpel® or LigaSure™, for quick removal of the gland once the venous drainage was controlled. **Danny**

Phaeochromocytoma — postoperative considerations

Management in an intensive care environment will help detect and appropriately treat hypotension. *Hypoglycemia* may occasionally occur in the first few hours after resection of a phaeochromocytoma, but this is easily treated. Due to **significant fluid shifts** (caused by dropping peripheral vascular resistance) in the peri-operative period and the need for rapid fluid infusions to maintain the circulation, a significant (dilutional) **drop in hemoglobin** level (by several grams/dL) is often seen and needs to be taken into consideration when evaluating the patient for possible postoperative bleeding. **Recurrence of phaeochromocytoma** is uncommon. However, our practice is to screen all patients who have had surgery by measuring urine and/or plasma biochemistry on an annual basis to enable early detection of any recurrent disease. **Malignant phaeochromocytomas** are very rare and only diagnosed when local infiltration or metastases are present — histology is unreliable in diagnosing malignancy.

Adrenal hypercortisolism

Cushing's syndrome (hypercortisolism) may be exogenous (due to steroid administration) or endogenous (excessive production). The latter is often due to a pituitary tumor (**Cushing's disease**) secreting ACTH that drives the adrenal gland to hypersecrete cortisol — ACTH-dependent hypercortisolism. Other causes include adrenal **adenomas** or **carcinomas** that autonomously secrete steroids (ACTH-independent hypercortisolism) — **adrenalectomy** is indicated for the treatment of these lesions. **Bilateral adrenalectomy** is sometimes required in ACTH-independent adrenocortical hyperplasia (which can affect both adrenal glands) and occasionally in patients with ACTH-dependent (pituitary or ectopic) adrenal disease where treatment of the tumor producing ACTH has failed.

A few points:

- Surgeons should understand that **these patients are at a higher than usual risk of complications** such as local/systemic infection, wound dehiscence and venous thromboembolism partly because of chronic steroid excess and partly due to the associated morbidity such as obesity, diabetes, hypertension and other cardiovascular problems.

- **Peri-operative steroid cover** with high doses of parenteral hydrocortisone (100mg q6-8 hourly) is required to enable the body to cope with increased steroid requirements. In patients having a **unilateral adrenalectomy** for cortisol excess, the contralateral adrenal is suppressed and this may take weeks to years to recover function. The peri-operative steroid dose is gradually tapered to physiological doses and these are maintained until there is biochemical evidence of recovery of function in the other adrenal (in patients having a unilateral adrenalectomy). Patients having **bilateral adrenalectomy** will need steroids lifelong. Close cooperation with, and advice from endocrinology colleagues are an integral part of multidisciplinary care and are invaluable in these situations.

- **Patients discharged** on replacement steroids (either to compensate for contralateral adrenal suppression following unilateral adrenalectomy or those who have had bilateral resections) **have a two-fold increased long-term mortality compared to the general population**. They should be warned of the risks of non-compliance to steroids and the need to seek medical help even for otherwise simple illnesses such as gastroenteritis and upper respiratory tract infections. Several non-specific symptoms (such as nausea, fatigue and anorexia) are associated with steroid insufficiency, but if untreated, sudden and severe deterioration in general health and hypotension can occur. Our practice is to provide them with a **'steroid' bracelet** or card advising carers of their adrenal status and warning of the risk of fatal adrenal insufficiency if not appropriately treated. Patients are also given a hydrocortisone syringe for self-injection if medical help is not readily available.

Conn's syndrome

Patients with Conn's syndrome (primary hyperaldosteronism where the source of aldosterone excess is unilateral) have surgery primarily to enable easier control of their blood pressure. Conn's adenomas are typically small and these patients often have bilateral adrenal nodularity. Lateralization of the side of adrenal aldosterone hypersecretion on the basis of cross-sectional imaging alone is therefore unreliable. We would therefore routinely perform selective venous sampling to determine the side of pathology before subjecting patients to an adrenalectomy. **Pre-operative treatment** of blood pressure typically requires a combination of antihypertensive agents and usually includes aldosterone antagonists such as spironolactone. This may be over a period of a few weeks before surgery. Any coexisting **hypokalemia** is also corrected before surgery. Patients should be warned that although blood pressure control will improve in the vast majority of patients following surgery, a significant proportion will still need antihypertensive agents in the long term. Postoperative weaning off antihypertensive agents is best done in close collaboration with physicians.

Adrenal cancer

Adrenal cancer is very uncommon and constitutes only a small proportion of patients undergoing adrenalectomy for functioning or non-functioning lesions. It is more common in patients with adrenal masses over 6cm, but cross-sectional imaging is unreliable in predicting malignancy unless obvious features of malignancy such as local invasion or metastases are present. A PET scan is increasingly being used as a predictor of malignancy in large, incidentally detected adrenal lesions. A high suspicion of malignancy influences the operative approach — I avoid laparoscopy in these situations due to the need to avoid capsular rupture during surgery. These tumors may be functioning or non-functioning; the former group usually have cortisol excess and need to be approached in a manner as described previously. During surgery, a detailed assessment of local invasion should be undertaken and *en bloc* resection of adjacent viscera needs to be considered. Surgery is the mainstay of treatment and inadequate surgery/resection carries a worse prognosis.

In conclusion, I hope I have been able to emphasize that a sound knowledge of the pathophysiology of endocrine disease is crucial to ensuring favorable outcomes. It is said that less than 20% of operative competence is related to 'technical skills' and the rest is related to cognitive and interpersonal skills — this applies to endocrine surgery more than any other. If in doubt, the non-specialist surgeon involved in the care of such patients should seek advice from experienced or specialist colleagues — this may be before, during or after the operation. Above all, the surgeon who undertakes endocrine surgery has to be a physician first — when you appreciate the medical aspects of the disease, it stops being so boring!

Let me finish with two aphorisms by a great endocrine surgeon: Jon Van Heerden.

> **"Meticulous surgical technique: a touch of a lady; allergic to blood."**
>
> **"If the superior (parathyroid) gland is missing, look inferior to the inferior for the superior; and if the inferior is missing, look superior to the superior for the inferior gland."**
>
> **Jon Van Heerden**

Chapter 22

Vascular surgery

Paul N. Rogers

As surgeons keep their instruments and knives always at hand for cases requiring immediate treatment, so shouldst thou have thy thoughts ready to understand things divine and human, remembering in thy every act, even the smallest, how close is the bond that unites the two.

Marcus Aurelius

If all surgery is dangerous, and it is, then vascular surgery is particularly dangerous! There are several reasons for this: the major nature of much of the surgery, the implantation of prosthetic material, the extensive comorbidity of the typical patient population. As a consequence the potential for catastrophe exists at every stage, ranging from calamitous early intra-operative hemorrhage to fatal late prosthetic graft infection. **When one considers that much vascular surgery is performed for prophylaxis, and therefore on asymptomatic patients, the occurrence of any complication is a matter of particular concern and any major mishap is a tragedy**.

In the golden age of vascular surgery — when giants walked the earth — if such an era truly existed, when the specialty was expanding and new techniques and graft materials were being developed, it was regarded as little more than *anatomical plumbing*. At that time, our understanding of the complex nature of vascular physiology and its interaction in turn with the pathology of atherosclerosis, with which most vascular surgery is concerned, was woefully inadequate. **As experience has accumulated, however, we have belatedly recognized, in some quarters anyway, that the presence of a blocked artery (and possibly some symptoms) is not in itself an indication for intervention.**

Medical practitioners in general tend to overestimate the benefits of what they do and also underestimate the risks of any intervention. This is particularly true of surgeons. Consider the following scenario.

The peri-operative mortality of aortofemoral bypass is frequently quoted as being between 2 and 5%, based on published case series. Some independent audits put it as high as 7%, and knowing what we do about publication bias we can be fairly sure that in some series it will be even higher than this. Now imagine a patient with intermittent claudication due to aorto-iliac disease visiting the doctor and requesting that something be done to alleviate the symptoms. The doctor then explains that a new drug has been developed that cures claudication completely with a single dose, but it has one drawback. The problem is that some patients have an unpredictable idiosyncratic reaction to the drug so that seven pills in every hundred kill the patient. Now, says the doc, do you feel lucky — or would you prefer to continue limping?

Should we really be offering aortofemoral bypass for claudication?

Before proceeding I have to warn you that this chapter cannot be 'exhaustive'. Vascular surgery represents a wide-ranging specialty and entire texts on "complications of vascular surgery" are available. Thus, this chapter won't deal with DVT, endovascular surgery, trauma, mesenteric vascular disease and chronic upper limb ischemia. What it will do, however, is to provide you with a 'different perspective'. So I hope you will continue reading.

Pre-operative considerations

A few key points

Patients must be optimized. All patients with documented arterial disease should already be treated with an antiplatelet drug — usually aspirin — and a statin. **Aspirin and statins should be continued peri-operatively, but clopidogrel should be stopped 7-10 days before operations on body cavities**. I do not stop clopidogrel for neck or limb procedures; some other surgeons do. Those patients already on beta-blockers should continue these medications but there is no compelling evidence that these compounds should be started in those not already taking them. Other medications should be continued as normal. Diabetic control should be satisfactory. Get the patients to stop smoking (fat chance!).

Selection is crucial. Arterial disease is a multisystem disorder. Always assume that the patient has coronary and cerebrovascular disease even if this is not clinically evident. Imagine that the typical vascular patient is like a house of cards; everything just in balance but not in great shape. **Any intervention must be seriously considered in light of the possibility that any misadventure will cause the whole edifice to tumble down.** The balance between risk and benefit is perhaps more difficult in this subspecialty than in any other. The threshold for repair of an asymptomatic abdominal aortic aneurysm (AAA) may be a maximum anteroposterior diameter of 55mm in a fit patient. What is the threshold when the patient is not so fit, but yet not so unfit as to make surgery out of the question? Somebody has written: "indications can be stretched like chewing gum or the brain of surgeons. Unfortunately arteries are not as pliable…"

Elective major vascular surgery is not for the isolated part-timer. While the surgery itself may be within the technical capabilities of the surgeon, there are many other factors that influence outcome. Studies of large-volume institutions have shown that the whole 'package of care' has a significant bearing on results. Peri-operative medicine (anesthesia!), critical care and other medical disciplines (cardiology, nephrology, etc.) have important roles to play and this factor becomes even more evident when the *failure to rescue* (FTR) rate is analyzed. **If you don't have the necessary support in your institution either change the environment or refer the patient elsewhere.**

When you ask a vascular surgeon to justify unnecessary surgery he'll cite from the following: we tried to save his leg, he had rest pain, his aneurysm was painful, she had TIAs, and always — the family wanted us to do whatever we can… and so forth.

Carotid surgery

The man is as old as his arteries.

Thomas Sydenham

We know that **symptomatic** patients with significant (>70% stenosis) internal carotid disease benefit from surgery (endarterectomy). We also know that those with minimal disease (<30% stenosis) do not. The position of those in the intermediate group is not so clear, and in fact it seems likely that their likelihood of benefit is related to the complication rate of the surgeon. The same could be said of those with significant asymptomatic stenosis. Surgery is said to reduce the ipsilateral *relative* risk of stroke by 50% per annum in these patients, and this sounds like a worthwhile benefit until you realize that the *absolute* risk reduction is 1% per annum. **A benefit of this magnitude is easily wiped out by surgery that is less than perfect, and indeed some argue that this benefit may already have been removed by the improvements in medical care that have occurred since the crucial randomized trials, on which these recommendations were based, were carried out**. Please remember that even in symptomatic disease the number needed to treat (NNT) to prevent one event is of the order of five or six: this means that the large majority of patients do not benefit from intervention — we just don't know which ones!

So what has this to do with prevention of complications you may ask? Two things are important: correct patient selection, and properly informed consent for surgery. Selection is concerned with three main issues:

- The symptoms are relevant (recovered stroke, TIA, transient retinal ischemia) and appropriate to the side of the stenosis.
- The stenosis is accurately measured and severe enough.
- The patient has no intercurrent disease that might prevent them from living long enough to benefit from intervention (life expectancy of at least five years or so).

Informed consent is always important but here the issues may be difficult for the patient to grasp. They must understand the concepts of risk and odds, and they must, crucially, understand that the surgery will not improve whatever symptoms they may still have from a previous stroke. **I find it useful to check understanding just before the procedure by asking "Why are we doing this operation?" and "What bad things might happen as a result of this operation?" The answers are sometimes astonishing — from patients who have been extensively counseled by several doctors already!**

Elective AAA surgery

> *To refuse to treat any aneurysm... is unwise; but it is also dangerous to operate upon all of them.*
> **Antyllus, second century A.D.**

This is like carotid surgery in that it is a prophylactic procedure. Selection is crucial. Patients must have the physiological and psychological reserves to withstand major surgery. Most patients can be assessed for 'fitness' for surgery by history and physical examination, aided by a few simple tests: blood count, serum biochemistry, ECG (EKG). Those who have demonstrable defects in cardiac or respiratory function, or whose reserve cannot be assessed due to an inability to exercise (e.g. from arthritis), may require additional cardiopulmonary testing. If significant cardiac disease is found then this should be managed based on standard clinical indications; the presence of the AAA is irrelevant. **Resist the temptation to make the patient 'fit for surgery' by cardiac intervention**. Informed consent is again an important part of the pre-operative routine. **The patient must understand the risk of death**. I recall a surgeon who counseled patients extensively on the risks of impotence but failed to mention the possibility that the patient might not survive. Perhaps this was a manifestation of his personal priorities…

Never forget that most patients with aortic aneurysms die with them unruptured!

Emergency AAA operations

In ruptured AAA the operation is commonly the beginning of the end with the end arriving postoperatively.

The diagnosis is what matters here. A typical history — collapse with back or abdominal pain, hypotension — and a pulsatile abdominal mass is all that is required. Don't delay with CT unnecessarily. The advent of endovascular aneurysm repair (EVAR) has changed this advice for some patients in some centers: stable patients may go to CT to assess suitability for EVAR. **Otherwise it's off to the OR directly.**

As always, futile surgery should be avoided. Those with extensive comorbidity are unlikely to survive. In particular, a chronic need of supplemental oxygen, severe cardiac disease and dialysis-dependent renal failure are powerful indicators that surgery is not appropriate. In addition, the patient's attitude to major lifesaving surgery may not be predictable. It is important to ask: "How do you feel about a big operation? Without it you will almost certainly die." Surprisingly often from elderly patients the answer will be "Well, doctor, I've had a good life and my dear wife passed away a couple of years ago…" Note that it's important to say "almost certainly die", because a very small number of patients do not die immediately and some may even leave hospital alive without an operation! Leave yourself some wriggle room.

Don't let the anesthetist put the patient to sleep until you are 'prepped and draped' and ready to go. Occasionally, relaxation of the abdominal wall on induction removes the tamponade that stops the AAA from continuing to bleed and the patient crashes. Rapid access to the abdomen to clamp the aorta is then essential!

Bypass surgery for intermittent claudication (IC)

Don't do it! This is the best advice. The natural history of intermittent claudication is benign. Very few patients with IC end up with an amputation and there is no evidence that early intervention reduces the risk of this possibility. Indeed in some circumstances the converse is true. Femoropopliteal bypass with prosthetic material roughly doubles the risk of eventual amputation. **Studies of exercise versus angioplasty versus surgery in the management of IC suggest that the eventual outcome (after years) is similar**. These patients should be managed first of all by carefully assessing and controlling their risk factors; smoking cessation is probably the key. Antiplatelet medications and statins should be started. They should have the diagnosis and its natural history explained and they should then be encouraged to walk within the limits of their disability in the expectation that the symptoms will improve gradually over many months.

Here I should point out that I believe that percutaneous angioplasty, particularly of the iliac arteries, is a reasonable undertaking for IC. But interventional radiology is not surgery and it's not what this book is about.

Critical limb ischemia

Here your hand is forced. Without successful revascularization a major amputation is likely. It is probably better to start with percutaneous angioplasty if both this and surgery are possible. If surgery is necessary it is very important to pay great attention to optimization as these patients are often a very unsteady house of cards indeed. Good angiographic images are essential for planning. Vein mapping pre-operatively may help in the selection of a suitable conduit. If the patient has infected necrosis or ulceration, then ensuring they are 'soaked' in antibiotics may diminish the risk of graft infection.

Remember: the patient does not need a functioning graft to sit in a wheelchair or lie in bed; an amputation stump would do.

Acute limb ischemia

There are two big questions here:

- Is the limb viable?
- Is the cause likely to be thrombosis or embolism?

Before considering these it is useful to administer heparin. This might be expected to do two things: reduce any tendency of the thrombosis to extend and also diminish the risk of further embolism.

Viability is determined by clinical examination (remember the "5 Ps of limb ischemia" from medical school?). Is there neurological dysfunction? What is the capillary filling like? Is there any muscle tenderness? Are the symptoms and appearances improving or not? If the limb is clearly viable you have some additional time to assess, investigate and perhaps observe. If not viable you must decide if it is salvageable or not. Fixed lividity, 'woody' muscles and contractures indicate a non-salvageable limb.

The separation of thrombosis and embolism can be difficult. Pointers to **embolism** as the likely cause are a clinically detectable source of embolism — recent MI, atrial fibrillation — the absence of a history of IC, and normal pulses in the contralateral limb. **Thrombosis** is more likely in patients with an obviously arteriopathic history and abnormal pulses in the other leg. If there is uncertainty then a delay to allow angiography to be done is the solution. The reason for this is that a simple transfemoral thrombectomy is often insufficient for the management of thrombosis. **Furthermore, some patients with thrombosis are best treated by intra-arterial thrombolysis if the viability of the limb is threatened, and so involvement of the interventional radiologists early is helpful**.

Patients with an obviously embolic event can often be taken directly to the OR for a 'simple' local anesthetic embolectomy. Always ask for anesthetic assistance with this even if a GA is not likely to be required; administration of some sedation is often necessary, and it's better that monitoring of this is done by someone who is not engaged in opening an artery.

Upper limb ischemia is much less common than leg ischemia. Often, if the limb is viable, then a period of close observation will be rewarded with an improving situation. The arm has a fairly rich collateral blood supply around vessels where emboli might lodge, particularly the elbow. With the passage of time these collateral channels open to such an extent that embolectomy can be avoided. This is a good thing since the results of transbrachial embolectomy are not universally satisfactory due partly to the small size of the vessel.

Venous surgery

> *Varicose veins are the results of an improper selection of grandparents.*
>
> **William Osler**

This essentially concerns treatment of varicose veins (VV). It's not clear that varicose veins cause symptoms in many of those who have them. The prevalence of VV in the population steadily rises with age, and with careful assessment exceeds 40% in those over 45 years of age. Oh sure, many patients attend the doctor with 'VV symptoms', but these symptoms are almost as common in those without varicose veins. There are, of course, many studies extolling the virtue of VV surgery and demonstrating the improvements in quality of life (QoL) that can be obtained. These QoL scores are designed specifically to address 'VV symptoms' and the improvements associated with surgery. This association may be the placebo effect of surgery, or it may be that patients are content that the appearance of their legs is improved — because this was what was really bothering them all along! **In any event it seems likely that any health gain after VV surgery will be small — the key word here being** *cosmesis*!

Another way of looking at the VV problem is to consider litigation associated with it. In the UK it is still the most common surgical treatment to be associated with successful litigation. This may seem surprising for what is essentially superficial surgery. However, it is my view that the problem relates to the fact that since most of these patients don't have anything very seriously wrong with them to begin with, they are extremely sensitive to <u>any</u> problems that arise as a result of treatment.

So how do we deal with this minefield? I suggest a three-pronged approach. Firstly, give the patients a correct appreciation of where the role of surgery sits (try to put them off having anything done); secondly, explain in great detail what undesirable effects there may be (try to put them off having anything done); finally, avoid complications in those who do have surgery.

What is the role of surgery? Surgery is never 'necessary'. Veins will recur. Symptoms may not be better. There will be scars.

What bad things might happen? DVT. Neuritis. Scars. Recurrence.

If, after all this, the patient still wants treatment, you have many tools from which to choose: conventional surgery — saphenofemoral or saphenopopliteal ligation, stripping of the long saphenous vein (LSV) and stab avulsions (phlebectomies); thermal ablation of the LSV (laser or radiofrequency); ultrasound-guided foam sclerotherapy (UGFS). Each of these methods has their protagonists and the debate will linger for a while yet. I propose to confine my later observations to conventional surgery — the important complications are mostly the same anyway!

In summary, your pre-op interventions should be focused on ensuring that the patient has a very clear understanding of the limits and risks of intervention. They must opt for treatment with their eyes wide open. This is cosmetic surgery (well almost always...).

Intra-operative considerations

It is useful when carrying out any procedure to be aware of the common, and not so common, problems that you can cause. By keeping these in mind during the conduct of the surgery and specifically avoiding them, you can reduce their incidence.

We mentioned already that much vascular surgery is prophylactic in nature; we are trying to prevent problems. **The decision to operate in the first place has been based on a careful assessment of the risk/benefit ratio. In some cases as the operation proceeds it becomes apparent that this ratio may not be what we thought. In other words if you encounter unexpected difficulties it may be advisable to abandon — oh yes, to ABANDON — the procedure rather than continue and expose the patient to unacceptable risks**. It's better to have a post-op patient with an unrepaired AAA than an addition to the hospital's mortality statistics.

In difficult procedures always think of the step *after* the next one — "If this doesn't work, what then?" Don't commit to any step without considering the next option in case your plan doesn't work. Always leave a way to the exit in good order.

Some advice applies to vascular procedures in general. **Use optical magnification**; I find 2.5x loupes adequate. This is essential for carotid endarterectomy and distal bypass work. In practice, when you have become familiar with loupes, they can be usefully deployed in any operation — with subcutaneous bleeders, for example, you can diathermy precisely the relevant vessel instead of reducing the surrounding countryside to a charred shambles. Even if you have perfect vision your view will be enhanced and the surgery improved. And anyway your vision will eventually deteriorate so why not get used to them now?

Use prophylactic antibiotics when prosthetic material is implanted. These should be appropriate to the local circumstances, but should at least cover *Staphylococcus aureus*. There is no need to continue antibiotics postoperatively. But you know this already...

Carotid surgery

Don't injure the nerves

The first at risk is the **mandibular branch of the facial nerve** which can be caught by a carelessly placed incision (it hardly seems possible, yet...). It's useful to leave the lower part of the earlobe visible when draping the patient to allow accurate placement of the incision. At the upper extent of the skin incision the **great auricular nerve** is often encountered; it can almost always be preserved, but in a minority of cases sacrifice is necessary and leaves little morbidity. Other cutaneous nerves must be divided. Deeper in the wound, at the upper end, the **hypoglossal nerve** is often seen crossing the internal carotid artery (ICA). It passes inferiorly and then swings anteriorly across the vessel. The angle of the nerve is frequently held in place by a small artery passing posteriorly from the external carotid artery to supply the sternomastoid muscle. The nerve may be freed if access to the more distal internal carotid is required by carefully ligating and dividing this small artery; this allows the nerve to move in an anterosuperior direction. **Be careful with any retractor used by your assistant at the upper end of the wound**; ensure that this is placed superficial to the plane of the nerve. The last nerve to be avoided is the **vagus**, lying in the groove between the carotid and internal jugular vein; injury to this may cause a **recurrent laryngeal nerve palsy**. A self-retaining retractor placed to hold the vein back may easily catch the nerve if care is not taken.

Don't cause embolism

"Dissect the patient away from the carotid." I attribute this quote, heard second hand, to Sir Norman Browse — a meticulous vascular surgeon who practiced in London. The principle is clear; the vessels should be disturbed as little as possible during dissection to avoid dislodging loose atherothrombotic material from the stenosis.

The current standard of care for symptomatic carotid disease is that surgery should be carried out as soon as possible after the index event. We know that this means that there is an increased likelihood that fresh thrombotic material will be present in the carotid at the time of surgery. Some intra-operative strokes are due to embolism of this material. Try not to send clots to the brain!

Shunting is controversial. It seems unlikely that the exact role of shunting will ever be finally determined. Some surgeons always shunt, some selectively and some never. If you use a shunt infrequently then at least make yourself familiar with its use. Insert it carefully and avoid distal trauma. Don't persist in efforts to cannulate the distal ICA if the shunt will not pass easily; complete the operation expeditiously without a shunt in the knowledge that only a small minority of patients need it anyway. When releasing the clamps to allow blood flow in the shunt, do it slowly so that any bubbles in the shunt may be identified and the clamp reapplied before the bubbles embolize.

Patching

Patching is good. Recurrent carotid stenosis is made less likely. It probably doesn't matter what material you use. The small risk of infection associated with prosthetic patches is matched, more or less, by the risk of vein patch rupture.

Avoid hematoma

Meticulous hemostasis is essential because all patients will be on antiplatelet medications. Most hematomas are due to venous problems so be sure to ligate all veins securely and pay particular attention to the manner in which the confluence of veins forming the **common facial vein** is managed. Individual ligation of the tributaries is often preferred to mass ligation of the confluence itself.

AAA surgery

Vascular surgery is peculiar because, above all, it is mainly surgery of ruins.

Cid dos Santos

Don't injure the veins

Inspection of the pre-op CT should warn you about abnormal venous drainage that may cause problems. **In particular, look out for a retro-aortic left renal vein, and if this is present then take great care when applying the aortic clamp**. If division of a normal anterior left renal vein is necessary to gain access to the *juxtarenal aorta*, then be sure to ligate the vein securely as far towards the vena cava as possible; this preserves the collateral venous drainage from the kidney and prevents renal venous hypertension. Other veins at risk of injury are the iliacs. **These can be damaged if attempts are made to encircle the iliac arteries**. It is better to confine isolation of the common iliac arteries to clearing the front and sides of the vessels and then applying clamps in an anteroposterior fashion.

Avoid injury to the iliac arteries

In the presence of extensive arterial calcification it may be difficult to find soft 'windows' in which to apply atraumatic vascular clamps. **When this happens it is better to use balloon tamponade to control back-bleeding**

from the legs and pelvis. It is more effective to do this with small Foley catheters rather than Fogarty embolectomy catheters because the balloons of the latter are thin-walled and burst easily when inflated against shards of calcified atheroma. Foley balloons are more robust. The catheters can be removed immediately before the last couple of stitches in the distal aortic anastomosis.

Minimize embolism

The other thing to do before final closure of the arterial anastomosis is *flush* the aortic graft and the iliac vessels in turn. Irrigate the lumen with heparinized saline to remove any loose debris and clots. These maneuvers may help to reduce the incidence of embolic occlusion of the femoral vessels and may also make trash foot less likely. Other strategies to avoid embolism include clamping the iliac arteries before the aorta and avoiding multiple attempts at clamp placement.

Use systemic anticoagulation in elective cases

3000-5000 units of unfractionated heparin are given by the anesthetist just prior to cross-clamping. This makes intra-operative distal thrombosis less likely. **However, in ruptured AAA cases, the administration of anticoagulants to a patient who is in danger of bleeding to death seems unwise**. Instead, once control has been obtained and the aorta opened, local anticoagulation of the distal circulation via the iliac arteries by instillation of heparinized saline seems a sensible compromise.

Look after the gut and the spleen

Try to operate with the small bowel and transverse colon packed away *inside* the abdomen. If you must exteriorize the gut always cover it with moist packs. Don't let traction on the transverse colon and mesentery damage the spleen. **At the conclusion of the procedure, just before closing the abdomen, inspect the sigmoid colon**. Is it well perfused? Do you need to improve the left side mesenteric circulation by re-implanting the previously ligated inferior mesenteric artery?

Stay out of the groin if possible

Groin wounds are notoriously problematic. The skin folds are moist and the adjacent perineum is an excellent source of contamination. Wound infections are frequent and although they may be relatively minor the potential for infection of underlying graft material is considerable. **I need hardly mention the possible consequences of aortic graft infection. Most AAAs can be repaired with a simple tube graft but if this is not possible then an aorto-iliac reconstruction is better than an aortofemoral bypass because it avoids groin wounds**. Late graft infection is twice as likely after aortofemoral reconstruction compared to aorto-iliac surgery.

Tunnelling grafts to the groin can lead to disaster

If you are forced to take a bifurcated graft to the femoral arteries then please be aware that the retroperitoneal tunnels must be made with care. Ureters can be injured and there are documented cases of the graft on the left side being tunnelled through the sigmoid colon (!). **To avoid ureteric injury don't overdo any dissection of these tubes since skeletonizing them injures the blood supply. Be careful not to include them in sutures when closing the retroperitoneum. And finally, tunnel the graft behind them.** Before we finish discussing graft tunnelling I should mention that without sufficient care it is possible to tunnel femorofemoral crossover grafts through the bladder (beware of patients with previous low abdominal surgery) and there is at least one documented case of an axillofemoral graft traversing the hepatic flexure of the colon. You have been warned.

Pay particular attention to abdominal closure (or non-closure [1])

The metabolic defects that cause AAA formation also appear to make these patients more prone to incisional hernia formation. Some surgeons now advocate prophylactic implantation of mesh to prevent this. I said "some" and this doesn't include me.

Bypass for occlusive disease

> *You do not sleep too well the night before a bad AAA — you do not sleep well the night after a distal bypass.*
> **Angus G. Maciver**

We already said not to do bypass surgery for claudication. But if you choose to ignore this advice and find yourself sucked into doing it, there are a number of factors you must keep in mind. **Use vein, not prosthetic materials, for lower limb bypass.** We know that the use of prosthetic materials roughly doubles the subsequent risk of eventual amputation. Don't be tempted to go below the knee if you plan on an above-knee fem-pop bypass and then find the popliteal artery unsuitable at that level. Rather abandon the procedure instead.

In critical limb ischemia (CLI) greater risks are justified. Vein is always preferable as a conduit, but it is acceptable to use prosthetic material if no suitable vein can be found (have you looked at the arms for suitable vein?). *In situ* vein and reversed saphenous grafts give equivalent results, but I find it easier to suture a small vein to a small artery! When a prosthetic graft is used then some kind of vein patching at the anastomosis is desirable — whether

---

[1] Always consider leaving the abdomen open (laparostomy) at the end of operations for ruptured AAA, thus avoiding the abdominal compartment syndrome. Always ask: can I, should I, close this abdomen? Non-closure can be a lifesaving decision.

you prefer a Miller cuff, a Taylor patch or a Wolfe boot is up to you. The addition of one of these anastomotic modifications improves the patency rates of the bypass. **Make sure that your graft isn't twisted or kinked!**

Remember: when dissecting the vessels in a patient with CLI that the survival of the limb depends on small collateral vessels. Don't damage these with unnecessary dissection. Be meticulous.

Acute limb ischemia

Do the embolectomy under LA if possible — usually it is. Think carefully about the location and orientation of any arteriotomy. A classic embolectomy arteriotomy is transverse, but if restoration of blood flow is not guaranteed and a bypass might be necessary, then a carefully judged oblique incision might give you better options.

In the leg always consider the need for a fasciotomy. It is said that if you think about it you should do it; this is obviously nonsense since it implies that a fasciotomy must always be done. Factors to consider are the duration and severity of the ischemia. A long period of profound ischemia makes reperfusion swelling more likely and the need for fasciotomy greater. **If a fasciotomy is done it should be a proper four-compartment one; this can be done readily through two carefully placed incisions**. Look it up! Temporary loose suturing of the skin with a subcuticular darn of monofilament material can permit gradual closure of the wounds postoperatively, reducing the need for eventual skin grafting.

Varicose vein surgery

Clearly identify the saphenofemoral junction; expose it. Don't confuse the veins and arteries (seriously!! — the superficial femoral artery has been stripped more than once). Don't injure the femoral vein. Ligate the junction flush and securely. When stripping — and you should do this — do so from groin to knee level; not to ankle as this greatly increases the risk of injury to the saphenous nerve.

The saphenopopliteal junction lies deep to the fascia. Follow the vein until it is obviously going down into the popliteal fossa. Be careful of the nerves and watch your assistant's retractor.

Postoperative considerations

The best-laid schemes o' mice an' men gang aft agley.
Robert Burns [2]

Recent nationwide audits have revealed that hospitals with similar complication rates can demonstrate different mortality rates. This is explained by the phenomenon known as failure to rescue (FTR) mentioned previously in this chapter and in ⟳ Chapter 2. This is usually a reflection of the hospital's process of care. It is generally accepted that individual surgeons do not have the ability to make big changes here but as the patient's chief advocate it's your job to ensure that any deficiencies in this process of care are mitigated by your attention to detail in the postoperative phase. **In vascular surgery patients these deficiencies are usually to be found in a lack of critical care facilities and delayed recognition and treatment of postoperative complications**.

Carotid surgery

A postoperative stroke is misery for the surgeon and patient. Both know it is possible but that doesn't lessen the grief. What is to be done about it? If it is apparent in the recovery room, the question of early re-exploration of the carotid arises. **The ready availability of duplex examination means that you know whether or not the vessel is patent**. If it's occluded then many surgeons advocate an immediate return to theatre to re-establish flow in the vessel; good results are reported from this strategy. Some surgeons do not re-explore and many of their patients also recover. Who is correct? The literature does not help. Make up your own mind.

Cerebral hyperperfusion syndrome is characterized by ipsilateral headache, neurological signs and seizures; it is caused by an increase in cerebral perfusion of over 100%. It is much discussed but there is no specific treatment and rapid blood pressure control is the only useful intervention.

AAA surgery

Good pain management, correct fluid balance and early mobilization are the goals here. **Don't flood the patient with i.v. fluids in a misguided effort to get a 'normal' hourly urine volume; 30ml per hour will be just fine**. Start oral fluids immediately and diet soon thereafter if the patient is tolerant of it.

---

[2] A Scottish poet. Translation: the best made plans often go wrong.

You'll have to back off from this if an ileus develops. The aim is the so-called "enhanced recovery after surgery" (ERAS), but this is just a modern over-inflated term for good, sensible surgical practice. Don't forget to reinstate DVT prophylaxis that may have been deferred pre-operatively.

The early postoperative phase is when the **risk of hemorrhage** is greatest (but it was dry when you closed…). Close monitoring is essential. If your patient has an epidural catheter in place for postoperative pain relief don't assume that this is the cause of any hypotension. Always suspect bleeding. **Always think about the abdominal compartment syndrome — measure intra-abdominal pressure!**

Another early but fortunately rare problem is **colon ischemia**. Rectal bleeding is the clue. This is more likely to occur after surgery for rupture because of the greater likelihood of peri-operative hypotension. The ischemia may be mucosal only (ischemic colitis), or transmural (colonic infarction). The former will recover with supportive measures while the latter mandates a second laparotomy and Hartmann's procedure. CT helps to differentiate.

There are many other potential 'medical' problems after AAA surgery that will require the assistance of your local cardiologist/nephrologist/diabetologist in addition to the intensivist with whom you already work closely. **Don't hesitate to get these folks involved, but don't let them take over and do foolish things**.

Bypass for occlusive disease

Early postoperative problems related specifically to the surgery are bleeding and graft failure. There are of course many other problems related to the extensive comorbidity in this group of patients — acute coronary syndrome, stroke, chest infection, yada yada — but I don't propose to extend this chapter unnecessarily with the tedium of their management. **Arterial bleeding is a straightforward problem: you have failed to perform an anastomosis correctly, missed a side branch of the vein graft or torn the vein with the valvulotome. Go and fix it!**

Immediate graft occlusion

You can't make a palpable pulse more palpable.

This is a more annoying problem. **There are many possible reasons for failure of the graft to run (think — inflow adequate? Runoff OK? Graft** technically satisfactory?), **but if you believed that the operation was worth performing in the first place then revisiting the OR at the end of a tiring day to salvage the situation is the correct thing to do**.

Re-exploring the graft at the likely site of trouble (you know where that is), or at the easiest point of access if you really cannot understand why the thing isn't working, is the right approach. Usually a simple graft thrombectomy is all that is necessary. Occasionally you realize that an anastomosis is no good and it has to be redone with a patch, or the graft has to be extended to a different site. Consider the possibility that the graft may be kinked or twisted (only if inserted by another surgeon, because surely you will have avoided this problem by careful initial surgery). Intra-operative arteriography may be useful in ensuring that everything is as it should be.

Of course, at the end of the procedure, examine the feet and document peripheral perfusion, pulses and/or ABIs. Do it yourself. I remember not a few cases when residents or nurses documented perfect peripheral pulses in perfectly ischemic limbs — the imagination tends to be active at night.

Late occlusion

Late graft occlusion is usually due to either neointimal hyperplasia at one or other of the anastomoses or to progression of arteriosclerosis upstream or downstream. This is the fate of many bypass grafts. Often there are no major consequences — a return of IC, a brief spell of 'ischemia' that resolves spontaneously or indeed nothing at all. **In some cases, however, acute limb ischemia or critical limb ischemia are the consequences**. Now something must be done or a major amputation may ensue. **Angiography is essential**.

If the limb does not require <u>immediate</u> revascularization (because of profound ischemia), then an attempt at intra-arterial thrombolysis may be possible. The criteria for undertaking this are now fairly well established: viability of the limb must be threatened, occlusion of the graft must be recent (within four weeks), there must be no contraindication to thrombolysis (recent surgery, bleeding tendency, active peptic ulceration, etc.), and the patient must be aware of the risk of stroke which is the major potential complication. **If thrombolysis is not an option then surgical graft thrombectomy should be attempted or insertion of a new graft considered**.

Sometimes revascularization is not the correct therapy — angiography will reveal that the underlying disease has progressed to an extent that precludes further successful surgery and then amputation may be the only option.

Occasionally the surgeon will know from previous acquaintance of the patient that revascularization is not possible — the previous, now failed, graft was the 'last chance saloon'. **Always remember: a fresh wound of a failed bypass graft procedure is not a prerequisite to amputation** (■ Figure 22.1).

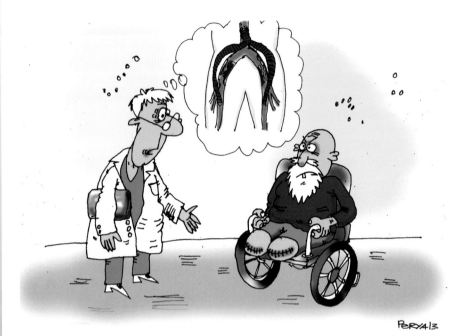

Figure 22.1. The old man: "So doc, do you still think the bypass to help my walking was the right idea?"

Graft infection

This subject requires a section of its own because infection of a vascular prosthesis is a disaster. It may occur early or late. It almost always necessitates removal of the graft to eradicate the infection. There are some exceptions. The groin sinus that was seen so often in the past when aortofemoral bypass was frequently performed for claudication was an indicator of, probably localized, low-grade infection. Often it did not progress and the patient continued happily for years with an irritating, benign discharge from a small sinus. This is uncommon nowadays because aortofemoral bypass is much less frequently performed and also because colonization and infection with the much more virulent MRSA is endemic. **MRSA infection of an aortic prosthesis is usually fatal!**

Extirpation of the infected graft

When presented with a graft infection and the affected patient is fit for surgical management then extirpation of the graft is your only option. **Excision of the whole graft is usually necessary but in some cases it may be possible/acceptable/advisable to leave a small stump of graft attached to a vessel**. This can be done if several criteria are fulfilled: the residual graft stump is fully incorporated; it is distant from the obviously infected portion of the graft; dissection of the involved vessel would be difficult and might threaten its patency. Similarly, if the affected graft is a bifurcated prosthesis, then it may be that only one limb is involved; in this situation removal of the affected limb, taking care to prevent contamination of the uninvolved, tissue incorporated, contralateral limb, may be possible.

There are several additional management options after graft excision has been accomplished: do nothing else; replace the graft _in situ_; replace the graft by another, routed differently. Curiously, removal of grafts inserted for limb salvage does not always result in loss of the limb affected, even if no replacement graft is inserted. It is almost as if a (sometimes short) period of enhanced perfusion is sufficient to permit development of collaterals that subsequently allow the limb to survive unaided. Whatever the reason, it is frequently possible to remove infected femoropopliteal, femorofemoral or axillofemoral grafts without replacing them. **However, if it's clear that the limb will not survive without further revascularization, then another attempt at bypass, if possible, is warranted**.

Aortic grafts are different. It is essentially not possible to remove these without some kind of replacement. The options are: _in situ_ replacement with an antibiotic-bonded graft (sealed Dacron® soaked in rifampicin); replacement with a silver-impregnated graft; replacement with cryopreserved allograft; extra-anatomic bypass — bilateral axillofemoral — which can be simultaneous or staged; replacement with superficial femoral vein. There are no data to support the superiority of one approach over another. It seems to this author, therefore, that in this desperate situation the simplest option is the best — _in situ_ replacement. Satisfactory long-term results have been reported by several authors.

Aorto-enteric fistula (AEF)

While we are discussing desperate situations it is relevant at this point to consider another presentation of aortic infection — aorto-enteric fistula. This occurs infrequently but may happen at any time after an aortic graft. The usual site is the proximal aortic anastomosis which lies adjacent to the duodenum and eventually erodes into its lumen. The presentation is usually with upper GI hemorrhage and the diagnosis should be strongly suspected in anyone who presents with this and who has had previous aortic surgery. The patient usually has a low-grade fever and raised inflammatory markers (WBC and CRP). UGI endoscopy shows no other relevant pathology — but if you slide the scope down into the distal duodenum you may find yourself looking at the graft! **CT is usually diagnostic showing both fluid and small bubbles of gas around the graft**. (PET CT can further contribute to diagnosis by showing the inflammatory reaction around the aorta, in equivocal cases.) Mortality from traditional open surgery, with graft excision and replacement, is very high as these patients are often desperately ill. **Recently, the advent of covered stents has led some to suggest that closure of the fistula endovascularly may be the best initial option — to buy time until the patient is stable and a definitive repair can be carried out**. This procedure obviously complicates any eventual surgery and the temptation will be to leave the stent graft in place and hope that residual infection might be managed by antibiotics. This seems a fanciful notion, but I suppose it might allow patients who would otherwise die to survive for a while longer.

And finally...

Vascular surgery requires a commitment and attention to detail that makes it different from many other surgical specialties. Often you are required to go to the hospital NOW! Long procedures are sometimes rewarded by complete failure — perhaps a deceased patient from a ruptured AAA or a call to go back and revise an occluded graft in the middle of the night. Sometimes too you must go and fix a mess that is not of your making — bleeding caused by other specialists who don't have the skills to correct the problems they have created, and then while you struggle at 2am they sleep soundly, unaware of the crisis. All this must be accepted with equanimity (and a moderate amount of cursing...) if you are to have a contented life in this complications-laden discipline.

"Remember that all is opinion."

Marcus Aurelius

Chapter 23

Bariatric surgery

Ahmad Assalia

Severe obesity restricts the movements and maneuvers of the body. It compresses blood vessels causing their narrowness. Breathing passages are obstructed and the flow of air is hindered leading to nasty temperament... on the whole these people are at risk of sudden death... they are vulnerable to stroke, hemiplegia, palpitation, diarrhea, fainting... any physical effort they make will weaken them.

Avicenna

Once practiced by few surgeons and hardly mentioned in the old textbooks of surgery, bariatric surgery has undergone a revolution in the last two decades — actually, since the consensus statement in 1992 by the National Institute of Health (NIH, USA) stating that morbid obesity is a surgical disease because of the high failure rate (~95%) of dietary and pharmacological interventions. Initially, it was looked upon as a kind of 'weird surgery', shunned by the so called 'surgical giants' and respected institutions. This was followed by an era of ambivalence: "OK... let's start doing it because others do that... there are so many 'fatties' out there who can build up our surgical volume... a nice income and a chance to practice advanced laparoscopic surgery... we do not want to stay behind!" And so on.

But what now? Now it's considered to be one of the 'hottest' and 'sexiest' domains of general surgery — in the USA bariatric interventions are the most commonly performed general surgical procedures in teaching hospitals! Why is this?

First, because obesity is a worldwide epidemic, increasing in incidence everywhere (well, you know which country has the world record ☺). Second, a large body of data has accumulated proving that obesity surgery is safe (well... almost) and effective (well... usually) compared to non-surgical measures. Third, following the minimal access revolution, the vast majority of bariatric procedures are completed laparoscopically — with all its apparent advantages. Fourth, there has been a huge investment and (aggressive) promotion by the industry (*bariatric industry*) — for obvious commercial reasons. Fifth, despite the reluctance of endocrinologists, it is accepted to be the best remedy for type 2 diabetes mellitus associated with obesity — the so called **diabesity**. Sixth, there is now much research into bariatric interventions and consequently journals dedicated to bariatrics are now in the mainstream of surgical literature — who would believe it? — some with high impact factors!

However, the public and the media, and even the medical community — including, I suspect, some of the Editors of this book — still look at every major complication and mortality associated with bariatric surgery with a magnifying glass. Many still feel that patients and particularly surgeons do have a choice — that this is not 'must do' surgery but something similar to cosmetic surgery, which in many cases can and should be avoided ("if only they would eat less..."). These are obviously misconceptions...

We have to remember that we are operating on a severe and chronic disease and not on healthy people with overweight! Therefore, it's legitimate to have complications and there will be always many of them. After all, we are doing complicated gastrointestinal (GI) surgery in obese people, very often with much comorbidity.

The morbidity and mortality depend on the type of procedure and the experience of both the surgeon and the institution. In general, the more complex the procedure the greater are the chances of morbidity and mortality. Mortality rates range from 0.1% for lap-band procedures to 0.2-0.8% for sleeve gastrectomy and gastric bypass, and around 1% following biliopancreatic diversion. The total morbidity rate is estimated to be 10-12% for sleeve gastrectomy and gastric bypass with major morbidity of 3-4%. These are more or less the official estimates; but there is always a 'real world' out there... with its 'hidden graveyards'...

Pre-operative considerations

Bariatric surgery entails the same risks of 'surgical' and 'medical' complications that are typical for any upper GI surgery — I do not wish to repeat what has been preached to you elsewhere in this book.

Bariatric interventions are always *elective* and we can postpone them if necessary. We have the luxury to select our patients properly and prepare them for surgery. We shouldn't listen to patients nagging and demanding an immediate surgery because "He/she can't take it anymore!" Once the obese patient has decided to undergo the surgery (after many years spent accumulating their fat layers), he/she wants to do it right now! Of course, we shouldn't surrender to the pressure.

There are several **basic points** that I wish to emphasize:

- **Obese patients have many related diseases, but even in the absence of such diseases one has to consider them 'unhealthy'!** They impose special anesthetic and medical challenges — the higher their BMI, the greater the surgical risk, a fact well known from non-bariatric general surgery. There is an increased incidence of respiratory, cardiac, infectious, thromboembolic and wound complications. Some of them may have latent, undiagnosed cardiac disease which could lead to postoperative cardiac events and even death. In brief, they deserve a thorough pre-operative work-up and a systematic anesthetic assessment.

- **We should encourage pre-operative weight loss, which has been shown to decrease complication rates**. If our patient has an extremely large liver (due to deposition of fat), we should put him on a low-carb diet for at least several weeks in order to achieve liver volume reduction and minimize technical difficulties posed by the enlarged liver. **We shouldn't have to struggle with huge livers during surgery and we shouldn't hesitate even to make this a prerequisite for the operation!**

- **The patient should prove that he/she has the right motivation for such an operation — that he will adhere to the postoperative dietary regimen!** At the beginning of my bariatric career, I admit that I was much less selective and didn't care much about this point. I believed that everything is doable and was perhaps afraid that patients will seek another surgeon or facility for their operation. This caused me not a few intra-operative difficulties and avoidable complications. After acquiring the right experience, and realizing that (for the meantime ☺) there are more than enough obese patients, I understood that the policy of insisting on pre-operative weight loss in the extremely obese and those with a huge liver truly pays off!

- **We should make maximal efforts to control chronic comorbidities**. Again, we have the time to do this. The *diabetic* patient should be controlled optimally — as we already know uncontrolled diabetes is associated with high postoperative complication rates. Patients with obstructive sleep apnea should be treated with CPAP devices (in order to treat pulmonary hypertension) and they should understand that it's crucial to bring their own machines with them to the hospital.

- **Some complications could be routinely prevented (or minimized), such as DVT/PE** by administering anticoagulation prophylaxis, preferably combined with sequential compression devices. This is basic and should be part of the peri-operative protocol.

- **We should choose the procedures that we are familiar with and avoid those with which we have insufficient experience**. I could share with you numerous 'stories' about what happens to morbidly obese patients undergoing the 'newest' lap bariatric procedure by a surgeon who has just started to climb the 'learning curve'. I could, but I won't… I bet that you know a few as well.

- **Try to tailor the operation to your patient and not the patient to the only procedure that you master!** If you think that the patient needs an operation with which you don't have enough experience, then ignore your ego and refer him to another surgeon with the right experience. For example: failed 'lap-band' procedures in patients with severe metabolic complications and/or gastroesophageal reflux and who are 'sweet eaters' are probably better converted to bypass surgery rather than sleeve gastrectomy. Also, failed vertical banded gastroplasties are better converted to gastric bypass (or even better, biliopancreatic diversion) rather than sleeve gastrectomy. If the patient desires an operation (about which he read online…) that in your judgment is not the right option for him, do not hesitate to refuse to operate on him, with the knowledge that he will finally find the surgeon who will agree to do the surgery…

- **With re-do surgery, we always have more complications!** Therefore, we should try carefully to select the patients and choose for them the right revisional procedure. In case we are confronted by a **hostile surgical environment** (e.g. an 'impossible' gastroesophageal area due to complicated previous 'lap-band' or vertical banded gastroplasty procedures) we should formulate in advance an alternative plan — with the patient being informed before the operation about any possible alternatives to be taken during surgery.

- Finally, in this **era of defensive medicine**, we should talk to the patients (more than once), explain and inform them in detail about all potential risks. We have to ensure that patients fully comprehend that this surgery is done for a serious disease and is not a cosmetic procedure devoid of complications. They should understand exactly what are the realistic expectations — for example, that it is very unlikely that the super obese lady will ever become a super model

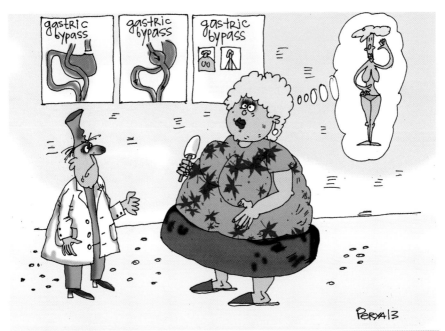

Figure 23.1. "Dottore, which of those operations would you recommend?"

(■ Figure 23.1). **Write down and carefully document these talks!** You will not regret this because you can never know when you will have to defend yourself against allegations that the patient was not properly informed (e.g. "he was told it's a simple procedure with almost no complications...").

Intra-operative considerations

There is no substitute for a perfectly executed surgical technique. The patient will pay the price for a lengthy and cumbersome procedure after the operation. Proper positioning of the patient and ideal trocar layout will further enhance the safety of the undertaking.

The following are a few preventive tips for each of the commonly practiced procedures (see Figure ■ 23.2 to refresh your memory).

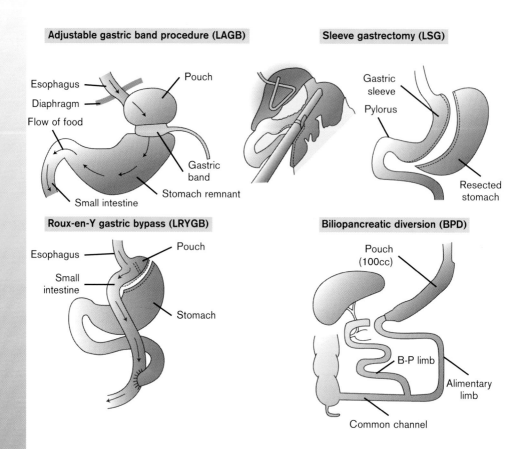

Figure 23.2. Common bariatric procedures.

Laparoscopic adjustable gastric banding (LAGB)

The creation of the path around the upper stomach should be atraumatic and along the anatomical planes. By doing this, we will avoid injuring the stomach or the lower esophagus. An elegant technique will avoid hemorrhage from the liver or spleen. The addition of gastrogastric stitches above the band seems to be superfluous, if the correct plane is kept, avoiding entrance to the lesser sac.

Laparoscopic sleeve gastrectomy (LSG)

The two most common and potentially life-threatening complications to be prevented are bleeding and leakage from the staple line — the latter tends to develop most commonly just below the gastroesophageal junction (*angle of His*).

Bleeding

Care should be taken when transecting the *short gastric vessels* during mobilization of the upper fundus and to avoid injuring the splenic vessels and the upper pole of the spleen. The stomach is a highly vascularized organ and the staple line tends to bleed, thus meticulous hemostasis should be ensured while transecting the stomach and creating the sleeve. The correct staple height should be used: longer staples in the antral area (4.2-4.8mm) and shorter in the fundus (3.5mm). Additional optional measures to consolidate hemostasis at the staple line include: hemostatic clips, over-sewing the staple line with a running suture, and the application of local hemostatic materials such as Surgicel® (oxidized cellulose) or biological glues.

The use of various reinforcement materials for the staple line is controversial, but it seems that it achieves better hemostasis; however, so far there is no proof for lowering the incidence of leaks. Applying biological glues over the staple line has not been scientifically proved but 'it looks nice' — a 'sedative' for the surgeon? And finally, **an important tip: make sure the blood pressure of the patient is high enough before concluding the operation — I specifically ask the anesthesist to raise the blood pressure deliberately in order to test hemostasis of the staple line**. In some patients who developed postop bleeding you swear that you have left the staple line looking as dry as the Sinai desert! So what happened? Most probably, the blood pressure during surgery was a bit low but when the patient woke up, perhaps because of some pain, the blood pressure spiked and the stapler line started bleeding! **The message: in the highly vascularized stomach with long staple lines, never leave the abdomen before making sure the blood pressure is high enough to simulate the postoperative scenario of pain and stress**.

Does pre-op DVT prophylaxis increase the bleeding rate? Probably yes, but not to the extent of causing life-threatening bleeding. You should not omit DVT prophylaxis for fear of bleeding.

Leaks

The importance of using the correctly sized staples on different parts of the stomach has been mentioned above. **It is also important not to interrupt the blood supply of the lesser curvature while mobilizing the posterior wall and taking down adhesions from previous failed procedures** (to which, unfortunately, many of our patients have been subjected). It is also important to create a straight staple line — not a frickin' ZIG-ZAG! I make a special effort to avoid thermal injury to the upper posterior fundus in particular, believing that this could produce leaks.

Even with a perfect technique — aren't we all perfect? — we still witness an incidence of leaks around 1-2%. The addition of over-sewing or reinforcement materials to the staple line hasn't been proved to reduce leakage rates significantly.

What about drains? Most surgeons would leave a 'prophylactic' closed suction drain along the staple line hoping that it would alert them to postoperative bleeding and **early leaks** (during the first two days). **Since the consequences of leakage are potentially horrendous and since drains might detect them early, and in some cases even treat them by converting them to controlled fistulas, it seems that the routine use of drains is justified.** I use them.

Narrowing of the 'gastric tube'

Albeit rare, stenosis of the gastric tube typically occurs at the angular notch (the *incisura* — the transition point between the body and antrum, near the 'crow's foot') or in places where over-sewing of the staple line included too much tissue thus further tapering the already narrow gastric sleeve. **To prevent this from happening we should be careful not to fire the stapler too close to the calibrating tube near the angular notch and not to take overly deep 'bites' when over-sewing the staple line — always over the calibrating tube!**

There is no magical size for calibrating tubes. In spite of the notion that the smaller the calibrating tube, the smaller the gastric sleeve and the more the weight loss, there are no hard data proving this beyond doubt. If you wish to create a small and tight gastric sleeve for more restriction, then use smaller tubes (32-36 French), with the knowledge that you might get more stenosis, more bleeding (stapling is closer to the vessels of the lesser curvature), and probably, more leaks (unknown reason, but possibly due to higher sleeve pressure). **Using tubes of 36-42 French seems to be a safer option, which I prefer**.

Stenosis and even occlusion of the gastroesophageal junction or the esophagus itself are very rare complications of careless stapling during the last steps of the sleeve resection. Proper technique and keeping the calibrating tube in place should prevent such disasters.

Laparoscopic Roux-en-Y gastric bypass (LRYGB)

This procedure shares some of the complications seen after sleeve gastrectomy, but in addition, it has its own specific complications related to the construction of two anastomoses — the Roux-en-Y **gastrojejunostomy** (GJ), and the **jejunojejunostomy** (JJ).

Bleeding

The same principles outlined above apply here as well when creating the gastric pouch. However, bleeding could originate also from the division of the small bowel mesentery, the staple line in the small bowel, the omentum or from the trocar sites. Bleeding could be intraluminal from the constructed anastomoses (GJ and JJ should be constructed with the correct staple height of 3.5mm). Obviously, one has to check for bleeding before closing the enterotomies through which the stapler has been inserted and, if present, achieve hemostasis with sutures. The same principle applies in hand-sewn anastomoses.

Leaks

This is the Achilles' heel of this operation! The more anastomoses one creates the higher the risk of this dreaded complication. The leak can develop from the gastric pouch itself, the JJ or GJ anastomosis, but **most susceptible to leakage is the last mentioned anastomosis**. Good blood supply, healthy bowel ends and tension-free construction reduce the risks of leakage of any GI anastomosis (Chapter 6, section 1) and this applies here as well. Surgeons have tried various anastomotic methods during LRYGB — hand-sewn versus stapled (linear vs. circular), but no method has been shown to be superior to the others. Most surgeons test the integrity of the GJ anastomosis by instilling methylene blue into the gastric pouch or even use intra-operative endoscopy. If a leak is detected, it should be repaired with sutures and the test repeated. **I leave a drain near the GJ — most surgeons do**.

Patients surviving anastomotic leaks commonly develop anastomotic strictures. However, it seems that the use of linear staplers or larger circular staplers (25mm) rather than the 21mm ones has the potential to lower the incidence of anastomotic narrowing.

Prevention of late small bowel obstruction (SBO)

The mesenteric defects created during the operation are known to be prone to internal herniation causing strangulating SBO. Thus, most authorities advocate closure of these defects during the initial operation. Lately, however, there have been some reports describing the technique of an **antecolic, antegastric right-oriented Roux limb to fashion the gastrojejunostomy** (without closing the defects) with a very low incidence of obstruction (~1%). Bringing up the small bowel to the stomach for the GJ in the antecolic position rather than through the mesocolon avoids a potential internal hernia and thus reduces the incidence of SBO.

Some surgeons still do not close defects routinely. Several reasons are cited: closure of defects could be time consuming and not accurate;

sometimes SBO develops even after closure of the defects; and anyway most obstructive episodes will give us the grace of some time to diagnose and treat. I personally utilize the above mentioned technique without closure of defects and have an incidence of delayed SBO of around 2%.

Prevention of gastric remnant dilatation

One has to take care not to damage the vagal innervation of the bypassed stomach (the portion distal to the pouch) and to avoid stenosis of the JJ anastomosis.

Laparoscopic biliopancreatic diversion with or without duodenal switch — BPD/BPD-DS

This is a more complicated and less popular bariatric procedure, practiced in few centers across Europe and North America, using malabsorption as the main mechanism for weight loss. The classical BPD (Scopinaro's procedure) entails distal gastrectomy and creation of a duodenal stump, with all its potential consequences. The BPD-DS involves sleeve gastrectomy and duodeno-ileostomy ('duodenal switch'). The most **distal anastomosis** (entero-enterostomy) is constructed at 50cm from the cecum in the classical Scopinaro procedure and at 100cm in the DS version. Precise measurement of the bowel and determining the length of the common channel designated for absorption are very important in order to achieve proper weight loss and prevent nutritional deficiencies.

All the intra-operative considerations described above also apply here for the prevention of bleeding, stenosis, leaks and delayed SBO.

Re-operative bariatric surgery

Again, we must tailor the repeated bariatric procedure to the previous one which has failed. Here are a few points:

- **Following LAGB**, it would be wise to remove the band and wait 2-3 months for the upper stomach and its vicinity to recover and then perform LSG or LRYGB. **Although patients (and the surgical ego) push us to get the job done (e.g. remove the band and add LSG or LRYGB) in one go, the staged approach has proved to be safer!**
- Sometimes, the upper stomach appears unsuitable for stapling because of previous staple lines (e.g. vertical banded gastroplasty) or local scarring and deformity due to failed LAGB. In such cases one

may have to change the plans and do a BPD procedure with all the stapling performed on a healthy and previously untouched stomach.

- **If the anatomy is judged to be very problematic, or serious complications are encountered, then converting to an open procedure or even aborting the surgery could prove to be a wise option**. Always remember: it's better to have a live and still obese patient rather than a dead one with a completed procedure!
- **Talk to your patients about all of this before the operation**: they have to be aware that operative plans are not written in the Bible or the Koran, that they may be waking up with something else done… or nothing at all.

Postoperative considerations

The potentially **life-threatening complications in the early postoperative period are pulmonary embolism, hemorrhage and anastomotic leaks**. Therefore, all our attention is focused to detect and manage these complications early.

Leaks

This is the most dreadful complication which constitutes a major cause of morbidity, death and lawsuits in this population. **The leaking sites are specific to the type of operation**:

- Leakage after **LAGB** is rare (less than 0.1%) but could originate from the posterior wall of the stomach or the lower esophagus — representing excessive operative trauma during creation of the 'tunnel' or insertion of the band.
- Following **LSG** it occurs from the staple line — in most cases from the upper portion of the stomach (near the *angle of His*). Analysis of multiple studies revealed an average leak rate for LSG of 2.8% (range 0-5%).
- After **LRYGB** a leak can originate from <u>multiple sources</u>: one of the two anastomoses (GJ or JJ), the staple line separating the gastric pouch and the bypassed stomach or even — and this applies to any laparoscopic procedure — an accidental intestinal perforation. **The most common site for leakage is the GJ anastomosis**. High-volume 'dedicated' bariatric centers claim leak rates of around 1-2% but the real figures 'out there in the community' are higher — around 5%.

Diagnosis

The spectrum and clinical features of anastomotic leaks in the UGI tract have been detailed in ⟳ Chapter 6, section 3. **In morbidly obese patients the immensely thick layers of fat which insulate the peritoneal cavity tend to muffle the abdominal signs of leak, so early diagnosis depends on obsessive vigilance and compulsive suspicion!**

> We should suspect an anastomotic leak in any patient developing dyspnea, tachycardia, with or without fever, abdominal tenderness and signs of sepsis. We have to remember that abdominal pain and peritoneal signs are not reliable features in this group of patients and that most of the findings are <u>non-specific</u> and easily confused with an acute cardiac event or PE.

Always suspect and immediately follow with a preconceived plan of diagnostic steps:

- Electrocardiography, blood tests for troponin levels, arterial blood gases and even CT angiography of the chest should be obtained to rule out cardiac ischemia or pulmonary embolism — this is particularly important in patients presenting with mainly non-abdominal complaints: respiratory distress accompanied by tachycardia.
- **In the majority of such cases emergency abdominal imaging is procured.** UGI contrast studies (fluoroscopy) may miss the leak in a high percentage of cases (~50%) and thus **our procedure of choice is a CT of the abdomen/chest** with oral contrast, looking for extravasation of contrast, and large amounts of free gas and fluid. At the same time, atelectasis, pneumonia and pulmonary emboli (i.v. contrast should be given as well) could be diagnosed or excluded.
- **In some patients an empiric abdominal exploration may be the only appropriate diagnostic (and therapeutic) modality!** Those are the cases where you have ruled out cardiac or pulmonary problems, imaging is negative or inconclusive, and drains are dry... but the patient is SIRSing or septic. One has to remember also that even in developed countries, the majority of hospitals lack CT scanners able to accommodate extremely obese patients. Therefore, making and confirming the diagnosis in such patients rests on clinical judgment and re-exploration. If the original procedure was laparoscopic, the patient is hemodynamically stable and you have the required skills, then re-explore laparoscopically. **By now you know that converting to open — or opening from the start — is not a sin!**

Treatment

As detailed in ⤳ Chapter 6, sections 1 and 3, the treatment should be tailored to the clinical situation. **If the leak is contained or controlled and the patient is not septic, it can be treated conservatively with fasting, broad-spectrum antibiotics and intravenous nutrition.** The patient would be lucky if a drain has been left behind and the leak is controlled through it. If the leak is presented as a drainable abdominal collection, then placement of a (CT-guided) percutaneous drain is the desired treatment.

Leaks can develop '**early**' (first 1-2 days), representing a technical failure, but most (the 'classic' ones) develop '**late**' — after five days and usually already when the patient has been discharged.

Early leaks can be detected by drains during hospital stay, but occasionally, as is the case in every other leak in the GI tract, they do not show up in the drain. **If the leak is detected in the drain (discharge of intestinal juice, oral methylene blue, high amylase levels, etc.) and the clinical set up is suggestive of a <u>controlled leak</u>, then the strategy of NPO, TPN, antibiotics is the recommended one, followed by endoscopic trials (with endoscopic clips, fibrin sealants and stents) to control the leaking point.** This approach should result in clinical resolution in up to 60-80% of cases. It may require several endoscopic interventions and the course could last several months. One has to be patient as these leaks are well controlled and they are low output.

In cases where the leak is not contained/controlled or the patient is SIRSing or septic with peritonitis, laparoscopic or open re-exploration is mandatory. In less dramatic circumstances get a CT scan and consider percutaneous drainage. In cases where the leak is not accessible by the percutaneous route, proceed with operative drainage — either laparoscopic or open as discussed above.

The basic rules in re-exploration are cleaning the abdomen and drainage (source control). You have already read in ⤳ Chapter 6 that attempts at closing the leak are usually futile and your aim is to achieve a controlled fistula. However, if you operate within a day or two after the operation and the tissues appear 'adequate' you may try to repair the leak with a few sutures — occasionally it will hold but usually it won't... ☹.

Finally, insert a **gastrostomy tube** in the bypassed stomach in LRYGB patients. A **jejunostomy tube** (distal to the jejunojejunostomy) should be considered if the leak originates from the *bypassed stomach* or the jejunojejunal anastomosis in LRYGB patients. A feeding jejunostomy could be of value also in leaking LSG and LAGB cases. Use your common sense!

A few specific points:

Controlled leaks following LRYGB tend to close spontaneously within weeks in most patients. On the other hand, **leaks after sleeve gastrectomy** are more resistant to conservative therapy needing endoscopic interventions and even surgical interventions in up to one-third of patients. Why is this?

The prevailing hypothesis is a poor blood supply in the upper part of the gastric sleeve and the elevated intraluminal pressure within the sleeve as compared to a better blood supply and the absence of high pressure in the gastric pouch after gastric bypass. **The recommended endoscopic treatment of leaks after LSG includes**:

- **In the 'early' post-leak phase (~40 days)**: insertion of a stent, which has to pass the incisura angularis, thus keeping the gastric tube in the correct axis and lowering its pressure. The mean duration of stenting is approximately four weeks.
- **In the 'late' post-leak phase (>40 days)**: in patients failing to respond to stenting or referred later, some experts would recommend pneumatic dilatation of the sleeve (again, to reduce intraluminal pressure) and endoscopic septotomy — dividing the ridge of tissue between the sleeve and the mouth of the fistula, draining the chronic peri-sleeve abscess into the lumen.
- **Operation for failed percutaneous and endoscopic treatments of leaking LSG**: this is the last resort. In brief, the options are converting the LSG to a LRYGB if there is a possibility to create the gastric pouch proximal to the fistula — anastomosing the small bowel to the opening of the proximal gastric fistula (after debridement of course). The most radical option is a **completion gastrectomy** with a Roux-en-Y esophagojejunostomy.

Leaks from the bypassed stomach following LRYGB are treated with drainage and gastrostomy — both drainage and gastrostomy can be done percutaneously by the radiologist.

Leaks from the JJ after LRYGB should be managed according to the principles outlined in ⮌ Chapter 6, section 4.

Late leaks

Late leaks usually present as well-defined, localized abscesses with fever, abdominal pain, intolerance to oral intake and occasionally some respiratory distress. CT of the abdomen is diagnostic and in most cases percutaneous drainage will be applicable and sufficient. If not then surgical re-exploration will be needed.

Bleeding

Bleeding could be intraluminal or intra-abdominal. The former presents as GI bleeding, especially following bypass procedures involving the construction of multiple anastomoses, but does occur rarely following LSG. After LRYGB it usually originates from the GJ. It resolves spontaneously in most cases but if it continues or results in hemodynamic compromise, then **open re-exploration** with direct control of the bleeding site is imperative. Access to the anastomosis may be gained either through an enterotomy in the Roux limb or by dismantling the anastomosis. Endoscopic hemostasis is probably inadvisable in the immediate postoperative period although it deserves a trial in experienced hands.

Intra-abdominal bleeding following LRYGB or LSG is usually self-limiting and does not require surgical intervention. Re-exploration is indicated if hemorrhage is hemodynamically compromising: over-sewing or clipping of the bleeding site at the staple line (or other bleeding location) usually solves the problem. Occasionally, a hematoma gets infected and presents as an intra-abdominal abscess which requires drainage (see ⮌ Chapter 3).

Pulmonary embolism (PE)

Obesity is a known risk factor for DVT and PE. Its incidence in the bariatric population may be as high as 1%. This risk should be modified either by the administration of pre-operative low-molecular-weight heparin (LMWH) or sequential compression devices (SCD) — some would use both modalities. The real incidence with the routine use of prophylactic anticoagulation is nowadays reduced to 0.1-0.2%. **The standard of care dictates that anticoagulation should be continued for 2-4 weeks after surgery.** This is the policy practiced by most surgeons. Nevertheless, there are some surgeons who do not use it because of a perceived high bleeding rate and they claim a very low incidence of DVT/PE with the use of SCD only. The placement of an inferior vena cava filter is recommended in patients with a prior history of DVT or PE.

The **diagnosis** is made clinically in the patient with tachycardia, dyspnea and hypoxia and should be confirmed by CT angiography of the chest which is currently considered the most reliable diagnostic test. As previously stated,

PE could be confused with leaks and even CT angiography of the chest could be equivocal. Therefore, occasionally, tests to rule out leaks should be performed like adding a formal CT of the abdomen with oral contrast. The treatment of PE is beyond the scope of this chapter.

Procedure-specific complications

Below are a few additional complications typical to specific bariatric procedures.

Bypass procedures

Acute gastric dilatation

This very rare complication can be dramatic. Dilatation of the *bypassed stomach* may occur spontaneously, as a result of obstruction at the 'downstream' jejunojejunostomy or secondary to the interruption of the nerves of Latarjet during the creation of the gastric pouch. You should suspect this in patients who develop hiccoughs and abdominal bloating accompanied by tachycardia; hemodynamic compromise may follow in extreme cases (**remember: massive acute gastric dilatation produces the abdominal compartment syndrome**). A plain abdominal radiograph often shows a large gastric bubble with an air-fluid level. But if the stomach is filled with fluid, the radiograph may not be helpful — CT is then diagnostic. **Treatment is by urgent needle decompression of the excluded stomach (image-guided if time allows) or surgical gastrotomy.** If there is no obvious improvement or in cases of hemodynamic instability, suspect gastric blowout! An urgent laparotomy is then mandatory. The patency of the jejunojejunostomy (an obstructed anastomosis could be the cause for the dilatation of the excluded stomach) should be verified in every case by an UGI study or during surgical exploration (contrast injected into the gastrostomy tube in the excluded stomach).

Small bowel obstruction (SBO)

SBO is a notorious complication of bariatric bypass procedures. This is not the 'early' postoperative SBO dealt with in ⟳ Chapter 8 but a 'late' SBO developing months and years after the procedure. Following weight loss and disappearance of visceral fat, the mesenteric defects created during the initial surgery become large enough to allow internal herniation of intestine. With the antecolic technique, two potential defects are created: between the cut edge of the Roux limb mesentery and the mesocolon (*Petersen's defect*) and at the jejunojenostomy. With the retrocolic technique, there is a mesocolic opening through which the Roux limb is brought up to the gastric pouch (■ Figure

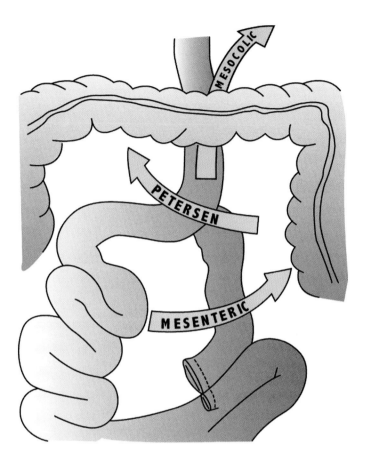

Figure 23.3. Sites of potential internal hernias after gastric bypass procedures.

23.3). Notably, the adhesions which could prevent internal herniation by fixing the loops of bowel in position are minimal after laparoscopic procedures.

The occurrence of SBO after RYGB could be treacherous. The symptoms are usually vague — intermittent, crampy, mid-abdominal pain with or without distension. Because of the altered foregut anatomy, nausea and vomiting are usually absent. Multiple episodes may occur with only transient symptoms (spontaneous 'in and out' herniation). **Hence, the diagnosis of internal hernia should be suspected in every patient after RYGB presenting with unexplained abdominal pain! In the non-emergency situation we must also rule out symptomatic cholelithiasis (common after bariatric surgery) and a marginal ulcer developing at the GJ anastomosis.**

Only a minority of patients present with obvious features of SBO with increasing abdominal pain, tenderness, and some degree of distension. Plain abdominal radiographs are usually non-specific. **Contrast-enhanced CT is the study of choice** (if not available then UGI contrast study is an alternative), but even CT can occasionally miss the pathology if symptoms subside spontaneously due to the small bowel movement in and out of the defect. **The bottom line is this: do not be misled by the vague presentation of SBO in the post-bariatric patient. Use CT liberally and proceed to the operating room as soon as possible before the incarcerated intestine within the internal hernia becomes compromised**. Even if abdominal imaging is non-diagnostic and symptoms vague consider diagnostic laparoscopy to reduce the herniated small bowel (if found) and close the mesenteric defects. Open exploration would be needed if the patient is hemodynamically unstable, there is necrotic bowel, the anatomy is 'confusing', or visualization is poor due to dilated small bowel loops.

Stomal stenosis and stomal ulceration

Stricture of the gastrojejunostomy is not rare; sometimes it is the consequence of healed leakage. Its incidence depends on the technique of creating the anastomosis: circular stapler, linear stapler or hand-sewn. The incidence could range between 1-2% up to 15-20% with small-caliber (22mm) circular staplers, with patients presenting with dysphagia, nausea and vomiting and at times odynophagia. Upper GI endoscopy is diagnostic and offers treatment with balloon dilatation. Occasionally, there is an associated **marginal ulcer** which should be treated with acid suppression. Persistent ulceration, especially if combined with some weight gain, should raise the possibility of a **gastrogastric fistula**. The diagnosis is achieved by UGI series and the management is surgical: disconnection of the pouch from the fundus using a stapler.

Stenosis of the gastric tube after LSG

This is rather rare and could be seen either early or late. The early form is the result of creation of a gastric tube that is too narrow — the stapler line having been tightly over-sewn. Patients complain of severe dysphagia, odynophagia and vomiting. UGI study confirms the diagnosis. Treatment is conservative, with endoscopic dilatation started some six weeks after the operation. In severe persisting cases conversion of the LSG to LRYGB should be considered.

Obviously, **the sleeve can dilate over time**. If this occurs then patients will gain weight. This is considered not a complication but a failure of the procedure which could be managed with conversion of the sleeve to LRYGB. And in fact some experts recommend using such a planned 'staged approach' in the high-risk 'super-super-obese' patients — start with LSG and follow with LRYGB...

Lap band procedures

Band slippage
This means that the gastric fundus slips proximally underneath the band. The clinical presentation can be subacute or chronic but occasionally is acute and dramatic due to ischemia of the gastric wall. Symptoms and signs include epigastric pain, reflux, vomiting, dysphagia, or even acute obstruction. An UGI contrast study is diagnostic in almost all cases, demonstrating that the band has moved downwards with a large pouch above it. **Immediate band deflation followed by laparoscopic exploration should be performed with reduction of the herniated stomach. Some surgeons would reposition the band provided the gastric wall is not ischemic and because they "believe in bands". The others (the smarter ones like me ☺) consider this a severe complication and a justification to remove the band and plan another bariatric procedure...** Rarely, when diagnosis and treatment are delayed, gastric wall necrosis develops and has to be treated appropriately — you know how...

Band erosion
In most cases, the presentation is subacute or chronic but it could manifest as an acute infection of the port site or intra-abdominal infection. Band erosion into the stomach occurs in 1-2% of cases. Patients can be asymptomatic, or they may rarely present with an acute abdomen. Diagnosis is made by endoscopy or an UGI study. The former visualizes the eroded band lying inside the stomach; on the latter you may see that the contrast is around the band passing freely without delay.

Late port-site infection combined with weight gain (as a result of alleviation of the restriction of food after erosion) and occasional epigastric pain, should raise suspicion of band erosion. As previously mentioned, this may cause an intra-abdominal abscess. **Treatment requires removal of the entire band system and repair of the gastric wall**. This can be done laparoscopically in most cases; however, some have advocated endoscopic removal. In the case of an acute perforation with associated abscess, laparotomy and closure of the perforation and wide drainage should be performed.

Infection of the port site usually presents as superficial surrounding cellulitis which should respond to antibiotics. With deeper infections (manifesting with recurrence of the infection, persistent drainage, or peri-band fluid on imaging) removal of the port is necessary. In some cases, even removal of the entire LAGB system might be required to eradicate extensive infections. These principles apply also to late infections of the port site.

> "For the vast majority of patients today, there is no operation that will control weight to a 'normal' level without introducing risks and side effects that over a lifetime may raise questions about its use for surgical treatment of obesity."
>
> **Edward Mason**

Dr. Mason of Iowa City, a pioneer of bariatric surgery (if you visit Iowa you will understand why...), spoke from his own experience: he saw bariatric procedures emerging and vanishing. So who remembers today the small bowel bypass operations, so popular some 30 years ago that entire chapters of its numerous complications had to be written? Will this chapter be thus obsolete 5-10 years from now? Let us hope so! **Moshe**

Chapter 24

Trauma

Ari Leppäniemi

Trauma laparotomy is like fishing. Often you get what's expected — one or two nice fish but nothing spectacular. Sometimes you get nothing, but it was nice to be out there and enjoy the atmosphere. Then one day when you least expect it, the big one hits. Immediately you know "this is it"! This is what you have been preparing for the whole of your life as a fisherman (or trauma surgeon). You need all your skills, patience, good decision-making and a bit of luck to land the big one. And whatever the outcome, you have to live with it for the rest of your life...

The key to reducing the risk of complications after trauma is to minimize delays to interventions aimed at aborting the natural course of the physiological deterioration caused by the anatomical tissue destruction. (Sigh!) Sounds complicated? Not really. Trauma to a major blood vessel can cause bleeding that, if not controlled in time (or stops spontaneously), will lead to exsanguination. Another type of blood vessel injury (intimal tear with subsequent thrombosis) can lead to end-organ ischemia, cellular death and loss of organ mass and function (or loss of extremity). A hole in the bowel or urinary bladder, for example, will lead to chemical and later to bacterial peritonitis and if treated too late, when systemic sepsis has settled in, can kill the patient. And even the commonly missed small bone extremity fractures can cause significant morbidity and loss of function when missed initially and discovered late.

A delay in diagnosis leads ultimately to a delay in treatment. Whether the injury is missed initially during diagnostic work-up, or is not recognized during surgical exploration, **a missed injury should spell "complication"**. Of course, technical mistakes during surgical reconstruction of tissue defects are another source of complications but they are not specific to trauma and are mostly discussed elsewhere in this book. Finally, trauma management is not just about operative surgery; the way we manage the physiological insult caused by trauma by giving too much or not enough fluids or blood products, for example, can lead to complications down the road — think of coagulation disorders, infections or abdominal compartment syndrome.

Pre-operative considerations

Tissue injury caused by an external mechanical (burns, electric or chemical injuries are not dealt with in this chapter) energy source can result from blunt or penetrating trauma. The main difference is that **penetrating trauma** will cause a hole in the skin and injure those organs that happen to be in the path of the knife blade or bullet (bullets do not always follow a straight line). High-energy missiles can cause tissue destruction up to 30cm away from their tract by inducing temporary cavitation that causes tissue damage by distension and friction. Obviously, short-range shotgun injuries or multiple bullet or stab wounds cause more injuries than a single penetrating agent.

The **blunt trauma** mechanism is more complex and causes tissue damage by direct compression (contusion, bursting), shearing forces and rapid deceleration. More often than not more than one organ or organ system is injured, and the exact localization of the organs at risk is more difficult. **Thinking about probabilities (and using your clinical experience) and applying a systematic approach to a trauma patient are the keys to success**.

Pre-hospital care

> *Failure to promptly recognize and treat simple life-threatening injuries is the tragedy of trauma, not the inability to handle the catastrophic or complicated injury.*
>
> **F. William Blaisdell**

Trauma care starts at the scene and pre-hospital care is an integral part of trauma care (or the "trauma chain of survival" as the Norwegians have said so nicely). But even so, pre-hospital care is just one part of a comprehensive and systematic approach and organization of all aspects of caring for trauma patients — from pre-hospital care through to evaluation and treatment, and ending with rehabilitation. **Inclusive trauma systems** cover the systematic approach to all trauma patients (including patients with minor injuries), whereas **exclusive trauma systems** concentrate on dealing with major trauma. This usually means that major trauma patients are treated in trauma centers. The modern key word is *regionalization* when trauma care within a specific geographic region is organized in a systematic way which usually means that patients with major injuries are transported directly to a major trauma center that has the facilities to deal with all kinds of injuries. **And there is considerable evidence to show that trauma systems save lives — the estimated survival benefit is about 15-20%.**

Conventional wisdom in trauma care favors the concept of the 'golden hour' — the time frame where all major problems induced by trauma should be diagnosed and at least temporarily managed. The reality is, however, more complex. One way of approaching this complexity of the management of trauma is to ask: **why do trauma patients die?**

Trauma patients die of bleeding, brain injury or (late) complications (infection and/or multiple organ failure). But going one layer deeper, the patient dies *early* due to lack of oxygen (think cells, especially in the brain), either because it does not get in (airways blocked), does not get into circulation (problems with respiration such as pneumothorax), or is not transferred in sufficient amounts to vital organs (circulation). **Thus, the initial ABC-approach (A for airways, B for breathing and C for circulation) makes sense.**

A & B...

The indications and proper techniques for pre-hospital intubation or other forms of securing **airways** are beyond the scope of this book, but it is sufficient to note that one way or the other, securing an airway is a crucial step in any medical emergency. Proper methods to secure adequate **breathing** are more controversial. Recognition of a true or potential *tension-pneumothorax* and needle decompression are in the armamentarium of most pre-hospital care providers but the effectiveness of needle decompression especially when placed in the high anterior mid-clavicular line is questionable. Cadaver studies have shown that in obese or athletic individuals, the standard size needle reaches the pleural space only in about 50% of the time, and that **placing the needle laterally around the 5th intercostal space in the mid-axillary line is more effective**.

C...

Major bleeding can only come from a major blood vessel, a large parenchymal organ, such as the liver (well, it comes from vessels inside or near the liver anyway) or a major fracture such as the pelvic bone or femur. A large proportion of patients who die immediately after an airplane crash, for example, have an aortic rupture, and they bleed to death in no time. Sometimes the bleeding from the aorta is contained by the adventitia and surrounding tissues, opening a window of opportunity (please forgive us for using the cliché!) to repair the injury before it bursts and leads to uncontrollable bleeding and death.

On scene and in the pre-hospital phase in general, there are two kinds of bleeding: controllable and uncontrollable. Bleeding from an extremity wound or a scalp laceration can be at least temporarily controlled by external compression, either locally or proximally (in the extremity only! I have seen an attempt to control bleeding from a neck wound by tightening the necktie... ☺). Recent experiences from war have rehabilitated the use of **tourniquets** and the new and easily applicable tourniquets (even put on by the injured themselves with one hand) have gained popularity in the civilian world. MAST (military anti-shock trousers) suits on the other hand seem to be doomed to the archives of history, but never say never... Finally, a new generation of local hemostatic dressings used by the military has made inroads to pre-hospital care and seems to benefit at least the pharmaceutical companies, and maybe the patients...

Internal bleeding from visceral or vascular injuries cannot be controlled in a hospital lacking surgical and/or angiographic facilities. There was a period in history where the wisdom (expressed by Walter B. Cannon in 1918) of **not trying to restore normal blood pressure and circulation until the bleeding source is controlled** was forgotten, and aggressive pre-hospital and pre-operative fluid resuscitation was considered the standard of care. Obviously, no circulation (oxygen) for more than a few minutes will lead to cell death, first in the brain and later in other vital organs. To manage the trade-off between maintaining sufficient perfusion, and not 'popping the clot' and causing more bleeding by restoring normotension, new strategies have been introduced into pre-hospital fluid resuscitation, such as **hypotensive resuscitation**, 'small-volume' or 'limited' fluid resuscitation, 'permissive hypotension' and even whole concepts such as '**scoop and run**' (in opposition to the previous *stay and play*). In urban areas, the scoop and run policy which means getting the patient to the nearest trauma center as soon as possible is the most popular and a Canadian study has shown that, paradoxically, the presence of doctors on scene actually makes the prognosis worse, probably because they tend to do more interventions and increase the scene time. Obviously, in rural areas, or if the patient is trying to die on you on the spot, some interventions are needed — if they can be performed on scene (such as securing the airway). Some linguistic enthusiasts (or people who cannot make decisions) have even coined terms like "play on the way"... **In the end, they all try to do the same thing; keep the patient (and the vital organs) alive until definitive care can be applied, i.e. surgery to control bleeding and restore circulation** (we need the help of our anesthetists here).

The use of **hypertonic saline** for fluid resuscitation in trauma can rapidly restore part of the lost volume and improve perfusion with a relatively small-volume infusion (for example, 250ml of 7.5% hypertonic saline combined with dextran expands the blood volume by 3-4 times the infused volume), and it also has beneficial immunological effects compared with Ringer's lactate. The potential disadvantages caused by the osmolar charge, such as hyperosmolar coma, hypernatremia lasting for more than a few hours or hemolysis, have not been confirmed in clinical studies when concentrations of or below 7.5% have been used. **The systolic blood pressure to aim for is around 60mmHg but in patients with brain injury it should be higher**. It is interesting why its use is still limited in many parts of the world. I guess civilization spreads slowly...

Hemoglobin-based oxygen-carrying fluids (HBOCs) have shown great promise for the last 25 years, and still do... but have not found their place in clinical use. **Recombinant Factor VIIa** gives a thrombin burst and promotes coagulation but its beneficial effects in trauma patients except for marginal reduction of blood transfusion needs could not be shown in two randomized studies. Its routine use in trauma is not recommended, and it is also very expensive.

The latest innovation is **hemostatic resuscitation** and is rooted in the discovery that tissue injury itself causes early coagulopathy, and the sooner it is reversed the better. Besides, as one of my surgical mentors used to say, "the patient is not bleeding Ringer's lactate...", so maybe we will see the arrival of whole blood transfusion in pre-hospital care, perhaps Mark 2, freeze-dried blood, just add water...☺. For more on massive transfusion see ⮑ Chapter 3.

Emergency department care

*In any emergency setting, confusion is a function of the cube
(n^3) of the number of people involved.*

Clement A. Hiebert

*If you arrive in the ER and don't know what to do, start putting
in tubes until somebody arrives who knows.*

Rip Pfeiffer

When a seriously injured trauma patient arrives at the hospital, the **trauma team** (that was activated based on the information from the scene) is waiting for the patient and will perform a series of evaluations and interventions following a predetermined and practiced model (like the pit stop in Formula 1...). The team leader (preferably a surgeon) runs the show and the rest of the team (most commonly consisting of another doctor/anesthetist, another surgeon, 2-3 nurses and radiologist/technician) performs **simultaneous** tasks including the **ABC** (airway, breathing, circulation) sequence and a **primary survey**. Unless the patient is dying on the spot, the team waits to get the information from the pre-hospital care providers about the injury: **M**echanism, detected **I**njuries, vital **S**igns and **T**reatment (the **MIST formula**).

A primary survey usually takes a few minutes. While doing the A, **protection of the cervical spine** is included in the protocol. **B might require placement of chest tubes (suspicion of tension-pneumothorax based on clinical assessment of tracheal deviation, distended neck veins and auscultation) before chest X-ray!** Adequacy of *circulation* is assessed by evaluating mentation, pulse, blood pressure and peripheral perfusion (temperature and skin color). **External bleeding** is temporarily controlled. **In penetrating injuries of the anterior chest (and sometimes outside the 'cardiac box'), the possibility of cardiac tamponade must cross your mind.** Distended neck veins should alert you, but might not be there because of hypovolemia. The rest of the *Beck's triad* (*hypotension* is self-explanatory but *muffled heart sounds* you only see mentioned in textbooks, not found in a noisy emergency department...) is not so helpful, whereas ultrasound (**FAST** — focused abdominal sonography for trauma) will tell you if there is blood in the pericardium. If found in significant amounts (anything more than 'tiny', 'small', 'minimal' or 'trace' that may be due to imaging artifact) and the patient has the clinical picture of pericardial tamponade (the FAST can also be false negative!), an emergency pericardial decompression is needed. **Forget the needle, it does not work, or if you get a lot of blood, you probably have put the needle through the heart wall...** Ken Mattox has given valuable advice: "The only thing the ED personnel should do with a patient with pericardial tamponade, is to wave to the patient on his way to the operating theatre..."

Emergency room thoracotomy is controversial and almost never used in blunt trauma patients in whom it is futile. In patients with penetrating trauma presenting in extremis, a rapid left anterolateral thoracotomy to relieve cardiac tamponade, control intrathoracic sources of bleeding (such as from lacerated lung), perform open cardiac massage and/or cross-clamp the thoracic aorta to reduce bleeding from major abdominal injuries, can sometimes save a life (it has never worked for me for the last two indications…). **However, as a general rule, surgery is best performed in the operating theatre, and it is the best place for a severely injured patient who is bleeding**.

The **primary survey** should be completed with **D** (*disability*, i.e. rapid assessment of neurology) and **E** (*exposure* of all wounds and body parts). If the patient requires no further immediate intervention, the team proceeds with a **secondary survey that includes a systematic assessment of all potential injuries going from head to toe**. Nasogastric and urethral catheters, pelvic binders to reduce bleeding and stabilize the pelvis, and temporary splints for extremity fractures may be inserted or applied. **Imaging studies** (cervical spine, chest and pelvic X-ray) are performed although more and more centers skip these in favor of a **CT scan** (**pan-CT** including head, neck and torso). And that's where the danger is (well, in addition to the radiation dose)!

The prevailing concept is that if the patient is hemodynamically 'stable' or responds to fluid resuscitation (the bleeding might still be continuing…), he/she can undergo a CT evaluation. If the CT is in the ED and can be rapidly performed, that's fine. But if you have to take the patient to a radiology suite some distance away, you might end up with **ABCTD** (AB CT and Death). It is not unusual to have a bleeding patient collapse in the 'tunnel of death'.

It's all about decision-making. There are only a few places where the patient can go from the ED — the OR, ICU, radiology, ward (or floor as the North Americanos would say) and one even gloomier place we try to avoid… **A patient who has severe surgical bleeding belongs to the operating room**. The location of penetrating injury and FAST examination will show you which cavity has to be addressed first. Stable patients with continuous arterial bleeding from solid abdominal organs (liver, spleen, kidney), pelvic fracture or in some cases from vascular injuries in difficult locations (subclavian, vertebral arteries) are elegantly treated with angiographic embolization or placement of a (subclavian) stent graft, if interventional radiologists are available without significant delay. Patients with injuries causing organ dysfunction and/or requiring invasive monitoring need intensive care, either postoperatively or when managed non-operatively.

Non-operative management

The current trend of **non-operative management** of solid abdominal organs started with splenic injuries in pediatric patients, and today virtually all (the co-editors warned me "never say never" but this is true in our own center) *pediatric* splenic ruptures are managed non-operatively. In adults, about 85% of blunt liver and spleen injuries are managed without surgery, sometimes requiring angioembolization to control bleeding from intraparenchymal arterial branches. **Hemodynamic instability is a contraindication for non-operative management but almost all other patients with blunt liver/spleen injuries can undergo a trial of expectant observation**. A CT scan (with i.v. contrast) shows the extent of the injury and possible extravasation (source of arterial bleeding that might be treatable with angioembolization), and equally importantly, may alert to the possibility of associated injuries that require surgical treatment.

A patient with a significant injury managed non-operatively is best treated in the place where hemodynamic monitoring is available (high-dependency unit or ICU), but obviously patients with less severe or isolated liver/spleen injuries do well in the ward as well. Whether absolute bed rest is needed for the first few days is controversial but I do feel uncomfortable with the idea of a jelly-like clot around the spleen being shaken when the patient walks around…

Non-operative treatment can fail for two reasons: a known injury that fails to heal or an unknown (missed) injury that causes problems later. Non-operative management of liver injuries fails in about 10% and in about 30% for splenic injuries, mostly because of continuous or recurrent bleeding.

Remember: a restless, pale patient, dropping hemoglobin-value, distended abdomen…, it is better to have a look — with your eyes, as radiation therapy does not stop bleeding… and yes, get blood!

Who needs surgery now?

Whether a patient suffers from penetrating or blunt trauma, the most important pre-operative consideration in trauma patients is: **who needs surgery now?** There are numerous management algorithms for trauma and there is no need to repeat them here (all textbooks and manuals have them). The key is to identify organ injuries requiring surgical (or other) intervention. In patients with abdominal trauma, bleeding from a solid organ or vascular injury must be stopped, critical organ perfusion must be secured, leakage from a hole in a hollow organ (or main pancreatic duct) must be controlled, and anatomical integrity of the abdominal wall and diaphragm restored. While **major bleeding** is usually diagnosed clinically (and location/cavity in blunt trauma verified with ultrasound), organ ischemia and especially hollow organ perforation are more difficult to diagnose until they cause symptoms (might take hours or longer).

Missed injuries

Missed injuries are the most common cause of complications in trauma. The most frequent **missed injuries** are *fractures* (cervical spine, extremity bones) followed by *abdominal* (gastrointestinal or urinary tract), *head* (subdural hematoma, mandibular fracture) and *chest* (hemo- or pneumothorax, rib fracture) injuries. **About 50% of missed injuries are associated with sloppy clinical evaluation, such as ignoring minor symptoms and signs, inadequate physical examination or misinterpreted information**. One-third are related to imaging (missing findings, inadequate investigation or interpretation). Patient-related factors (altered consciousness or hemodynamic instability) are rarely the cause but must be taken into consideration during clinical examination. **A tertiary survey or a comprehensive general physical examination with reviews of all investigations including radiographs and blood results will detect about 90% of initially missed clinically significant injuries when performed within 24 hours**. I usually do that the next morning in the ICU or ward on trauma patients whether they have been operated on at night or not. Start with the head, go through the torso (including the back) and finish with the extremities; **your hands and the stethoscope are all that you need!**

Some specific injuries

Blunt bowel injuries

Blunt bowel injuries are rare (less than 1% of all blunt trauma admissions) and easily missed during clinical examination. A pre-operative delay of as little as five hours increases morbidity! All algorithms state that peritonitis is an indication for laparotomy, but it rarely develops rapidly and the initially subtle signs are easily missed in the noisy, busy ED full of action, and in obtunded patients, already receiving analgesia. Besides, traumatized patients may have a tender abdomen from other causes such as abdominal wall contusion. **CT scans are getting better in detecting bowel injuries** (free air, thickened bowel wall, *unexplained free fluid* in the absence of solid organ injury) and should be used instead of plain X-rays or ultrasound in hemodynamically stable patients. **Retroperitoneal perforations of the duodenum and colon can be tricky — rely on CT!** Isolated **mesenteric injuries** are almost impossible to detect early unless causing significant hemorrhage. Once, I decided to operate on a blunt trauma patient because he needed so much opioid analgesia even though clinical examination and CT scan did not show anything special. The patient had two large mesenteric lacerations with 1.5 meters of ischemic, but not yet necrotic, small bowel…

Pancreatic injuries

Pancreatic injuries are fortunately rare but often missed. Detecting a transected pancreas on CT is not easy and sometimes the initial CT is normal even in the presence of a major duct injury. I never understood what "high-index of suspicion" means but I guess here is when you need it… ERCP is not available at night and MRCP (if available) is often not helpful. **So, if in doubt, wait until morning for ERCP or have a look with your own eyes**. Many studies have shown that elevated amylase levels are not a reliable sign of a pancreatic injury. But…, if the amylase levels are high, I would have a closer look at the pancreas on CT! Repeat the CT if needed…

Diaphragmatic injuries

Diaphragmatic injuries show up on a CT scan if one of the abdominal organs has herniated though the hole into the chest. On the right side the liver protects the hole somewhat, although I once did a laparotomy and could not find the liver… Finally, it was discovered in the chest and you could hear the sucking sound when my hand went up the dome of the liver and pulled it back into the abdomen through the big hole in the diaphragm. Stab wounds in the left flank have a relatively high risk (about 17%) of diaphragmatic perforation; it does not show up on CT (unless there is herniation), contrary to what my radiology colleagues say, and might be the **only indication for an exploratory *laparoscopy* in abdominal trauma**.

It's decision-making time!

Remember that it is what you decide to do that makes the difference to the patient, not what you write in the notes (well, for lawyers this might be so…). The key question is: who needs surgery now? **And here is a simple, Finnish, algorithm-free approach to abdominal trauma — but most of these principles would apply, more or less, to the rest of the world as well**.

Operate on patients:

- Who have bleeding that causes hemodynamic instability (use FAST to determine where the major bleeding is).
- With abdominal gunshot or close-range shotgun wounds unless they are low-energy *tangential* wounds (you still need to explore the bullet wound!). In some high-volume trauma centers, hemodynamically stable patients with abdominal gunshot wounds (especially in the right

upper quadrant) and no peritonitis undergo CT and are treated non-operatively if no 'surgical' injuries are detected. In our place the risk of a significant organ injury after a penetrating gunshot wound is about 90%. Would you take a chance?

- With anterior abdominal stab wounds that penetrate the anterior fascia (determined by wound exploration with a finger, obvious evisceration or radiology). These patients have a 60% chance of an organ injury requiring surgical repair. However, in many places such patients are managed, selectively, without an operation, based on CT findings or repeated clinical examination. We Finns tend to be more aggressive...
- Who are asymptomatic with stab wounds, especially to the left thoracoabdominal region; they can undergo a laparoscopy to rule out an occult diaphragmatic injury.
- Who have an organ injury on CT that requires surgical repair.
- That are 'sick' and you have no good explanation for it.

Having said this I admit that our Finnish protocol is not written in stone (although our practices on abdominal stab wounds are based on two randomized studies from our department and many retrospective ones...) and there are people around the world who would 'smoke the fish' differently. More frequent use of CT or just expectant observation is fine if you think it is better to 'wait and see' than 'look and see'... Laparoscopy (in stab wounds it avoids a negative laparotomy in about 55% of patients) seems attractive but 'running' the bowel reliably is not easy and it does not see into the retroperitoneum...

Always ask: is there anything I can do pre-operatively to reduce postoperative complications? Start antibiotics in all penetrating injuries and when contamination is likely. The type of antibiotics needed depend on local conditions. For the abdomen I use simple things like cefuroxime and metronidazole... Make sure you have blood and blood products available. **Don't over-resuscitate the patient with crystalloids**. And go through your operative strategy while scrubbing... **And now we are going fishing!**

Intra-operative considerations

This section deals with abdominal injuries. In most places thoracic injuries are managed by cardiothoracic surgeons, head injuries by neurosurgeons and bone and joint injuries by orthopedic surgeons. The days are gone when one surgeon had the competency to operate everywhere in the body — at least in major western hospitals receiving patients with severe trauma. I used to work in developing countries and in field hospitals with the International Committee of the Red Cross doing the best I could (including delivering anesthesia with ketamine, the true friend of a surgeon — it does not drop blood pressure and you don't even need to intubate...), but I would not dream of doing craniotomies or fracture surgery today in my hospital. Of course, in **rural areas**, you might need to do a lot of things if you are by yourself, but that's another story...

The standard incision for trauma laparotomy is the long midline incision extending from the xiphoid to the pubis. If needed, you can add a transverse extension all the way to the back that gives you a reasonable access to every part of the abdomen and retroperitoneum (my definition of *single-port surgery...* ☺). The only exception is a patient with a scarred midline from a previous operation and the need for fast access. In that case you can start with a transverse incision. Although one of my mentors used to say that "it's easier to operate when the incision is placed over the organ that is to be removed", this does not apply to trauma. Don't fool yourself that a bullet hole that went in through the right upper quadrant only injured the liver. (Well, if you have a pre-operative CT and you are SURE that you know what the injured organs are, you can use a more aptly placed incision...)

Once you are inside the abdomen you always have two choices: is this patient 'healthy enough' so that I can explore and repair all injuries systematically and definitively, or is the degree of physiological derangement so severe that the patient would not tolerate that — which means that you have to shift into **'damage control' mode: you go away to fight a battle another day**. In fishing terms: cut the line and let your trophy fish slip away... with your most expensive *Rapala* lure in his mouth ☹...

Damage control

Packing a liver injury was first described by James Pringle (yes, the same guy who got famous for the Pringle maneuver) in 1908. He actually used perihepatic packing in four patients, one of whom survived the initial operation but died four days later from pulmonary embolism. At autopsy the bleeding from the liver (and the right kidney which he also packed) had stopped. William Halsted used the same technique but inserted rubber sheets between the liver and packs to prevent the packs from adhering too tightly to the liver and causing rebleeding when removed (I think he got this one wrong, but again nobody is perfect...). In any case packing was forgotten for about 70 years and attempts at bailout before definitive repair of all injuries was considered the equivalent to "losing one's surgical manhood"... Then in 1983, Harlan Stone and co-workers showed that it actually saves lives, and the rest is history... The term "damage control" comes from the Navy (not stopping a ship that has been hit to become an easy target, but containing the leaks with whatever means available and moving to the nearest port for definitive repair) and was coined by Mike Rotondo and Bill

Schwab in Philadelphia. **Adoption of the damage control philosophy probably represents the biggest change in trauma surgery during the last 50 years**.

Who needs damage control surgery?

It is not the anatomy (severity of the injuries) but physiology that counts! If the patient is acidotic and hypothermic and has already bled a lot, think of damage control. Don't wait for the coagulopathy to settle in, that means that you are already late! Other things I find useful, especially when called to help in an ongoing operation, is to know **how many units of blood the patient has already received. Anything with two digits should make you worried...** And to prevent you from losing track of time (happens easily when you encounter tough injuries and need to do some mobilization), asking your favorite nurse to tell you every 15 minutes that "another 15 minutes have passed, doctor" (with that very specific tone...), helps your decision-making. The textbooks say that damage control surgery should not last for more than one hour but I rarely can achieve that. I think 1.5-2 hours is more realistic...

Don't let the 'blood brain barrier' stop you talking to your anesthetist; he or she knows better what the patient's physiology is. And the good anesthetist has already started from the beginning worrying about coagulation and has given the patient coagulation factors and platelets... The current fuss about the best ratio of plasma and packed red cells (1:1 or something else) is probably nonsense, just start early with the fresh frozen plasma (and platelets and fibrinogen) and keep giving them when giving blood. The only rational way to find out what the patient actually needs (is he coagulopathic, fibrinolytic or just about right?) is by the use of a **thromboelastogram** (TEG) in the OR but this needs a bit of sophistication. But once you have learned how to use it, it is of great help! Google it up!

Increasing the temperature of the OR has long been considered useful (to the patient, not the surgeon), but like many ideas that seem so good in the armchair, it actually doesn't pass the test of scientific evaluation as it has been shown recently that OR temperature has very little effect on the patient's temperature (forget the extremes of course).

How to conduct a damage control laparotomy

The first priority is to stop bleeding, major bleeding is always visible and really bad bleeding is audible...

If you encounter an abdomen full of blood, the textbooks say to proceed with *four-quadrant packing*. What it really means is that initially you just put packs *everywhere*, around the liver, the spleen, pelvis, etc. Before putting the packs in, just scoop out most of the blood (suction usually gets blocked) and insert the packs. Once you have the situation under control (talk to the anesthetist!), start removing packs gently beginning from the least likely place to bleed, and deal with the bleeding sources.

There are not too many major bleeding sources in the abdomen, think big vessels or the liver. Like most things in life, there are two possibilities: you can control the bleeding directly or you need to do some dissection to get there.

Bleeding from the liver is usually easily visible and in blunt trauma most often comes from the right lobe. Temporary control of the bleeding from the liver can be achieved with bimanual compression followed by appropriately placed packs. At this stage you seldom need to mobilize the liver, but that might become necessary later (see below). This **temporary perihepatic packing** stops the bleeding in most cases. If the patient is in a bad shape, think of **definitive perihepatic packing** (and packing other places such as the left upper quadrant, pelvis, root of the mesentery, etc.). **Don't put the packs into the liver tissue through the crack but try to restore the contour of the liver by placing packs above, below and laterally**. In most cases it is not wise to mobilize the liver before packing but sometimes you need to dissect the right lobe free to achieve enough compression with the packs. Start at the lower margin of the right lobe and free the adhesions to the superior part of Gerota's fascia, proceed laterally and go around the liver, dividing its ligaments close to the capsule until you are able to bring the right lobe almost to the midline. **Don't pack the liver too tightly and with too many packs, you might compress the inferior vena cava**. Utilize the rib cage and the lateral abdominal wall to get enough support for the perihepatic packs.

Major vessel injury

Although packing controls bleeding from the majority of sources, it does not stop **bleeding from major arteries**. You need proximal control of the bleeding artery (and distal as well). The bad news is that most of the major arteries are *retroperitoneal* which means that you need to do some dissection to get there. The good news is that major arterial bleeding usually manifests as a *growing hematoma*, not overt bleeding that hits your face (the patient with that kind of injury dies before getting to the OR). The location of the hematoma gives an idea what vessel is bleeding. A detailed description on how to access various major vessels in the abdomen is beyond the scope of this book, but here are the basic rules:

- **Central supramesocolic hematoma** — think proximal abdominal aorta and the major branches (celiac, superior mesenteric artery) →

proximal control above (left thoracotomy) or just below the diaphragm → access with **left visceral rotation** by mobilizing the spleen, tail of the pancreas and left hemicolon to the midline (the left kidney is usually left in place but can also be included).

- **Central inframesocolic hematoma** — think infrarenal aorta or inferior vena cava → compress inflow to the aorta by placing your assistant's hand just below the diaphragm to compress the aorta against the vertebra → access with a quick **Cattell and Braasch maneuver** by mobilizing the right hemicolon, going around the cecum and dividing the left lateral edge of the mesenteric peritoneum all the way to the ligament of Treitz, and then lifting the whole bowel package up and exposing the infrarenal parts of the aorta and inferior vena cava, control with clamps (the aorta) or direct compression with small pieces of gauze on a clamp ('sponge on a stick') which works very well with the inferior vena cava.

- **Lateral retroperitoneal hematoma** — think kidney and renal vessels → access by mobilizing the ipsilateral hemicolon and on the right side the duodenum (the Kocher maneuver) → direct control with clamps and manual compression.

- **Hematoma around the iliac vessels or within the hepatoduodenal ligament** (hepatic artery or portal vein) — access through the hematoma but remember the need for proximal control.

- **Hematoma behind the liver** — think retrohepatic inferior vena cava... **if it does not expand, leave it alone and pack it! For God's sake do not open it!** Forget atriocaval shunts; there are more papers published on it than patients surviving the procedure. If the hematoma grows, call your hepatic surgeon friends to help. If they are not available or far away, **AND you have practiced it before**, aim for hepatic vascular isolation by putting a clamp on the inferior vena cava below the liver but above the renal veins (easy), clamp the hepatoduodenal ligament — the Pringle maneuver (easy), and dissect your way around the suprahepatic IVC (very difficult) or go into the pericardium and clamp the vena cava there (quite difficult). Otherwise, practice the 2Ps — pack and pray!

- Once you have temporarily controlled bleeding from major vessels, you have three options: **repair, ligate or insert a temporary vascular shunt**. Sometimes direct suture repair is the best way to treat an arterial injury. A temporary shunt is acceptable if repair is impossible or you are in a hurry. Ligation is a good option to almost all veins if you have no time to repair. I have ligated the infrarenal vena cava and the common iliac vein in desperate situations and got away with it.

After the first round of packing and vascular control, check the physiology and time and decide on the next step. If the patient is cold and acidotic and has received a lot of blood, just check the packs and reinsert them if necessary. If they look good and control the bleeding, don't touch them. **If the patient is fine, you may consider proceeding to definitive repair** (details to follow below).

Bleeding from sources other than major vessels or the liver can be managed with packing although sometimes a quick splenectomy or nephrectomy (check the other kidney!) is a better option. **Remember that removing a badly injured kidney is not cancer surgery**. Just mobilize the kidney along its lateral surface, clamp the vessels and tie the ureter and you're done. (However, a non-expanding perirenal hematoma after blunt trauma is best left alone. Exploring the hematoma usually leads to an unnecessary nephrectomy.) Sometimes **extraperitoneal pelvic packing** is used to control (venous) bleeding from a fractured pelvis, but angioembolization is often needed for arterial bleeding control.

Controlling contamination is your next priority. Multiple holes in the bowel can be stapled or closed with a quick suture. Badly damaged, ischemic segments or segments with closely located multiple holes should be resected, and bowel ends closed with staplers or simply tied with umbilical tape. **Don't do any anastomoses!** Holes in the gallbladder (rare) and urinary bladder (common) can be closed with a continuous single-layer suture. If you see a divided ureter, just tie it and leave the suture ends long (it helps you to find the ureter later). Close the hole in the diaphragm and put a drain near a divided pancreas. If the common bile duct is divided, just insert a proper size tube through the hole ('I-tube') to drain the bile externally. <u>**Remember**</u>**: a pancreatic and common bile duct injury would be the only two indications for leaving a drain after damage control laparotomy.**

After controlling bleeding and contamination, have a quick look around to see that you haven't missed anything, and get the patient rapidly to the ICU which is the best place to correct acidosis, hypothermia and coagulation disorders. Leave the abdomen open! There are proponents of closing the abdomen after damage control in order to increase the tamponade effect. That is simply wrong. It does not help but makes things worse. Closing the abdomen after fluid resuscitation and multiple blood transfusions (visceral edema), and having the packs inside will be a perfect way to induce one of the common complications after trauma laparotomy — **abdominal compartment syndrome**. There are many methods of temporary abdominal closure. More sophisticated ones utilize one or other form of a negative pressure dressing — which by the way was first described (*BJS*, 1986) by one of the co-editors (Moshe). But if you don't have them or are in a hurry, use the good old Bogota bag. It was actually invented by Oswaldo Borraez in Bogota, so the real name is "Bolsa de Borraez". Take a sterile infusion bag or equivalent, cut it into one sheet (avoid sharp edges or cut them away) and suture the bag to the skin with a continuous suture (I use 2-0 Prolene®). Yes, to the skin and not the fascia which gets easily damaged with sutures. It is also good for the subcutaneous fat to be inside and not left outside to dry… this may be especially relevant in the USA where the guys who are shot or injured seem to be fatter and fatter… as the rest of the population ☺.

Definitive repair

When you do a trauma laparotomy in a patient who is physiologically fine and stable, you have the luxury of performing definitive repair to all organ injuries. You just need to find them first. There are many ways to explore the abdomen; use the one that seems logical to you and is easy to remember (you don't want to miss any injuries!). Some organs are easily visualized; others need some dissection to expose completely. Once you encounter an injury, you repair it and then move to the next one. **This is my sequence** (sounds almost like Frank Sinatra…) outlined below.

If you have temporary packs in, remove them carefully starting with the least likely site to bleed, scoop and suck out the blood and **eviscerate the bowel** to check the central inframesocolic retroperitoneum for hematoma, bile or anything else that should not be there, then move around in a systematic way:

- **Start with the right lobe of the liver**, the gallbladder and the left lobe, check both sides of the diaphragm and move to the spleen.
- **Palpate the left kidney** on the way down, look at the left iliac vessel area, the urinary bladder (and female internal genitalia), then the right iliac vessel area.
- **Check the right kidney** and go to the gastroesophageal junction. Inspect the anterior wall of the stomach, the pylorus and the first two parts of the duodenum.
- **Do a Kocher's mobilization** to inspect the posterior duodenum and the head of the pancreas and then move to the ligament of Treitz. If there are any indications of a possible injury to the third part of the duodenum (either in the pre-operative CT scan, or edema, bile stain, air bubbles or blood in the area during exploration), divide the ligament of Treitz and expose the third and fourth parts of the duodenum. You can slide your index fingers along the posterior wall of the third part of the duodenum from both sides and meet in the middle.
- If you feel a hole in the duodenal wall or bile is coming out when you withdraw your fingers, do the Cattell and Braasch maneuver (see above) which gives you an excellent view of the whole third part of the duodenum.

- **Then go through the small bowel and its mesentery** and make sure you see every bit of the bowel wall. Finally, check the cecum and follow the colon all the way to the rectum. Mobilize the ascending or descending colon to expose their posterior parts if in any doubt about possible damage there. Don't hesitate to mobilize the colonic flexures if needed.
- **Finally, open the gastrocolic ligament and inspect the posterior wall of the stomach and the body and tail of the pancreas.** Look for hematomas on the surface of the pancreas and don't think it is a subcapsular hematoma. It usually means that the pancreas is transected, and when you press the hematoma gently with your finger, there is no pancreas underneath! For complete visualization of the pancreas you sometimes must mobilize the tail (with the spleen) and dissect along the inferior pancreatic border.
- **Missing an injury to the main pancreatic duct is easy.** Forget the intra-operative pancreatograms by cannulating the papilla though a duodenotomy or distal pancreatectomy. They never work and create more harm. Visualizing the whole pancreas and having good luck is the best way to find (or exclude) a main pancreatic duct injury!

Going through all repair options and strategies for every organ injury would require almost another book (and there are many around) but here are some of the main points that might keep you out of trouble, organ by organ. The following may duplicate what has been written elsewhere in this book but heck — I want you to know how we, the Finns, do it:

- **If the liver does not bleed, leave it alone!** Small superficial bleeders can be sutured. Use absorbable monofilament with a big enough, non-cutting, needle and tie carefully just enough to stop the bleeding. In deep lacerations and through-and-through injuries, suturing carries a risk of continuous bleeding inside the liver (I have seen a patient dying of liver failure after massive intrahepatic hematoma). Think of other options such as angioembolization (if arterial bleeding) or perihepatic packing. Through-and-through holes can also be managed with internal tamponade through the hole using a Sengstaken-Blakemore tube — it can be self-made from an NG tube and a Penrose drain — filled with saline. Creating a bigger hole by extending the laceration with a finger-fracture technique (or some fancy tool) to gain access to bleeders and then suture them requires some experience in liver resection. **Obvious unviable peripheral pieces of liver should be resected.** Non-anatomical 'debridement' is all you need, anatomical lobectomy virtually never. If there is any sign of bile leak from the raw liver surface, leave a drain. **If you are not familiar with liver surgery, and simple procedures such as suturing or local hemostats do not stop the bleeding, the three most important techniques to know are packing, packing and packing...**

- Suturing small bleeding lacerations of the **spleen** is possible, applying the same principles as for the liver. Partial splenectomy and wrapping the spleen in an absorbable mesh look good in drawings, but in reality they seldom work. **Splenectomy is usually the best option!** After all, the lifelong risk of *overwhelming post-splenectomy infection* (OPSI) is much smaller (remember vaccination and antibiotic prophylaxis information for the patient) than leaving a badly controlled bleeding spleen behind.
- Suturing a lacerated **kidney** stops bleeding from the parenchyma; just remember to close any open intrarenal cavities with fine absorbable sutures first. Bad renal injuries, renovascular injuries and proximal ureteric injuries usually require a **nephrectomy** provided that the other kidney is there and of normal size. Leaving a non-functioning kidney (after renal artery injury) behind might cause problems in the future (hypertension) but of course it can always be removed later. For serious polar injuries, a *heminephrectomy* with a linear stapler is an option. Just remember to take your time when closing the stapler (count to seven) to allow approximation of the capsule to occur without tears. A badly lacerated left renal vein can be ligated as long as you do it proximally (on the caval side) to the gonadal vein junction. You surely know why… (if not then send me an email!).
- The management of **pancreatic** injuries is dictated by the presence or absence of injury to the main pancreatic duct and its location. To determine if the duct is intact, you have to see the whole pancreas (see above for exposure). If in doubt that the duct is severed (major laceration or transection, central perforation, macerated pancreas) treat it as one. **If the pancreatic duct is OK, just drain the peripancreatic area**. If the duct injury is left of the superior mesenteric vein, a distal pancreatectomy and splenectomy is what the patient needs. **In young patients with no other major injuries, you can do a splenic-saving distal pancreatectomy**. It just takes a little more time to dissect the pancreas away from the splenic vessels. However, when the injury to the duct is *proximal*, resection of the pancreas distally to the ductal transection site is associated with a significant risk of diabetes. Thus, under *favorable conditions*, I would do this: complete the transection of the pancreas at the site of injury, close the proximal stump (don't take too deep bites, the common bile duct is near!) and preserve the distal body/tail complex by anastomosing it with a Roux-en-Y loop of jejunum.

However, in most cases of pancreatic injury, the 'Tim Fabian method' is the safest: **"Treat the pancreas like a crayfish, suck the head… eat the tail"** (I hope you enjoy the metaphor) (■ Figure 24.1). In destructive injuries of the head of the pancreas (and duodenum and the papilla), you sometimes might need a **Whipple's procedure**. In

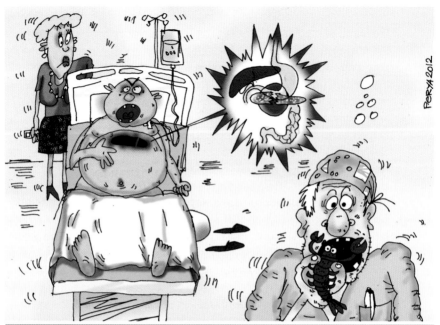

Figure 24.1. "Treat the pancreas like a crayfish, suck the head... eat the tail..."

those kinds of injuries your first priority is controlling the bleeding from nearby vessels. The **(staged) Whipple** is then more of a debridement procedure to take out the badly destroyed pancreatic head and duodenum, and the procedure is part of damage control. You can always (or have the pancreatic guys help you to) do the anastomoses at the second operation.

- **Missing a duodenal injury is asking for trouble**. After 24 hours the duodenal wall that has been soaking in bile resembles wet toilet paper; try to suture that (many tried... ☺) and see what happens. It always leaks. So, get there in time and it is like suturing any other part of the small bowel. I prefer a tension-free (Kocher!) two-layer closure. If you can place it transversely, fine, but diagonal or longitudinal closures are also OK if the injury requires that. Duodenal stenosis happens rarely and can be managed later on endoscopically. Always secure the duodenal closure with *decompression*. I prefer to use a soft *nasogastric* tube with extra side holes placed (before closing the hole) clearly past the injury site all the way to the duodenojejunal angle. A tube duodenostomy through a new hole (Witzel style) or a retrograde tube through a jejunostomy create a new risky hole and I only use them if I have to. For more complex duodenal injuries, the standard for years has been **pyloric exclusion** (closing the pylorus and performing a gastrojejunostomy) but according to recent studies it has few benefits over suture and decompression. If things really get bad (duodenal leak or fistula), I prefer **complete duodenal diverticulization** (antrectomy, vagotomy, Roux-en-Y gastrojejunostomy and biliary diversion with a T-tube), but that is very seldom needed. **All complex duodenal injuries require a feeding-jejunostomy that helps you start enteral feeding while waiting for the duodenal fistula to close.** Finally, ALL duodenal repairs should be drained with periduodenal drains. Why not put the drain in while you are there instead of having to go there again after a few days or rely on some 'Mickey-Mouse' drains inserted percutaneously... (more about the duodenum in ⮑ Chapter 6, section 3).

- A hole in the **stomach** needs suture repair, resection is hardly ever necessary. **In penetrating trauma don't forget always to look at the posterior wall!** The management of **small bowel injuries** is also straightforward: suture the holes or resect and perform an anastomosis. I prefer an old-fashioned end-to-end anastomosis with a two-layer continuous 4-0 absorbable suture, but it's your call. Whatever works best for you is fine. **Again: beware the stapled anastomosis if the bowel is edematous... and usually in severe trauma it will be!**

- **The colon** is another story. Although at least five randomized studies have shown that primary repair is safe in all colon injuries, **there is some evidence to support diversion in patients with multiple severe injuries, significant blood loss, concomitant urinary tract injury, etc., especially if the injury is in the distal transverse colon or splenic flexure where the blood supply is weakest.** Think what you would do if it were your sister, and do the same for your patient. A colostomy is not the end of the world, and having no colostomy gives little comfort if you are in a coffin...

- **Extraperitoneal injuries to the rectum** require proximal diversion. Presacral drainage does not help unless you already have an abscess. Having a look through the anus, suturing a distal hole if you see it, and cleaning the rectum (irrigation) from stool makes the postoperative course a little easier.

- Repairing a severed **ureter** over a stent with interrupted absorbable sutures and closing the **urinary bladder** with two-layer (some use one) absorbable urine-tight sutures is straightforward. I prefer a Foley catheter over cystostomy to 'protect' the repair.

- Even small holes in the **diaphragm** can cause severe problems if left undiagnosed. Most of the lacerations are small enough to be closed with two-layer (or a single one) non-absorbable suture repair. Large defects in the lateral portions can be fixed by dividing the lateral attachments and fixing the edges of the diaphragm higher up in the chest wall. Major central defects require prosthetic repair.

So, now you have repaired all injuries, cleaned the abdomen of blood and bowel content, irrigated it gently making sure you have *sucked out all fluid* (subphrenic spaces!), left drains (duodenum, pancreas, urinary tract, sometimes liver) and are ready to close. **There are some abdomens that you cannot close (leaving them open is a no-brainer) and some you should not close, because of visceral edema**. With modern temporary abdominal closure methods it is not a problem: leave it open! But if everything looks good and you think there is no need for a second look (vascular repair!), go ahead and close the abdomen with your regular technique. Being old-fashioned (and increasing my dinosaur points as my residents tell me) I use large interrupted sutures to close the fascia. I just hate to see the continuous suture cutting through the fascial edge and ruining the whole thing. A small hernia is better that a major wound dehiscence… [The other three Editors agree with the residents' diagnosis — dinosaur!]

Did you notice that I did not mention laparoscopy in this section at all (well once… only concerning diaphragmatic injuries), and there is no mention of robotic surgery either ☺ (■ Figure 24.2).

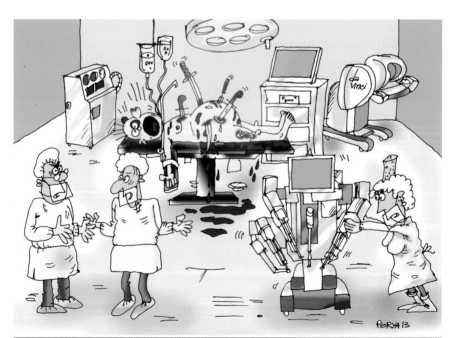

Figure 24.2. Surgeon: "WTF…???" Resident: "Sir, I thought you might try repairing the liver with the robot…"

Postoperative considerations

Your first concern after operating on a trauma patient is an **injury that might have been missed** when the patient was rushed to the OR. **Go to the ICU and do a tertiary survey (see above) as soon as possible but at the latest next morning**. [Moshe tells me that in "the old days", after an "intake" in Baragwanath Hospital, Johannesburg, they used to do the "post-intake rounds" on patients positioned in beds, between the beds and under the beds. Sometimes the 'missed injuries' were found under the beds but not always alive. I hope the situation in your trauma unit is better...] **Review all X-rays and go through the patient from head-to-toe**. A polytrauma patient might have small fractures, tendon injuries or a hemo/pneumothorax that was initially missed. Always worry about a possible head injury or vertebral injury, don't hesitate to do — or repeat if needed — a CT scan or any other investigation. **Remember that time is the best diagnostician: 24 hours after the trauma silent/latent injuries may declare themselves (e.g. blunt intestinal injury)**.

After a damage control laparotomy (when you have talked to the family, dictated the notes, had a cup of coffee, and changed your bloody clothes and underwear...), go to the ICU and talk to the intensivists about what you found and what you did. Check that there is no major bleeding (you left the abdomen open, right?) under the dressing. **If there is, or the intensivist suspects that the patient is still bleeding 'from somewhere', don't hesitate to take the patient back to the OR and repack — but make sure the patient is clotting before attempting repacking**.

Correction of acidosis and rewarming the patient after damage control surgery is crucial and need to be monitored closely (base deficit and lactate helps). Restoring organ perfusion without using too much crystalloid reduces tissue swelling and makes the postoperative course so much smoother and gets the patient ready for the planned reoperation and removal of the packs. **But when is the right time?**

Some trauma surgeons prefer to do the **second operation with definitive repair** as soon as the patient is stable, and the acidosis and hypothermia have been corrected. **But there is a trade-off: if you go there too early you risk rebleeding when removing the packs. Doing it too late might increase the risk of infection**. Trauma surgeons in Cali, Colombia (and they see a lot of trauma), have actually studied this and have come up with the optimal time point that is 48-72 hours. **After hearing about this, I became a 'two-and-a-half-day guy'**. I prefer to do the second operation during the day-time (at least in Finland the worst injuries occur at night-time — and at the weekend — perhaps something to do with our alcohol consumption habits...) and do it myself. But even if the same surgeon performs the second operation, it is important that the number and location of the packs are clearly recorded to make sure that they all come out. Retained sponges or packs are what make the lawyers really happy…

Removing the packs is not a minor operation to be delegated to the most junior surgeon — therefore do it yourself! It takes patience to remove the packs without causing rebleeding. Wet the most superficial pack generously with saline, wait (always have a couple of jokes ready) and remove them one by one, always making the next one wet first. Remove them by rolling gently (like removing a glove), not lifting up rapidly. When the last one on the surface of the liver is due, I use the tip of a large syringe to push it gently while irrigating at the same time. Once the packs are out you do what a man's got to do; do the anastomosis and other repairs, irrigate and close of course — if possible…

Abdominal compartment syndrome (ACS) can occur even with an open abdomen, or an abdomen that was closed at the second operation after damage control (tertiary ACS), but especially after the initial trauma laparotomy when all injuries were repaired and the abdomen was closed. **Intra-abdominal hypertension is like fever, if you don't measure it, you don't see it**. Measuring intra-abdominal pressure through a Foley catheter is easy and should be a routine after all emergency abdominal surgery, and especially in patients who have been in shock and have received a lot of fluids and blood products. **There is no specific value that requires decompression but anything above 20mmHg should make you worry**, especially if there is a concomitant new organ dysfunction that you cannot explain. If the urine output starts to decrease, airway pressure increases and the patient's hemodynamics are not stable (the **abdominal perfusion pressure [APP]**, i.e. mean arterial pressure minus intra-abdominal pressure, should be above 60mmHg), think of ACS! Try conservative measures first if you haven't yet (NG tube, rectal tube, stop enteral feeding, remove intra-abdominal collections by percutaneous drainage), consider removing fluids by hemodialysis, and if not helpful, open the abdomen again and leave it open. If the patient is trying to die on you in the ICU right now, do it at the bedside!

Managing the open abdomen with modern techniques is not a disaster and using the mesh-mediated vacuum-assisted closure technique (unfortunately it was first described by the Swedes but it works… ☺), or some of the other techniques (e.g. the Velcro-based patch described by Dietmar Wittmann), the delayed fascial closure rate approaches 90%. **If you don't get the fascia closed and there is enough skin to mobilize and close over the defect, this is your best option**. If not then wait until a little bit of granulation tissue forms over the bowel loops and put on a skin graft. **The 'planned hernia' will mature in 6-9 months and will then be ready for abdominal wall reconstruction**. If there is enough of the patient's own skin to close it in the midline, we start with the **component separation** (first described by Albanese from Argentina in the 1950s, later refined by Ramirez *et al* in 1990) and use an additional sublay mesh if needed. Very large defects require a friend in the plastic surgery department; our preferred technique is the microvascular (free) tensor fascia lata flap. If the defect is too big for component separation but there is enough original skin to reach closure at the midline, a standard mesh repair (I use the sublay technique) can be used. So far the role of a *bioprosthesis* is unclear but I have used them a few times in contaminated fields or after removing an infected (non-absorbable) mesh. Warn the patient about the high incidence of recurrent hernias or residual bulging that may resemble a recurrence.

Most of the complications after trauma laparotomy are managed in the same way as after other abdominal surgery. Postoperative bleeding may require interventional radiology (angioembolization) or reoperative surgery to arrest the bleeding. Anastomotic leaks are managed as after non-trauma surgery (see ⬭ Chapter 6). Postoperative abscesses, if clinically significant, are managed with percutaneous or surgical drainage. Bile collections need to be drained as well; sometimes ERCP will identify the leak site (usually in the liver after hepatic laceration) and it can be managed with a biliary stent. Persistent pancreatic fistulas after missed lacerations, with at least a partly intact main pancreatic duct (side-fistula), are best treated with endoscopic stenting, and this is the first-line treatment also of end-fistulas after distal pancreatectomy. However, if there is a complete transection of the pancreas that has been missed initially, the fistula might not close spontaneously unless the tail is removed. But patience is golden, since some of them heal spontaneously. Duodenal leaks require drainage, enteral feeding and patience (see above).

Non-abdominal complications, such as acute myocardial infarction, pulmonary embolism, etc., obviously can occur after trauma as well (⬭ Chapter 13). **Thrombosis prophylaxis should not be omitted for trauma patients and is very rarely the cause of recurrent bleeding** (although it is easy to blame it for bad surgical hemostasis). A retrievable vena cava filter is used in some trauma centers for the prevention of pulmonary embolism in the high-risk trauma patient who cannot receive anticoagulation.

Polytrauma patients used to get **ARDS** or TRALI (transfusion-related acute lung injury) especially after major resuscitation and/or pulmonary contusion. For some reason the incidence of ARDS has dropped dramatically, probably because of less aggressive fluid management, better ventilatory techniques and prevention of abdominal compartment syndrome. Retained hemothorax after thoracic trauma or thoracotomy needs to be evacuated early; empyema is a failure.

A negative laparotomy for trauma carries about a 20% complication risk, mostly pulmonary and wound complications. **But trauma is a surgical disease, so don't feel sorry if you operated as long as you had a good reason for doing so. Nobody gets it right every time!**

Ach, it has been a long lecture, I need a drink. All the rest you will find elsewhere in the book, for trauma is general surgery and trauma surgeons have to be the best general surgeons.

> **Doing trauma surgery with minimal complications is like smoking a fish. Make sure you have the equipment you need, be mentally ready, know the fish qualities, anticipate the unexpected... and watch the fire carefully. Interfere when the time is right, and do the right thing. And don't forget to reward yourself with a glass of chablis, if successful. They go together nicely... as does the post-fishing sauna (■ Figure 24.3).**

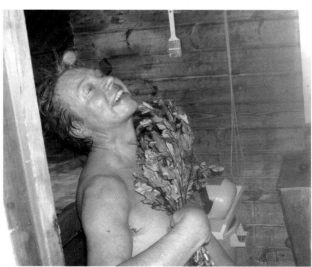

Figure 24.3. The Finnish surgeon's daily routine.

Chapter 25

Pediatric surgery

Graeme Pitcher

If an operation is difficult you are not doing it properly.
Robert E. Gross

Most pediatric surgeons will tell you the following about their patients: they have interesting and varied pathology; they are usually in the prime of their lives without the degenerative comorbidities of old age; you make a difference that will allow your patient's life expectancy to exceed your own; and they can easily be single-handedly picked up and put on the operating table where exposure is much easier and where you find pristine tissue planes. All of that is true. Surely we should rarely see complications in such patients!

The reality is that pediatric surgical patients often have multiple congenital abnormalities, are frequently on systemic immunosuppressive medications that complicate their wound healing and thus can be significant surgical challenges. Surgeons have to understand the anatomy, physiology and natural history of the often rare conditions in order not to fall into a multitude of pitfalls. This is particularly true for neonatal surgery. Very few general surgeons fully understand neonatal surgical conditions and even fewer have the experience necessary to operate safely on newborn babies. **Unless you have been specifically trained to operate on newborns, send the patient to a pediatric surgeon, no matter how far away.**

Parents also rightfully expect their otherwise healthy child to undergo a surgical procedure without any complications... so the pressure is on the surgeon! However, as in any type of surgery, complications will occur when operating on children and these are not always preventable. How the surgeon handles the communication around the complication is critically important. **The triangulated doctor-child-parent relationship is one of the challenges of pediatric practice**. A complication or setback at any stage of care must be communicated to the parents (and the child, if they can understand) in an honest and transparent manner as soon as all the facts are known. It is also important to provide parents with a very clearly communicated prediction of the expected course the patient may follow and what long- and short-term implications of the complication may be. **In my experience it is usually not the complication itself which gets the surgeon into deep water but the failure to address it promptly, and communicate honestly with the parents**.

Pre-operative considerations

Many complications can be prevented by proper planning. Make sure that your patient is correctly marked and consented. **Wrong side or site** surgery is particularly common with inguinal hernia repairs. It is easy to forget the details of a patient you might have seen some weeks before. Check your notes and examine the patient when asleep on the OR table to confirm the findings that you are operating for. Look for the subtle thickening of the cord that confirms that a hernia is on the side you think it is on! **Always examine anyone who has an emergency abdominal operation after they are anesthetized and before your prep the skin** — you will be surprised at how often you find something which changes your approach!

Anesthetic complications

Despite advances in the field of pediatric anesthesia and its development as a subspecialty, one has to recognize that in certain circumstances, the surgeon's role is relatively simple and that the greatest risk for serious morbidity lies with the anesthetic. This is certainly true in newborns, for whom the risk of anesthesia still remains greater than for older individuals. Serious anesthetic complications usually reflect poorly upon the surgeon too. With this in mind these are my thoughts for avoiding anesthetic morbidity:

- **Avoid any procedure under general anesthetic in the newborn period that can wait for later in life**. Non-life-threatening cysts, lumps, bumps and hamartomas should not be operated upon at this time. Circumcisions must be done only under local anesthetic in newborns (that is, if and when a Rabbi is not available ☺).
- Ensure that the **anesthetic colleague** allocated for the operation that you are contemplating has the necessary training and experience.

Children with congenital cardiac abnormalities, for instance, are a particular challenge. Don't embark upon any surgery on a child with cyanotic heart disease or single-ventricle physiology without a pediatric or cardiac anesthetist who is intimately familiar with such patients.

- **Don't do any operation in the middle of the night if it can safely wait until the next morning** [true in adults as well! — Editors]. This applies especially to appendectomies. Consider the patient with appendicitis in the ER at 2 a.m.: if the appendicitis appears to be 'uncomplicated', surgery can be done more safely with a fresh team at 7 or 8 a.m. If perforated and sick (having been lying at home for five days), the patient will benefit from administration of i.v. antibiotics and a few hours of fluid resuscitation and an operation in the morning. Besides, surgeons are arguably human too and we need our sleep.

- You may need to operate for some **'urgent' emergencies** which truly should not wait (■ Table 25.1).

- **Communicate well with the anesthetist**. Reach across the screen between you and the anesthetist which sometimes functions like the blood-brain barrier (and we all know which side the blood is on…). Keep an eye and ear on the monitors. If you are losing blood, make sure that your colleagues across the drapes know how much and why, and how much longer you expect it to continue.

Table 25.1. Conditions requiring urgent operation.

Condition	Comments
Testicular torsion	Simple operation — testicle saved by avoidance of delays
Unstable patient with internal bleeding	Never place such a patient in an ambulance or CT scanner
Compartment syndrome in a limb or abdomen	Decompression can save limb or life
Strangulated inguinal hernia	Incarcerated hernias can usually be reduced but if there are skin changes and intestinal obstruction suspect strangulation
Malrotation, volvulus	The acidotic sick infant must receive emergency surgery

Intra-operative considerations

Here are a few key points:

- **Hypothermia** is a common problem, especially when operating on small pre-term babies. Keep a warm OR, wrap babies and use a warming blanket such as a Bair Hugger®.
- **Children are smaller than adults** (no prizes here). To see properly you need magnification (even if your eyes are young and strong). 2.5x loupes are ideal for general use. Most pros use a set of 3.5x as well. Use them for **every** case!
- For the same reason a **headlight** is mandatory whenever you are doing an open procedure in a body cavity.
- **Laparoscopy in small children is very different to adults**. Don't do it unless you have been trained specifically — see below.
- **Operating room safety in a non-children's hospital**:
  - **make sure that i.v. access is secure** (to your satisfaction) prior to starting a case. A blood transfusion onto the drapes carries a

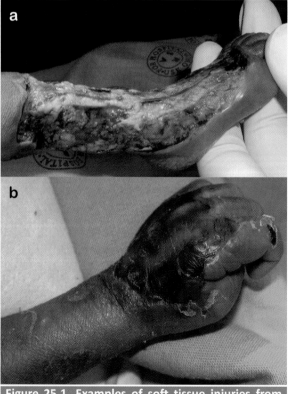

Figure 25.1. Examples of soft tissue injuries from extravasated i.v. lines in small children.

particularly poor prognosis and extravasation into the foot or hand of a small child can cause a nasty injury (■ Figure 25.1);

■ **electocautery pads**. Make sure the pad is big enough for the size of the child and that it stays as dry as possible (■ Figure 25.2);

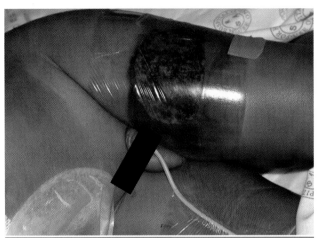

Figure 25.2. Burn caused by an electrocautery pad using a neonatal sized pad on a larger child, concentrating the current.

■ **skin prep** (particularly alcohol-based solutions) can injure the thin and vulnerable skin of the newborn (■ Figure 25.3);

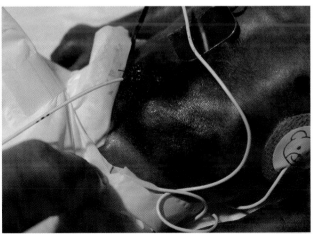

Figure 25.3. Skin burn caused by using alcohol to prepare skin for insertion of an umbilical catheter.

- use specially designed pediatric **oximetry probes** only (■ Figure 25.4);

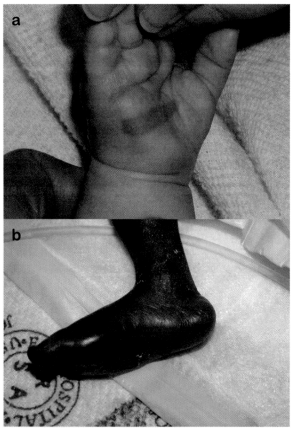

Figure 25.4. Partial pressure necrosis from the application of an adult oximeter probe transversely across: a) a child's hand; and b) foot.

- **don't use monopolar electrocautery on the penis during circumcision**. The current is conducted through a narrow structure and can cause necrosis and even loss of the entire organ! (The image I have could be too shocking for you…)
- **Children waking up after anesthesia** are typically afraid and sometimes uncooperative. Dressings, drains and tubes are at peril in this phase and need to be securely fixed to prevent the need for reinsertion and the parental, pediatric and institutional anxiety that is associated with it.
- **Keep the child anesthetized until dressings are secure and all tubes are secure**. Communicate with the anesthetist. The simpler the

dressing the better! Cyanoacrylate glue serves the dual role of a skin closure adjunct and dressing, and can't be ripped off. **For example**: when completing the simple operation of circumcision, the diaper should be in place before the patient awakes to avoid a frantic grasp for the pristine, newly operated and perfectly hemostatic organ — resulting in the need for a second anesthetic on the same day and suture replacement.

- The use of **locoregional anesthesia** techniques and good postoperative pain management go a long way to allowing safe and comfortable emergence from anesthesia.
- **Children's BMIs are rising**; in the US we accept this more readily than climate change, bringing with it challenges for surgeons:
  - pay particular attention to **positioning these large children and adolescents on the OR** table to avoid pressure complications, especially during long operations in the lithotomy position;
  - **thromboembolic complications are more common**. In obese, high-risk adolescents, consider the need for mechanical devices and heparin prophylaxis.

Postoperative considerations

Keep in mind:

- If you think a postoperative **ICU** bed may be necessary, it usually is!
- **Transporting sick babies to the NICU or PICU is dangerous**. Patients can extubate, important drains can be pulled out, infusion pumps and IVs can malfunction and so forth. Do everything to make sure that the trip is undertaken safely. An experienced nurse or respiratory therapist transport team prevents many problems. Always accompany your patient back to the unit.
- **Vomiting and aspiration is a common and potentially life-threatening complication**, especially in newborns and young infants who cannot protect their airways. Make sure that NG tubes are in the correct position and working well when needed.
- **NG tubes should be secured carefully** to avoid pressure on the nares, otherwise skin necrosis with longstanding cosmetic implications can occur.
- Ensure that **postoperative orders** are as simple and concise as possible:
  - **avoid overdoses due to miscalculated dosages** — decimal points are notoriously misplaced;
  - make sure **enteral medications** are clearly ordered and given that way.

- **Be cautious and circumspect with potassium replacement in children**. Most children tolerate mild hypokalemia without any problems and replacement can be dangerous (soft tissue injury at drip sites and iatrogenic hyperkalemia being the worst complications).

Complications specific to certain operations

The spectrum of complications in pediatric surgical patients is listed in ■ Table 25.2. A few of those listed in the Table are outlined below.

Table 25.2. Common complications in pediatric surgery.

Complication	Comments
Anesthetic complications	In babies, always consider if the surgery is worth the risk?
Laparoscopy	Entry injuries and port-site hernias
Plumbing dysfunction, displacement, dissatisfaction and dysphoria	Central venous catheters, infuso-ports, dialysis catheters (peritoneal and vascular) are all lifelines!
Superficial wound infection	Contaminated cases
Gastrostomy complications	Leaks, device displacement
Pyloromyotomy problems	Inadequate myotomy and mucosal breach
Nissen fundoplication faults	Early herniation, twisted Nissen
Incisional hernia	Big bites on little sheaths can prevent these
Common hernia pitfalls	Missed epigastric hernia, recurrence

The problems of laparoscopy in children

The complications seen are similar to those seen in adults (⊃ Chapter 9). The most feared is entry injury with visceral or great vessel damage. **This probably occurs more commonly than we think as it is rarely reported.** I have, for example, seen an aortic injury from an unrecognized entry injury in a boy undergoing laparoscopic appendectomy elsewhere — yes, it always happens elsewhere — which resulted in advanced ischemia of the lower limbs. For many operations the benefits of laparoscopy have not been clearly defined. **Often a small incision is much safer, particularly if you are less experienced.** Compared to adults (and the size of ports), body cavities are much smaller in babies and children. This makes port placement (especially initial) sometimes difficult and always potentially dangerous. Using a Hasson approach is by far the safest.

Babies tolerate high intra-abdominal gas pressure poorly. Use the lowest pressure (8mmHg or less) that allows exposure. Low flow rates also provide a margin of safety to prevent accidental over-inflation. Be very vigilant of this and decompress the abdomen if in any doubt. Babies with single-ventricle physiology rely on preload for cardiac filling. Avoid laparoscopy for these patients.

Ports have to be perfectly positioned just inside the abdomen and secured to the skin or fascia for longer operations. **In many cases you can avoid ports altogether** and place instruments directly into the abdomen via tiny stab incisions with a number 11 blade. This is safer and avoids a lot of frustration.

Port-site hernias occur more frequently than in adults. Hernias can develop even in 5mm port sites in small children if the fascia is not closed. This is particularly true close to the linea alba where the muscle is thinnest. **Place ports as laterally as possible so that they may have the greatest chance of healing without defects.** When using stab incisions without ports, ensure that the instruments are removed without pulling omentum into the wound.

Central venous catheter (plumbing) problems

I think that it is fair to say that no surgeon *enjoys* placing a catheter in a kid! We secretly see them as the worst manifestation of our role as technical service providers to the physicians who use them — but may not always understand them. The cost and morbidity of return trips to the OR for these usually sick children is considerable. The best attitude to the problem is to acknowledge how important these 'life-lines' for the patient are and to ensure accurate placement and function and avoid complications at all costs. Despite this they are the commonest cause for (usually petty) misery in pediatric surgical practice by far!

The commonest complications are:

- Incorrect catheter position:
  - too deep (can cause intermittent arrhythmias);
  - too shallow (can result in catheter flipping into brachiocephalic veins);
  - wrong catheter placed. Check with an oncologist or a referring doctor personally — don't rely on hearsay! — on which catheter to use: double vs. single lumen? Port-a-Cath® vs. Broviac®? Power port (for high-pressure injection for patients needing CT scanning)?
- Catheter kinked in tunneled track.
- Infant anticoagulated by using too much heparin flush.

My tips for avoiding problems after a career in causing them are:

- Always meet the parents pre-operatively and explain the details of the procedure and the accurate risks and benefits personally. Include all the plumbing problems in your description so that they do not come as a surprise.
- Pay extraordinary attention to every small detail of the procedure personally — don't leave it to trainees.
- Make sure you place the correct catheter type and diameter of catheter.
- Ensure platelet counts are adequate for the procedure (typically greater than 50,000) and transfuse if not.
- Avoid mechanical woes: check catheters for leaks, assemble Port-a-Cath® connections yourself, and ensure no kinks.
- Fix the catheter securely to the skin with a well-placed 'Roman sandal' -type stitch. Exiting catheters are best dressed with a pigtail type coil under an occlusive dressing so that traction on the catheter does not dislodge it.
- Never omit good fluoroscopy to check position.
- Always check function intra-operatively and flush with heparin. Do not inadvertently anticoagulate a small child with a flush. Consider using 10 units heparin/ml in small children instead of the usual 100U/ml to avoid this complication.
- Most importantly — when you have a problem, address it without quibbling. If the darned thing is not working adequately there is no alternative!

Pyloromyotomy

Babies with pyloric stenosis (and everyone in the hospital) seem to be getting younger and younger! The laparoscopic approach has also become increasingly popular. This remains a stressful operation (especially for the occasional operator) for the simple reason that patients are usually normal, otherwise healthy infants in whom we can reasonably expect a 'perfect' result. Despite this high expectation, complications still occur. These fall into three categories:

- Intra-operative complications — mucosal perforation or bleeding.
- Inadequate pyloromyotomy.
- Wound complications.

The operation can be done open or laparoscopically. Do it the way you are most familiar with — this is usually the safest. Laparoscopy affords great 'wound benefits' for these infants: cosmetic superiority, lower rates of infection and dehiscence, equivalent rates of intra-operative complications, quick recovery times and great parent satisfaction. **The only caveat is a higher rate of incomplete pyloromyotomy in some studies**.

If your patient has been vomiting for three weeks without the parents or a doctor thinking of the diagnosis (■ Figure 25.5) (yes this still happens all over the world!), make sure that the baby is well resuscitated and supported nutritionally before you operate. Peri-operative TPN is sometimes even needed

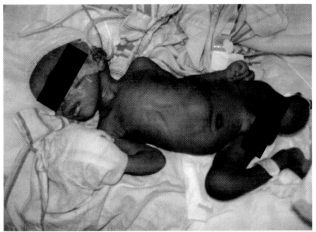

Figure 25.5. A dehydrated, severely malnourished child with delayed diagnosis of hypertrophic pyloric stenosis. Note the visible gastric peristalsis.

in these neglected cases and look out for *re-feeding syndrome* seen in severely starved patients who are suddenly fed again and exhibit hypophosphatemia, hypomagnesemia and sometimes even coma and cardiac failure.

Avoidance of complications

Only do a **laparoscopic pyloromyotomy** if you are very familiar with laparoscopy in babies. The open technique gives good reproducible results. Port insertion is probably the most hazardous part of the operation. Damage to the liver, although not well described in the literature (surprise!), does occur.

Usually the umbilicus can be dilated bluntly to accommodate the (3mm) camera port, which is then placed carefully within the peritoneal cavity. Subsequently, instruments are inserted under vision, *typically without ports*. Avoid placing these stab incisions too close to the midline or incisional hernias are possible in this thinner part of the abdominal wall. To avoid inadequate pyloromyotomy, the boundaries of the pylorus need to be well established by visualization as well as by palpation with the tips of the instruments. Start the pyloromyotomy in the middle of the thickened pylorus and work proximally and distally, taking care not to extend it too far distally where the risk of mucosal injury is higher. **I believe that it is easy to do insufficient dissection proximally and therefore I go to great pains to ensure that the myotomy extends well onto the gastric wall**. After completion, one must ensure that the two muscle halves easily move independently when grasped with blunt graspers and moved cranio-caudally on each other. Mucosal injury is best avoided by understanding the function of the knife or electrocautery tip you are using and proceeding slowly. The last stage of blunt spreading usually disrupts any residual fibers safely without risking the mucosa. **Inflating the stomach with air is useful to detect any mucosal injury**. The umbilicus is closed with a simple suture technique and the skin is closed with glue alone.

Management of complications

If you breach the mucosa don't panic! There are two choices:

- Close the breach directly with 6.0 PDS® fine sutures. Check that it is airtight with an air insufflation test. Or...
- Close the mucosa and muscle, rotate the pylorus through 90° and do a new myotomy at a new site. This time don't perforate!
- Both of these options can be done laparoscopically or after converting to an open procedure depending on skill and comfort level.

Bleeding from the cut muscle edges is usually of no consequence and will stop by itself. A touch of the cautery on a bleeding superficial vein is usually enough if you are obsessive.

Incomplete myotomy results in continued vomiting past 24 hours postoperatively. It is difficult to confirm the diagnosis with a test. Ultrasound does not help (the muscle is still hypertrophied) and a contrast study typically shows partial emptying. The decision to reoperate is clinical and usually happens after the baby continues vomiting for two or three more days in hospital, depending on the surgeon and parent's patience!

Unrecognized mucosal perforation is very unusual. The baby will look sick, tachycardic, febrile sometimes and vomit postoperatively. You can confirm it with a water-soluble upper GI study. This complication is best treated by reoperation, washout and closure as described above. Obviously, such leaks if missed or recognized late can be lethal!

Nissen fundoplication

The commonest clinical problem is incorrect patient selection. This is an operation, which works well for well-selected patients who are also well counseled and have realistic expectations. Cynics will add (do you know any solid surgeon who is not at least a little cynical?) that the patients with the best results are those with normal esophagi who didn't need the operation at all! Essentially, fundoplication should be used for four main groups of indications:

- Infants with **complications** of persistent reflux **despite maximal medical treatment**:
  - stricture;
  - aspiration, near SIDS (sudden infant death) attacks;
  - failure to thrive due to inadequate oral intake.
- Children with anatomic abnormalities such as hiatal hernias.
- Neurologically impaired G-tube-dependent patients with complicated reflux not responding to medical and feeding management manipulation.
- Older children and adolescents with symptomatic reflux where surgery is offered based on symptoms and treatment tolerance or failed medical therapy.

The Nissen fundoplication has become the gold standard anti-reflux operation for children. In some situations, incomplete wraps are preferable but these are few and far between. In short, don't do anti-reflux surgery if there is any alternative way of treating the child. If you are going to do it — do it well!

The commonest technical problems seen early after the Nissen procedure are incorrect wrap construction and wrap dislodgement and

the development of a para-esophageal hernia. The presentation will depend on the age of the child. Young infants will typically show feeding problems and retching as the only symptoms of wrap failure. If a young child was doing well after wrap and suddenly starts to have problems, get a contrast swallow (■ Figure 25.6). Incorrect construction includes: the wrap being too tight, an inadequate wrap with persistent reflux (rare), construction of the wrap around the stomach instead of the esophagus, and the creation of the 'twisted Nissen' (■ Figure 26.7).

The tricks I suggest to get the best possible Nissen fundoplication in a child are:

- Calibrate the diaphragmatic hiatus as well as the wrap to an appropriate caliber for the child's age: 22F for babies 2-4kg, 60F for adult-sized adolescents and discretion used for the sizes in between.
- The wrap should be no greater than 2-3cm in length and be constructed in a floppy fashion, i.e. without circumferential tension on the gastric fundus.
- Mobilization of the greater curvature by ligation of the short gastric vessels appears to minimize the risk of performing the wrap under tension; in particular, it prevents the rare complication of a twisted Nissen where the fundus (especially a portion low down on the greater curvature) is drawn across under tension and causes obstructive swallowing symptoms. The most extreme form of this causes a two-compartment stomach.
- When planning a Nissen fundoplication for the neurologically-impaired child — who should make up the majority of patients if you are doing the operation for the right reasons — you should give consideration to the need for a gastrostomy tube.
- Reoperative surgery can be challenging. Unless you are a very skilled laparoscopist, open redo Nissens are probably safer.

Gastrostomy tube complications

Common complications in pediatric surgery are the variety of mishaps (miseries) caused when you place a gastrostomy tube. The **PEG** (percutaneous endoscopic gastrostomy) approach has unfortunately made referring physicians feel that placing a G-tube is no longer a real operation and therefore safe. Nothing could be further from the truth. **PEGs have a higher complication rate than open placed G-tubes in small children**. The incidence of complications from injury to the colon and liver is much greater than with open operation. The child who recently was given a PEG tube who shortly after beginning feeds has immediate watery diarrhea and passage of feed in the stool has a **gastrocolic**

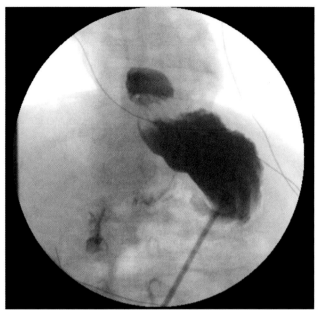

Figure 25.6. Paraesophageal herniation after a previous Nissen fundoplication.

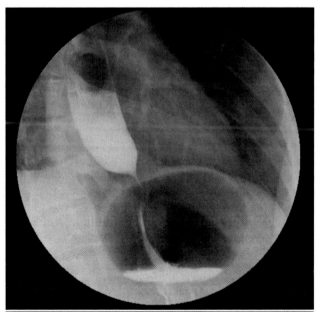

Figure 25.7. Creation of a two-compartment stomach or 'twisted Nissen'.

fistula. This needs to be repaired with open surgery (■ Figure 25.8). **The smaller the baby the higher the complication rate will be from PEG tubes — strongly consider doing a safe 'old-fashioned' operation**.

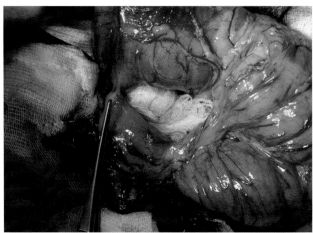

Figure 25.8. Fistula between the stomach and left transverse colon caused by transcolonic placement of a PEG tube.

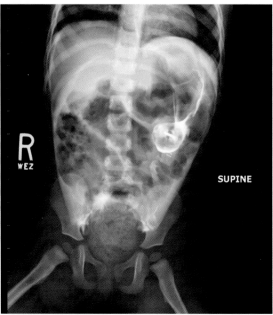

Figure 25.9. Intraperitoneal leak after insertion of a G-tube demonstrated by a water-soluble contrast study through the tube.

No matter how the tube is placed it can leak intraperitoneally and from the skin surface and in the worst case can cause a **necrotizing soft tissue infection**. They can block and stop functioning and can migrate up and out of their tracts. With growth they can ride up on the costal margin and need revision. Secure them well to avoid the child pulling them out postoperatively. If they leak intraperitoneally (■ Figure 25.9), stop feeds, re-explore, wash out and secure the leak efficiently (usually the tube can be preserved and reinserted). If they become displaced you can often reinsert them with an endoscopic approach using a PEG set and avoid reoperation. (See also ⊃ Chapter 6, section 3.)

Intussusception

In developed countries intussusception is a low-risk condition, easily identified by ultrasound and treated by air or hydrostatic reduction in the radiology suite in most cases. In many first-world hospitals such patients may not even see a surgeon during their treatment (a fact that makes me dysphoric and my mast cells degranulate...). In the developing world intussusception remains a high-risk condition that is diagnosed late, causes infants to be very ill and is usually treated by the surgeon with a significant proportion of babies needing resection of ischemic bowel. Complications related to air or hydrostatic reduction can occur in either setting. The most dangerous is without doubt perforation. **Candidates for air reduction must meet *all* of the following criteria**:

- Must be fully resuscitated, warm with a functioning i.v. line.
- Accompanied to the IR suite by a surgeon or member of the surgical team.
- Under the age of three years (older kids have a higher chance of lead point intussusception caused by pathology such as Meckel's diverticulum, polyp or tumor).
- No acute peritonitis.

If a pneumoperitoneum occurs during reduction — this is easily seen by extraluminal tracking of air on fluoroscopy, but to detect this the radiologist needs to screen frequently at times when high pressures are used — gas insufflation must be immediately stopped. If the baby is compromised then the abdomen should be decompressed with a large-bore cannula. **When things go wrong, they go rapidly and horribly wrong. Someone who can intubate and resuscitate an infant (not just your friendly radiologist ☺) needs to be there just in case!**

Incomplete reduction can occur. If the intussusception cannot be reduced (with certainty), then emergency operation is appropriate. Often the reduction goes smoothly but the radiologist is not convinced that the very last stage of reduction is complete. Don't be in a hurry to operate on babies under those conditions. If you do you will open many abdomens to find complete reduction. Rather wait 8-12 hours, evaluate the child's clinical progress and repeat the ultrasound. This will often save an unnecessary laparotomy.

Inguinal hernia and groin surgery

Open inguinal hernia repair remains the gold standard. Making a simple, safe extraperitoneal groin operation a difficult laparoscopic one, that requires deep anesthesia and muscle relaxation in a small child, makes no intuitive sense, and the data for laparoscopic repairs seem to support this. Keeping the anesthetic safe and simple reduces the risk for anesthesia complications, which are the most significant bad outcome for hernia operations in young children. Overall recurrence rates should be of the order of 1-2%. There is no substitute for experience in reducing the recurrence rates of infant hernia repairs. The operation can be quite demanding in a small baby with a large thin-walled sac.

Unilateral versus bilateral repair?

One of the commonest complications of infant hernia repairs is the development of a contralateral hernia after successful hernia repair. **In term, otherwise healthy babies or older children, this is expected to occur in about 5% of patients**. Ex-premature babies, those with excessive fluid in the peritoneal cavity such as children with ventriculo-peritoneal shunts or cirrhosis, or children with a discernable abnormality of the opposite side (e.g. cord thickening or large hydrocele) should receive bilateral repairs — especially if the baby has comorbidity which results in a higher anesthesia risk. Subjecting such babies to the risk of repeat anesthesia within weeks or months of the original operation is certainly not desirable. **Term babies, healthy older children and children with a normal contralateral examination can be treated with unilateral operations**. The role of laparoscopic evaluation of the contralateral hernia ring is controversial. I reserve it for older children whose parents do not want to take the risk of contralateral recurrence. Performing laparoscopy at the time of hernia repair on small fragile preterm babies requires deep general anesthesia with muscle relaxation and results in a greater anesthetic risk. Here, bilateral repair is much safer. Whatever your strategy, make sure the risk of recurrence is well communicated to the parents and they are satisfied with the approach you are taking.

Tips to avoid complications are:

- Make sure you are operating on the correct side. I follow the usual pre-operative marking recommendations but, in addition, always examine the patient on the table prior to making the incision and make sure the exam findings match the side operated on. Better safe than sorry!
- Make sure you use magnification. Even with young eyes the operation is much easier when you can see the structures well!
- Place your incision in a skin crease over the mid-inguinal point. This gives you good access to the deep ring where the important part of the operation is done.
- In babies with large sacs it is easier to deliberately open the sac than to try and keep it intact. You usually end up opening it anyway and the dissection is easier if you can reduce the content and do it all under direct vision.
- Define the sac edges clearly. Suture-ligate the sac securely.
- **If you can't find the sac, don't dig**. Breaching the fascia transversalis and injuring the bladder is by no means rare!
- Always open the sac of a girl to be sure that you do not do an inadvertent tubal ligation.
- When operating for hydrocele, make sure that you empty the scrotal sac by widely fenestrating it. Don't rely upon these emptying through the divided *processus vaginalis* or you will be aspirating them postoperatively in the clinic on unhappy boys, watched by even unhappier parents.

Umbilical and epigastric hernia repair

Umbilical hernias should be repaired if they have not closed spontaneously before school-going age. Complications are recurrence, which is rare (just close them soundly with good technique and it should not happen), wound hematomas (I use an adhesive plastic dressing compressing a small sponge to avoid this, although it is probably treating my own anxiety more than the patient) and infection, which can usually be easily managed. Warn parents that the belly button will not look like a perfect 'inny belly button' immediately postop. The swelling needs to subside for a few months!

An **epigastric hernia** is typically a tiny midline or slightly eccentric defect in the linea alba. It usually contains only a small nubbin of preperitoneal fat. These hernias are congenital defects and do not close spontaneously — they need to be fixed at some point. Closure requires identification of the defect and placement of a few absorbable sutures. Recurrence is most unusual. The only challenge or pitfall is accurate identification of the defect. **Make sure that the exact position of the hernia is marked when the patient is awake**. The hernia may be difficult or impossible to identify in an anesthetized child.

Make sure again that you are repairing the correct site. I have seen babies get their umbilicus closed unnecessarily when they actually had an epigastric hernia!

Incisional hernia

This can occur after any incursion into the peritoneal cavity. We now accept that in children all of these are technical complications and are almost always avoidable. The factors causing them in children are the same as in adults.

Some child-specific avoidance tips are:

- Occasional children's surgeons are prone to placing sutures too shallow in smaller children. This will fail. Small kids still need deep fascial bites! Like adults.
- In small babies, layered closure can result in shallow bites. Sometimes single-layer mass closure gives better results.
- Close the fascia with an appropriate suture gauge for the age of the child:
  - 4.0 for newborns;
  - 3.0 for infants;
  - 2.0 for age 1 to 3 years or 20kg;
  - 0 for older kids;
  - 1 for teenagers and older.
- Absorbable material such as PDS® or Vicryl® is preferred. If using PDS® in small children with thin skin, make sure the knot is well buried or else it will cause a bump that will bother (at least) the parent. It may even ulcerate the thin overlying skin.

Some years ago, shortly after the birth of our discipline, pediatric surgeons were known to have referred to themselves vainly as "the indomitable, attempting the impossible". I wonder whether this was used to justify the uncomfortable reality of frequent complications? The fact that we are now just another division of surgery providing routine clinical care is surely a sign of the incredible progress made in the last 50 years. Maybe in time we will cure the vanity too!

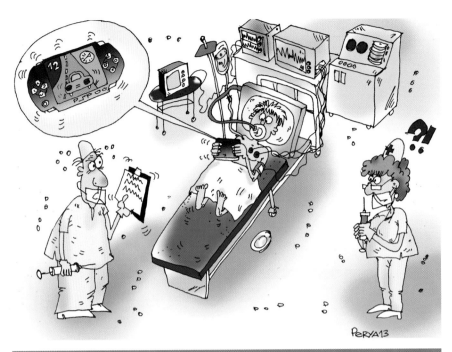

Figure 25.10.

I have never seen an anesthetized child playing Nintendo (■ Figure 25.10), but let us try and make the ordeal of operation for him as uneventful as possible so he can play with his toys on the way to the OR and as soon as possible after waking up from anesthesia!

And remember: children are not small adults!

Chapter 26

Urology

Zohar A. Dotan

You recognize a surgeon or an OB-Gyn because he has blood on his shoes, a urologist because he has urine on his, and an anesthetist because on his you see spots of spilled coffee.

Bernard Cristalli

General surgeons like to complain (or boast) that they "swim in s**t" every day. We urologists are luckier, for we have to swim only in urine! In this chapter I will discuss urological complications which are typically encountered — or created — by the general surgeon. I will try to teach you how to avoid s**t while swimming in urine ☺!

I do not recall a single month during my years of urology practice when I did not have to deal with a urological problem encountered by general surgeons. The insults made or encountered by accidental visitors to the urinary tract are generally produced by **two mechanisms: obstruction to the flow of urine or leakage of urine**. Urology is the art of mending pipes and fixing leaks, and those are the skills you need to deal with these problems (■ Figure 26.1).

Pre-operative considerations

Renal failure

Renal failure is defined as a glomerular filtration rate (GFR) of less than 60ml/minute. It is a relatively common condition that can affect up to 10% of the general population, **most of whom have mild to moderate renal failure**

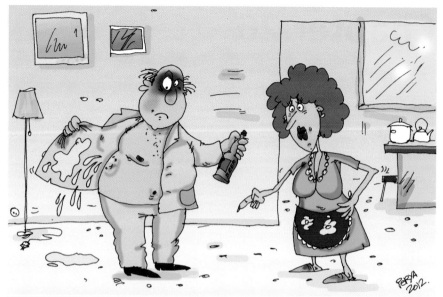

Figure 26.1. Patient urinating through a hole in his loin. Wife: "Did you spill beer on your pyjamas?"

that is asymptomatic. The diagnosis relies on laboratory results, mainly the serum creatinine (SCR) level. The relationship between SCR and GFR is not straightforward. Small changes in the SCR level may accompany large changes in GFR in mild renal failure. **Therefore, mild changes in the SCR level should be considered seriously during the postoperative course.** As a rule of thumb, renal failure should be suspected when the SCR level is 1.4mg/dL (124μmol/L) and above in males and 1.2mg/dL (106μmol/L) and above in females.

Medical students know that renal failure can be classified as pre-renal (the most common), renal and post-renal:

- **Pre-renal failure**: in the surgical patient this implies poor renal blood flow caused by shock or dehydration. Note that the **BUN/plasma creatinine ratio** (normally at 10-15:1) tends to be elevated (>20:1) in pre-renal failure.
- **Renal failure**: this means that the renal parenchyma is diseased, either chronically (diabetes, hypertension) or acutely due to acute tubular necrosis following profound shock for example.
- **Post-renal failure**: this implies chronic obstruction to the outflow of the urinary bladder (or rarely both ureters). **This interests the urologist.**

In cases where renal failure is newly diagnosed or suffers deterioration, post-renal causes should be ruled out by **urinary ultrasound**, including assessment of the post-voiding residual volume of the bladder. A volume of less than 150cc rules out the presence of *infravesical* (from the level of the bladder neck to the distal urethra) causes of renal failure in most cases (in rare circumstances, a small-capacity bladder can cause hydroureteronephrosis with a small residual volume). **The presence of hydronephrosis or hydroureteronephrosis is always abnormal and a urologist should be consulted**.

Hydronephrosis or hydroureteronephrosis

Hydronephrosis (HN) is defined as dilatation of the pelvis and calyces, and hydroureteronephrosis (HUN) as dilatation of the ureter, renal pelvis and calyces. **Dilatation of the collecting system does not always imply obstruction, although in the majority of cases it does**. Conditions such as vesico-ureteric reflux and other congenital disorders can lead to HUN. Causes of obstruction can be **intraluminal** (i.e. stone, blood clot), **luminal** (i.e. tumor, fibrosis), or **extraluminal** (i.e. retroperitoneal mass or tumor, retroperitoneal fibrosis). HN/HUN can be uni- or bilateral depending on the etiology. Unilateral obstruction is due to pathology at or proximal to the level of the ureteric orifice. The explanation for bilateral HUN is usually found in the bladder or below it (infravesical). **The main reasons for infravesical obstruction that leads to bilateral HUN are benign hypertrophy of the prostate, carcinoma of the prostate and urethral stricture**.

There is no correlation between the magnitude of the collecting system dilatation and the severity of renal failure, especially in the presence of dehydration. **If you have doubts about the significance of mild hydronephrosis, first correct any dehydration and then repeat the ultrasound 1-2 days later. Hydronephrosis combined with infection requires rapid intervention to save the kidney**.

When planning an elective laparotomy in patients with hydronephrosis consult your urological colleague first. Occasionally, drainage of an obstructed kidney should be performed — either by a **nephrostomy tube** prior to surgery, or at the beginning of surgery by **retrograde insertion of a ureteric stent**. This approach can improve the postoperative outcome even if the hydronephrosis is unrelated to the primary disease and it also provides the opportunity to correct the cause of hydronephrosis during the laparotomy together with the urologist.

Renal mass on pre-operative imaging

Renal tumors are not infrequently identified on imaging (ultrasound, computed tomography or magnetic resonance imaging) that is done for reasons other than renal pathology. **A renal 'mass' means a lesion that measures more than 15 Hounsfield units (i.e. it is not a cyst!) on CT and enhances following administration of intravenous contrast material.** The presence of a suspected renal mass should lead to pre-operative evaluation that includes contrast-based imaging (CT or MRI) when the initial detection was by ultrasound or a non-contrast CT.

The management of a renal mass depends on its size, the initial reason for imaging and the surgical procedure that the patient is scheduled to undergo. Most renal masses are primary renal tumors rather than metastatic disease or manifestations of infection. The natural history of small renal masses is 'benign', i.e. the growth rate is slow and they do not usually metastasize. The treatment is usually surgical and can be combined with other surgical procedures, if it fits the location of the initial surgery — upper abdomen or the retroperitoneum. The treatment of small renal lesions (less than 4cm) can be postponed until the surgical emergency or semi-emergency situation has been resolved. If the mass is larger than 4cm, the feasibility of simultaneous urological intervention should be considered in consultation with your trusted urologist.

Intra-operative considerations

Difficult catheterization

Urethral catheterization is frequently employed prior to the operation, mainly for the following indications:

- Pelvic operations.
- Operations longer than two hours.
- Major operations or 'ill patients' in whom the urine output has to be monitored.

Failure to insert the catheter is relatively common. The reasons include the presence of strictures along the urethra, false passages created in previous attempts at catheterization or lack of experience by the physician or nurse who performs the procedure. Benign hyperplasia of the prostate (a common cause for urinary retention) rarely leads to difficult catheterization.

Narrowing of the urethra is common in three locations:

- **Meatal stenosis** is easy to identify — there is an inability to insert the catheter beyond the distal 2cm.
- The **bulbar urethra**, the most common area for urethral strictures, is due to previous endoscopic urological surgery and sexually transmitted disease.
- **Bladder neck stricture** can develop following prostatectomy for benign disease (open or transureteral) and following radical prostatectomy or radiotherapy for prostate cancer.

The easiest option for **management** is to dump the bloody Foley in the trash bin and growl "get the urologist!" But what do you do if there is no urologist nearby?

It depends on the location of the problem. You can dilate a meatal stenosis with a narrow *Tiemann catheter* (10F, 1mm = 3F) and above. Another option is to insert a small-caliber metal sound and slowly dilate the narrowing to a size 24-28F. The procedure is done under local or general anesthesia. In cases of a more proximal stricture, your options are:

- Insertion of a small-diameter catheter.
- Retrograde insertion of a guide wire and dilatation of the urethra.
- Flexible cystoscopy, identification of the stricture and insertion of a guide wire followed by retrograde dilatation of the stricture.

The latter options should be done only by somebody trained in those procedures.

When transurethral catheterization fails, and the bladder is palpable above the pubic bone, insertion of a suprapubic catheter is the procedure of choice. I recommend the use of ultrasound guidance, especially in patients with a history of lower abdominal surgery. Inject local anesthesia 1-2cm above the pubic bone in the midline, then insert a needle into the bladder as a guide for location and depth; if urine is aspirated via the needle, an incision is placed at the needle site and the suprapubic catheter is inserted over a wire, using the Seldinger technique, or directly through a large-bore needle. The catheter is secured by inflation of the catheter balloon. Before removal of a suprapubic catheter, a urological evaluation should be made, to ensure the integrity and patency of the urethra. For more details about difficult catheterization see overleaf.

The 10 commandments for a difficult catheterization:

- **Identify the difficult cases prior to an elective surgery**: a history of difficult urination, prostatectomy, pelvic fracture or previous difficult catheterization. If there is a clue for a difficult catheterization, talk to the urologist.

- **Don't insert a catheter** with no clear indication for its use.

- **Maintain a strict sterile technique** despite the difficult catheterization. This will prevent urinary tract infection and sepsis.

- **Lubricate generously** with lidocaine gel at the beginning of the catheterization. Inject 5-10cc of lidocaine gel retrogradely into the urethral meatus with a syringe in your dominant hand, while the non-dominant hand presses the penile glans to prevent spillage of the gel.

- **Choose the right catheter** rather than taking the catheter you were given by the OR nurse. Catheters differ according to their diameter, form of the tip and the presence and size of a balloon. For the 'average' case use a 14-16F Foley catheter.

- **Avoid future urethral stricture**: don't use force to pass the catheter for it can cause a false route and *urethrorrhagia* (bloody discharge at the urethral meatus) that will make the catheterization more difficult, risking a future urethral stricture.

- **Try a smaller or different catheter** such as a *Foley-Tiemann* catheter or a *Coude* catheter.

- **Try passing a metal guide wire** with a flexible proximal end (as in the Seldinger technique for central line insertion). After the guide wire has passed the stricture and reached the bladder, a *Council* catheter (with a hole at its end) will slide over it. Don't forget lots of gel.

- **Call the urologist!** If all of the above failed, call the expert for help. He could opt for a flexible cystoscopy to pass the guide wire under direct visualization or insert a suprapubic catheter.

- **Don't remove a catheter after a successful difficult catheterization before urological evaluation**.

Misidentification of the ureter during exploration

In most retroperitoneal and many abdominal operations, identification of the ureter is needed, since the **best method of avoiding ureteric injury is to identify it along its course**. Sometimes the bundle of gonadal vessels is mistaken for the ureter — look more medially as you go caudally and remember: the gonadal vessels do not contract when pinched! The *right upper ureter* can be identified posterior to the ascending colon, cecum and appendix. The *left upper ureter* can be seen posterior to the descending colon, sigmoid and mesentery. When medial rotation of the colon and its mesentery is carried out, the ureter can be seen within the retroperitoneal areolar tissues lying on the psoas muscle. **The easiest location to identify the ureter is at the point where it crosses the common iliac vessels, usually at the bifurcation into the internal and external branches**. From that point, the ureter can be tagged with a vessel loop and followed toward the bladder. **The ureter should not be skeletonized from the adjacent soft tissue in order to avoid injury to its blood supply as this can cause ureteric ischemia and late stricture**. If you anticipate difficulty in finding the ureter, a ureteric catheter can be inserted via cystoscopy at the beginning of the procedure in order to help in its identification later on. Lighted ureteric catheters are available to the fancy laparoscopic surgeons among you.

Ureteric obstruction by a retroperitoneal/intraperitoneal mass

Evaluation of HN/HUN should be done as mentioned above. The involved kidney should be drained by a nephrostomy or ureteric catheter prior to surgery, if it is to be delayed for more than a few weeks from the diagnosis. During surgery, the ureter is identified and the involved segment is recognized. Occasionally, ureterolysis can be performed; if this is not possible for technical or oncological reasons, resection of the involved segment is needed. **An end-to-end anastomosis of the ureter is possible if only a short segment (<5cm) has been removed. For lower ureter involvement, reimplantation to the bladder is preferred**. Lower ureteral defects up to the crossing of the iliac vessels can usually be reimplanted to the bladder; occasionally the bladder should be dissected and fixed to the psoas muscle by a non-absorbing suture (*psoas hitch*). When a longer segment of the ureter is missing (or resected), the missing part can be replaced by a bladder flap that is created and anastomosed to the end of the ureter. Another option is an ileal ureter, i.e. an isolated segment of small bowel segment that can easily reach up to the renal pelvis. On the right side, the terminal ileum is used; on the left, a window in the sigmoid mesentery is created and the ileum is inserted through it along the left gutter. Obviously, such procedures require the expertise of a urologist!

A pelvic mass invading the urinary bladder

Invasion of the bladder by pelvic tumor or an inflammatory mass (e.g. diverticular) is not uncommon. Hematuria, pneumaturia, fecaluria and painful urination may all be described by the patient. Any bladder mass or perivesical mass is usually seen on the pre-operative CT. However, its absence does not exclude the presence of bladder invasion. Cystoscopy should be done prior to surgery, since it may change the pre-operative staging and modify the surgical procedure and its timing. If bladder involvement exists, the surgical options include partial cystectomy (a less extensive procedure) or total cystectomy or even pelvic exenteration. Resecting a cuff of bladder and performing a urine-tight closure in two layers with absorbable sutures is not a big deal but the two last mentioned procedures should be performed only by trained urologists. The ureteric orifices should be identified during surgery, and if you don't see them ask the anesthesia team to infuse a bolus of indigo carmine, and look for a blue jet.

Renal trauma

The Editors asked me to limit myself to complications. You will have to read elsewhere about the mechanisms, grading, diagnosis and management of renal injury.

Renal injury is more common after blunt than penetrating trauma. The majority are low-grade injuries — i.e. involving peripheral parts of the kidney and not the collecting system or the renal vessels. Complications of renal injury are:

- **Bleeding** — the most dangerous complication. The kidney blood flow is significant and injury can lead to hemorrhagic shock, especially after renovascular trauma. **Information about the other kidney is important**, and if it is found to be absent or small-sized during abdominal exploration — and nephrectomy is deemed necessary — an on-table IVP can be done in order to confirm the presence and the function of the contralateral kidney, before committing to removal of the injured kidney. **In most centers in this day and age, the contralateral kidney will have been assessed before the operation with a CT**. If discovered during the operation, most perirenal hematomas following **blunt trauma** should not be explored to avoid an unnecessary nephrectomy. **However, active bleeding, an expanding or pulsating perirenal hematoma, or a suspicion of major renal vessel injury requires exploration**. In this case, preliminary vascular control of the hilar renal vessels is not necessary — simply elevate the kidney from its bed and deal with the pedicle — as if you were doing a splenectomy. **For patients with an isolated renal injury and not in need of an operation, and those who bleed after surgery, angiographic embolization is the best choice! A penetrating renal injury detected during abdominal exploration is a different fish altogether**: you have to explore and do whatever necessary according to the amount of damage found: repair, partial or total nephrectomy.

- **Urinary leak** — can happen in a destructive (grade IV renal) injury of the collecting system. It can be observed as perirenal or peri-ureteric contrast material visible on abdominal CT, or present as a retroperitoneal urinoma. Treatment options include observation, internal drainage of the collecting system and percutaneous drainage of the urinoma.

- **Arteriovenous fistulas and pseudoaneurysms** rarely follow renal trauma or surgery. They are usually treated by arterial embolization, avoiding surgical exploration and the risk of nephrectomy.

Ureteric injury

The ureters may accidentally be tied or cut during retroperitoneal surgery, colorectal surgery, or gynecological procedures (hysterectomy and Cesarean section [C/S] carry a 1% risk of ureteric injury!). The anatomy of the ureters and their identification has been mentioned above — the segment which is most at risk is the lowest. Prevention of injury is crucial — when dissecting a complex colorectal mass or a large uterine tumor, define the ureters at the outset. When a difficult dissection is anticipated, retrograde insertion of a ureteric catheter can help to identify their course.

A careless technique and/or frenzied attempts to achieve hemostasis during hysterectomy or C/S puts the ureters at risk. During C/S the ureter is at risk when the lower segment uterine incision is extended, or tears, too far laterally. **In such a situation always think about the ureter, stay near the uterine wall, and avoid placing deep, blind sutures 'too far to the sides'**. In 'experienced hands' such an injury may be recognized, and fixed, during the operation. But commonly, the obstructing ureteric suture is diagnosed well after the operation when the patient develops hydronephrosis. BTW: some surgeons manage to injure both ureters during the operation: for example, look at this series from Ghana of 14 (!) cases of bilateral post-hysterectomy hydronephrosis, presenting as postoperative renal failure or anuria [1].

When **fixing an injured ureter** the treatment options depend on the location, the severity of injury, the length of the injured segment and the function of the ipsilateral kidney. A short, incompletely injured segment can be repaired over a ureteric stent with interrupted absorbable 4-0 sutures in a manner that will not narrow the ureteral lumen. For segments up to 5cm in length, an end-to-end anastomosis (uretero-ureterostomy) can be used following dissection of the distal and proximal ends. The anastomosis should be done with no tension (remember to *spatulate* the ureter's end in order to avoid anastomotic stricture — you place an incision along the distal part of the ureter in order to increase the diameter of the anastomosis) and a ureteric stent should be retained for approximately six weeks. For a distal ureter defect, reimplantation of the ureter to the bladder is a useful method. The bladder is mobilized and the ureter is anastomosed to the bladder following spatulation. A perivesical drain should be inserted at the end of the procedure (as in all cases of urinary reconstruction). The bladder is drained by a transurethral catheter for 5-7 days. **Cystography prior to the removal of the catheter can be avoided in selective cases** with no clinical features of leakage. If you are not sure whether what's dripping from the drain is urine or serum, then send a sample for creatinine level. Obviously it is advisable to keep the catheter and perform a cystography when leakage is demonstrated and following a complicated reconstruction. The ureteric stent, if used, is left for six weeks for maturation of the anastomosis. The upper ureter is the most difficult part to reconstruct — uretero-ureterostomy can be used for short segments as described above in an end-to-side anastomosis. Longer segments will be reconstructed by a *Boari flap* — a bladder flap that can reach the upper ureter territory — or an ileal ureter. **If the patient is unstable or you practice in the bush, simply close the injured ureter with a metal clip or a tie!** A day or two later insert a percutaneous nephrostomy tube followed much later by delayed reconstructive surgery (by a urologist!)

Bladder injury

Bladder injury may occur during pelvic procedures such as hysterectomy, C/S and sigmoid and rectal surgery. **Prevention includes insertion of a**

---

[1]   Mensah JE, *et al.* Delayed recognition of bilateral ureteric injury after gynaecological surgery. *Ghana Med J* 2008; 42(4): 133-6.

Foley catheter at the start of the operation but remember that even an empty bladder can be injured easily. For example, during *repeat* C/S the bladder may be adherent to the lower segment of the uterus, and be injured during elevation of the peritoneum which covers the lower uterus. When the two structures (peritoneum and bladder) are plastered together, or there is no time to separate them carefully, place your uterine incision higher than usual! **Remember that the head of the fetus when impacted deep in the pelvis tends to push the empty bladder upwards, almost out of the pelvis**. Keep this in mind: open the peritoneum as high as possible for what may look like peritoneum in the lower midline may be the bladder, and soon the Foley catheter's balloon will be looking directly at you...

It is important to identify the injury intra-operatively. In the case of a 'decent' sized bladder perforation, the bladder mucosa or the urinary catheter will be hard to miss, but if you are not sure ask someone to crawl below the drapes and fill the bladder through the catheter with saline and indigo carmine (or methylene blue). The margins of the injury should be marked by sutures and repaired with absorbable sutures (I do it in two layers). Finally, the bladder should be filled with saline to check watertightness. I would leave a drain along the repaired bladder but not everybody agrees that this is necessary. The Foley catheter should be left *in situ* for 5-7 days. Whether to obtain a routine **contrast cystogram** prior to removal has been discussed above. The (rare) leak which may develop is treated with prolonged bladder catheterization — the need for re-exploration and surgical repair is extremely rare.

Postoperative considerations

This is the place to remind you that unlike the GI tract with which you deal every day, the urinary tract is usually sterile. **And sterile urine leaking into the abdominal cavity is initially relatively silent**, until the abdomen swells up due to urine ascites and ileus or the urine becomes infected. In this situation the urine will be reabsorbed from the peritoneal cavity causing elevations in the serum BUN and creatinine. **If sampled, the ascitic fluid creatinine/serum creatinine ratio will be greater than 1.0, suggesting an intraperitoneal urine leak**.

Urinary retention (UR)

This situation ranges from an acute inability to void to chronic 'hesitancy and dribbling' with a large post-voiding residual volume. UR is more common after peri-anal procedures and/or spinal anesthesia — a history of pre-existing voiding dysfunction due to symptomatic prostate enlargement and previous episodes of urinary retention should sound a warning. **Medical therapy for symptomatic benign prostate enlargement (BPE) with alpha- blockers should not be stopped prior to surgery since this will increase the incidence of postoperative UR.**

The therapy of UR depends on whether it is acute or chronic, the volume of post-voiding residual bladder content, and the presence of acute renal failure or hydronephrosis. In the acute setting a urethral catheter should be inserted. Usually, when the cause of UR is BPE, catheter insertion is relatively easy. When it is difficult, think about the possibility of a urethral false passage (due to traumatic catheterization), a urethral stricture, lack of experience with the procedure or a wrong diagnosis — remember that UR is not the only explanation for a failure to produce urine!

Tips for managing UR:

- Make sure that UR is the diagnosis — rule out anuria or oliguria. Ask the nurse to get a 'bladder scan', which is now available in most places, to determine the bladder volume.
- If the diagnosis of UR is correct insert a Foley catheter to the bladder; don't use force to advance it as this may injure the urethra and produce urethrorrhagia and possible stricture. If you fail at that stage call the urologist (or if he is not available, insert a suprapubic cystostomy).
- The following steps should be done by the urologist:
  - insertion of a delicate metallic guide wire and slide the urethral catheter over it (Council type);
  - flexible cystoscopy — after reaching the bladder insert a delicate metallic guide wire and pass a urethral catheter over it (Council type);
  - insertion of a suprapubic catheter (see "Difficult catheterization" above).

Complications of bladder surgery

Partial or complete bladder resection may be associated with several typical complications:

- **Hematuria** — this is usually minor and is treated by adequate hydration and observation. Severe hematuria is treated initially with cystoscopic evacuation of clots and continuous bladder irrigation (CBI); if major or persistent, a reoperation may be necessary.

- **Urinary leak** — most cases of extraperitoneal leakage can be treated successfully with prolonged bladder drainage (use a Foley catheter of 18-22F). If the leak persists (as documented on cystography), urinary diversion by bilateral nephrostomy tubes may be necessary; but this is extremely rare, limited to severely diseased bladders — due to radiation injury for example. Intraperitoneal leakage should be treated by laparotomy to deal with the perforation.
- **Ureteric injury** — the common location for injury during bladder surgery is the ureteric orifices and the perivesical distal ureters. The management of distal ureteric injury is described above.
- **Small-capacity bladder** — the best way to avoid it is to anticipate the volume of the bladder following surgery. When extensive resection of the bladder is necessary, total cystectomy or augmentation cystoplasty (bladder enlargement with a loop of small bowel) should be considered instead.

Delayed ureteric injury

When a ureteric injury is missed during surgery or following trauma, the presenting symptoms can include flank pain, urinoma, urinary sepsis or renal failure. The diagnosis is established with abdominal CT (of course with i.v. contrast) — look for the presence of hydroureteronephrosis, extravasation of contrast, or a retroperitoneal/pelvic urinoma. Treatment options include drainage of the collecting system by nephrostomy or a ureteric stent. A delayed ureteric stricture leading to hydronephrosis and renal failure requires reconstructive surgery.

Scrotal swelling

Scrotal swelling developing after the operation may result from intrascrotal causes (e.g. epididymo-orchitis, hydrocele — hey, did you examine the scrotum before the operation?) or represent **scrotal edema**. The latter condition is not uncommon after perineal or prostatic operations. It may be secondary to abdominal wall edema or part of generalized anasarca — the dependent scrotum tends to swell up easily... even after traumatic insertion of a catheter. Scrotal swelling after operations for groin hernias is discussed in ➲ Chapter 15. Careful examination, supplemented, if necessary with an ultrasound examination, will provide the diagnosis. The

Table 26.1. Urological complications encountered by general surgeons. *Continued overleaf.*

Complication	Comments
Tying or injury to the ureter during retroperitoneal or pelvic surgery	■ If patient 'stable' — 'untie' or repair over a stent. ■ When diagnosis delayed (presence of hydroureteronephrosis) — drain the kidney by percutaneous nephrostomy and perform antegrade imaging. Endoscopic therapy is advised. ■ Delayed reconstructive surgery is reserved for failure of endoscopic therapy and long ureteral defects.
Missed ureteric injury following abdominal trauma	■ Drain kidney by percutaneous nephrostomy, followed by antegrade imaging to identify the lesion. ■ Endourology therapy — insertion of internal stent, if possible. ■ 6-8 days later, repeat imaging. Treat accordingly.
Bladder tear diagnosed during pelvic surgery	■ Repair in two layers, test for watertightness by filling the bladder. ■ Consider the use of a suprapubic catheter at the end of surgery. ■ Leave a perivesical drain. ■ Postop cystography in selected cases.
Bladder injury diagnosed following pelvic surgery or trauma	■ Perform a CT cystography. ■ Rule out associated abdominal/pelvic injuries. ■ Determine intraperitoneal vs. extraperitoneal bladder perforation. The latter one usually is treated conservatively, while the former needs to be explored and repaired.
Delayed hematuria after abdominal trauma	■ Common causes: renal and bladder laceration. ■ Clinically significant: missed renal laceration. ■ Treatment: angiography and selective embolization. In rare cases — surgery.

Table 26.1. Urological complications encountered by general surgeons.

Complication	Comments
Postoperative hydronephrosis	■ Drain the kidney by percutaneous nephrostomy or by retrograde stent. ■ Perform antegrade or retrograde imaging. Treat accordingly. ■ Delayed surgical reconstructive surgery is reserved for failure of endoscopic therapy and long ureteral defects.
Postoperative urinoma	■ Percutaneous drainage in symptomatic patients. The fluid should be cultured and the creatinine level should be determined. ■ Identify the source of the urinoma by CT with intravenous contrast. ■ Perform antegrade or retrograde imaging. Treat accordingly. ■ Delayed surgery is reserved for failure of endoscopic therapy and long ureteral defects.
Postoperative urinary retention	■ In the case of postoperative anuria, insert a urethral catheter or use ultrasound to determine the intravesical volume. ■ Rule out pre-renal causes. ■ In the case of urinary retention, identify patients with the diagnosis of bladder outlet obstruction. Treat accordingly.

majority of cases resolve spontaneously without any specific therapy. Thus, surgical drainage is very rarely necessary.

■ Table 26.1 will provide you with a summary of what I tried to convey in this chapter. To some of you this chapter may appear a little banal. For this you will have to blame the Editors.

> Treat the urinary system the same as your garden hose pipe — as the water goes in, it should go out: if not then fix or dislodge or stent and if desperate just drain and try again later.
>
> **Moshe**

> My old urology Professor, Olof Alfthan, used to say: "Drink a lot and urinate often..."
>
> **Ari**

Epilogue

Lessons learned from surgical complications

David Dent

The science of surgical complications has been extensively covered in the preceding chapters. In addition to this science there are other dimensions to surgical complications which may be called their philosophical and personal aspects.

Surgery is merely a craft, and surgeons merely journeymen/craftsmen. Some surgeons may have additional special training and knowledge in the sciences of immunology, oncology, or special experiences acquired in the sister profession of medicine. **However, the act of surgery — operating — remains a craft, and the gloved surgeon standing at the operating table is a craftsman**. As such, the surgeon-craftsman may be brilliant, or good, or mediocre, or just plain bad. This pungent fact is one that surgeons and the public prefer not to think about. There are good and bad tennis players, aircraft pilots, sculptors, violinists, auto repairers and plumbers. **So, too, there are good and bad operating surgeons**. It follows that the quality of the surgeon and their surgery will define the complications of their operations. It also follows that good surgeons have few complications, and bad surgeons have frequent complications. While the human body is amazingly forgiving of some errors, other, repeated or gross errors rapidly escalate into major complications.

As a whipping boy was punished for the misdemeanours of a prince, or a scapegoat sent into the desert for the sins of others, so surgical complications may be attributed to everything but the surgeon who caused them. A psychiatrist (incidentally, don't ever ask a psychiatrist for their opinion of surgeons) would call this **"displacement of guilt"**. This mechanism may be found, for example, in the academic hierarchy where the yes-sir, no-sir trainee will apologize effusively the instant the 'Supreme Leader' transects the common bile duct. The professionally appointed scapegoat for some surgical problems is the anesthetist, who in addition to providing anesthesia must bear certain professional responsibilities of guilt such as an apparent lack of relaxation in the patient, real or imagined. Instruments and apparatus, and their perceived shortcomings, are also a hardy standby for guilt displacement.

Some surgeons are reluctant to accept that their patient has a complication. While clearly obvious to other doctors, the nursing staff, and perhaps the cleaning lady, the surgeon enters into a stage of denial. Ignoring complications or pretending that misadventure did not occur is the worst course to take, and the situation usually compounds itself. **Some surgeons use trivializing descriptions**. Wound infection is dismissed as "a little redness", or as "serum ooze", or as "sutures being too tight". Hemorrhage may be "dampness" or "old blood". The bile from the drain is "old bile". Valuable time may be lost in this way, and correction and remedy delayed. **If it is true that there are big surgeons and little surgeons, denial is the mark of the little surgeon!**

A surgeon is an accomplished and easy fair weather friend to his patient. Surgical reassurance, bonhomie and good cheer are characteristic and legendary. A surgical complication, however, is foul weather, and in these circumstances the daily visits are painful for both the surgeon and his patient. **Full disclosure** of the problem is essential with the patient and the family. Apart from its ethical aspects, full and open disclosure is the major factor in avoiding litigation. It is a lonely siege for both parties as each day and visit passes, and as the complication may not get less, but perhaps worse. At this point there is a vital action the surgeon must take. Popular quiz shows have lifelines as difficulty escalates, and phone-a-friend is helpful to contestants. In surgery **a second opinion works wonders** in reassuring both the patient, and the surgeon. The second surgeon must examine the patient, review the investigations, and counsel the patient. This second-opinion surgeon will not experience a more grateful handshake and thank you than from a colleague that they have supported. In addition to this reassurance of equals, there is, or should be, a special interaction between the teacher and the young trainee when the trainee has a complication of their surgery. It is usually completely obvious that the trainee is going to present a complication on a ward round when instead of saying that the history was typical of appendicitis, as was the examination, they start a laborious and circuitous account of the history, and a most detailed account of the examination (the listeners' hearts sinking as the narrative proceeds), ending in a description of the error and the complication. **The teacher will have gained an ally and be a hero for life if they reassure the trainee, and walk with them through the difficult ensuing days of management**.

The greatest influence in the reduction of complications has been **surgical audit**, and the **morbidity and mortality (M&M) conference**. All credit must go to a surgeon who practiced a century ago: Dr. Ernest Amory Codman (1869-1940) of the Massachusetts General Hospital in Boston, and later at his own institution, the End Results Hospital [1]. Codman was a contemporary and friend of Harvey Cushing, and with George Crile and Charles Mayo was one of the prominent founders of the American College of Surgeons. Codman discussed the unvarnished truth, and stated "I am naturally disgusted with humbug, self-deception, hypocrisy, smugness, cupidity and injustice". His hospital issued annual reports of complications. For example, there was patient number 77, in whom Codman had ligated the common hepatic duct, leading to death: "I had made an error of skill of the most gross character and even [during the operation] failed to recognize that I had made it." **He classified errors into lack of knowledge or skill, surgical judgment, lack of care or equipment, and lack of diagnostic skill**. Much has evolved since then. Contemporary M&M conferences are held at many academic institutions in the western world. They may also be held at large surgical practices. Their goal is to educate and to modify surgical behavior rather than to be punitive. Even the Supreme Leader of academic departments should have their complications submitted to the same scrutiny and comment as those of the plebeian trainees. M&M conferences also identify system problems like those of waiting lists, outdated referral policies, and intra-hospital movement of patients. **However, a handful of polite show-case presentations do not make a true M&M conference!**

Those who swore the Hippocratic Oath, "I swear by Apollo the Physician..." are aware of the pantheon of Greek Gods that relate to medicine. If there were a god of surgery, it would be Asclepius — that specialist in emergency medicine and trauma — the Iliad recording that he removed arrows from the legs of several warriors. **The Greek Gods abominate *hubris*, which is arrogance, boasting and showing off**. Hubris is certainly found with surgeons, and certainly about their claimed lack of complications. The Greek Gods respond swiftly and viciously to hubris,

---

[1]   Neuhauser D. Heroes and martyrs of quality and safety. Ernest Amory Codman MD. *Qual Saf Health Care* 2002; 11: 104-5.

usually in kind, with *nemesis*. Examples of complications and surgical hubris might be "I have never, ever, had to return to the OR after a cholecystectomy", or "I have done well over a hundred laparoscopic inguinal hernia repairs without a *single* major complication". The originators of these statements are invariably seen looking extremely haggard, incommunicative, and thoughtful within the week.

The journey with a patient who has a complication is usually a road less travelled. It is an unexpected journey which may be short, but occasionally long and arduous. The long journey is a difficult journey, and the companionship of a second opinion will make it more tolerable. All surgeons make this journey. The chapters in this book have told us how to avoid the journey, or how to make it an easier one for both the surgeon and the patient.

> "I shall be telling this with a sigh,
> Somewhere ages and ages hence:
> Two roads diverged in a wood, and I —
> I took the one less travelled by,
> And that has made all the difference."
>
> **Robert Frost**

Index

Locators followed by 'n' indicate footnotes

AAA (abdominal aortic aneurysm) 434-5, 441-3, 445-6
       infected grafts 449-50
abandoning the patient, inadvisable 193-4, 197
ABC of pre-hospital trauma care 473-5
ABCDE primary survey 476-7
abdominal binders 150
abdominal compartment syndrome 150, 443n, 446, 486, 494
abdominal wall
       dehiscence 145-54, 212
       delayed or non-closure 83, 494-5
       temporary closure 151, 154, 443n, 486-7, 492
       weakness after removal of tissue for breast reconstruction 407
       see also hernias
abscesses
       anal 286
       anastomotic leaks 464-5
       at the wound site 78, 84, 86-7
       drainage 67, 68, 86, 356
       post-appendectomy 354-6
accessory bile duct of Luschka 317, 330
activities of daily life 18-19
adhesions 157-8, 173-4
adjustable gastric banding (LAGB) 456, 460, 461, 469-70
adrenalectomy 413-16, 417, 426-30
adult respiratory distress syndrome (ARDS) 236, 243-4, 495-6
age 17
       see also elderly patients; pediatric surgery
air leak test 98, 266-7
airways
       acutely compromised after thyroidectomy 419-20
       in trauma 473
albumin status 18, 206
aldosterone over-secretion (Conn's syndrome) 429-30
alpha-blockers 427
ambulation of patients 35, 162
American Society of Anesthesiologists (ASA) risk classification 19, 20
anal surgery 279-90
       fistula 280-1, 285-6, 289-90
       hemorrhoids 279, 282-5, 288, 290
analgesia 35, 162, 253-4
anastomoses, gastrointestinal 91-143
       colorectal 134-43, 261-2, 265-7
       esophageal 98, 103, 106-16
       gastric bypass 458-60, 461
       gastroduodenal 116-28
       intra-operative considerations 96-9, 108-11, 117-23, 137-9
       obstruction 97, 105-6, 166

postoperative leaks 99-105, 107, 111-16, 123-8, 129-34, 139-43, 266-7, 271-2, 461-5
pre-operative considerations 93-5, 106-7, 116-17, 135-6
small bowel 128-34
anesthesia
in anal surgery 283
in hernia repair 296
pediatric 498-9, 502-3
in the Third World 208
angiographic embolization/stenting 340, 371-2
angioplasty 436
antibiotics
in abdominal trauma 481
in appendicitis 350, 353-4
bile leaks 388
in breast surgery 394
C. difficile colitis 250
before colorectal anastomosis 136
in hernia surgery 308
in the ICU 241, 243
postoperative 70, 71, 87, 353-4
prophylactic 61-2, 70, 80-2, 83
for VAP 243
in vascular surgery 439
anticoagulants and antiplatelet agents 40-4, 50
bariatric surgery 454, 457, 465
prophylactic 206, 248-9, 454, 457, 495
trauma patients 495
vascular surgery 432, 442
antihypertensive agents 427, 429-30
antimotility agents 275
antipsychotic agents 254
aorta
aneurysm (AAA) 434-5, 441-3, 445-6, 449-50
trauma 474, 484-5
aorto-enteric fistula 449-50
aortofemoral bypass 432, 442, 448
APACHE II risk stratification 19-20
appendectomy 345-60, 499
ARDS (adult respiratory distress syndrome) 236, 243-4, 495-6
arm ischemia 437
arterial bleeding, in trauma 484-6
arterial surgery 431-3, 439
see also specific vessels
ascites 298
chylous 374
urinary 529
aspiration of gastric contents 159, 503
aspirin 41-2, 43, 50, 432
assistants
in rural practices 224-5
supervision of junior staff 192, 211, 536-7
atrial fibrillation 42, 271

axillary lymph nodes 402, 403-6

bariatric surgery 451-70
       bleeding 457, 459, 465
       leaks 457-8, 459, 461-5
       SBO 157, 459-60, 466-8
barium contrast agent 104, 140
behavioral errors in surgeons 24, 186-7, 536, 537-8
benign prostatic hypertrophy (BPH) 297, 530
beta-blockers 252, 427, 432
bile duct
       anatomy 317, 323-4, 330, 334-5
       iatrogenic injuries 315, 319, 323-4, 325, 334-7
       stones in 321, 324, 338-9, 341
       strictures 341
       trauma 486
bile leaks
       after gallbladder surgery 328, 330-4, 337
       after liver surgery 385-8
biliary dyskinesia 322
biliopancreatic diversion 456, 460
bilirubin 333
bladder, urinary
       iatrogenic injuries 304-7, 528-9, 532
       invasion by pelvic mass 526
       post-voiding residual volume 521
       suprapubic catheterization 523
       surgery on 530-1
       trauma 491
bleeding and hemostasis 39-55
       AAA surgery 446, 449-50
       adrenalectomy 427-8
       anal surgery 288
       anticoagulants/antiplatelet agents 40-4, 50
       appendectomy 356-7
       avoid if possible 30, 64
       bariatric surgery 457, 459, 465
       breast surgery 395
       carotid surgery 441
       cholecystectomy 326, 339-40
       drains 48, 68
       gastric 245
       hernia repair 300-1, 302-3, 308
       laparoscopy 175-6, 179-80
       liver surgery 381-3, 384-5
       pancreatic surgery 366, 370-2
       pelvic 52-3, 264-5, 486
       rectal 270
       trauma patients 50-4, 474-5, 477, 483-7, 488, 493, 526-7
       see also transfusions
blood pressure
       in adrenal disorders 427, 429-30
       in bariatric surgery 457

postoperative hypotension 49-50, 107
    in trauma patients 238, 474-5
blunt trauma 472, 477, 479-80
Bogota bags 486-7
bowel anastomoses 91-106
    colorectal 134-43, 261-2, 265-7, 271-2
    small bowel 128-34
bowel injuries
    colorectal surgery 257-78
    during hernia repair 300, 303-4
    intussusception 513-14
    during laparoscopy 176-7, 178-9
    trauma 479-80, 486, 487-8, 490-1
bowel ischemia 270-1, 274, 299-300, 446
bowel obstruction/stricture
    anastomotic 97, 105-6, 166
    colonic 258
    EPSBO 155-68, 356
    gastric bypass surgery 157, 459-60, 466-8
    laparoscopy 174
bowel preparation 136, 260
box-ticking 7-8
breast surgery 393-411
bridging therapy (heparin) 42-3, 50
burns
    diathermy-related 178, 210, 501
    radiotherapy 408
bypass surgery, vascular 432, 436, 443-4, 446-9
    see also gastric bypass surgery

calcium
    in parathyroid disease 421-2, 424, 425-6
    in thyroid disease 417, 421-2
carbon dioxide (CO_2), in laparoscopy 177
carcinomatosis, peritoneal 166, 364
cardiac anomalies (congenital) 499
cardiac complications
    of radiotherapy for breast cancer 409
    risk assessment 20
    tamponade 476-7
cardiac valves, mechanical 42
carotid surgery 433-4, 440-1, 445
cecum 359
celiac axis, stenosis 373
central venous catheters 235, 246-7
    pediatric 505-6
central venous pressure (CVP) 235, 383
cerebral hyperperfusion syndrome 445
cervical esophageal anastomoses 106, 110-11, 113-14
Cesarean sections 527-8, 529
CHAD scores 42
check lists
    hemostasis 47

in the ICU 233
pre-closure 32
pre-incisional 27
children's surgery 497-517
Child's scoring system 378
cholangiography, intra-operative 324-5
cholangitis 318, 341
cholecystectomy 315-43
cholecystitis 318, 320
acalculous 342
cholecysto-biliary-enteric fistula 319
choledocholithiasis 321, 324, 338-9, 341
chylous ascites 374
circumcision 502, 503
cirrhosis 317, 378-9
classification of complications (Clavien) 5
classification of risk 19-20
clopidogrel 41-2, 43, 50, 432
Clostridium difficile colitis 250-1
closure of the wound 32, 69, 83-4, 148-52
failure see dehiscence
clotting tests 40
coagulopathy 45, 53-4, 483
colon
in AAA surgery 442, 446
anastomoses 134-43, 261-2, 265-7, 271-2
C. difficile colitis 250-1
cancer 258, 259, 266, 279
in cholecystectomy 340
diverticulitis 360
ileus 166-7
inflammatory bowel disease 259, 262
intra-operative considerations 137-9, 261-9
ischemia 270-1, 299, 446
postoperative complications 139-43, 269-78
pre-operative considerations 135-6, 258-61
trauma 479, 488, 491
colostomy 137-8, 141, 258, 262-3, 267-8
closure 277-8
complications 83, 273-7, 278
common bile duct (CBD) see bile duct
common facial vein 441
communication 185
bariatric surgery 454-5, 461
disclosure 190, 196-7, 214-15, 536
with the family 26, 33, 190, 192, 193, 214-15, 498
in the ICU 254-5
in pediatric surgery 498
postoperative 33, 34, 214-15
pre-operative 26, 156, 190, 192, 207, 434, 435, 439, 454-5
community relations in rural practices 221, 227
comorbidities 17, 317
in obese patients 453-4

compartment syndrome
      abdominal 150, 443*n*, 446, 486, 494
      lower limb 444
complexity of an operation 22, 28-31
complications, definition and classification 3-5
computed tomography *see* CT (computed tomography)
confusion, sedative-related 253-4
Conn's syndrome 429-30
consent 189-90, 434, 435, 454-5
constipation 36, 287
contamination 62-3
contraindications *see* not operating
contrast agents
      ileus/EPSBO 161, 162
      leaks 104, 129-30, 140-1, 271
cosmetic issues in breast surgery 398-400, 406-7, 408
countryside practices 188, 217-27
creatinine 520, 529
critical limb ischemia 436, 443-4
critical view of safety 323-4
Crohn's disease 259, 262
cryoprecipitate 54
crystalloids 54, 237
CT (computed tomography)
      anastomotic leaks 129-30, 140-1, 271, 462
      bile leaks 333
      ileus/EPSBO 161, 162
      in rural practices 222-3
      trauma patients 52, 477, 478, 479
culturing of bacteria 71-2, 87-9, 240
Cushing's syndrome 428-9
cystectomy 530-1
cystic duct 317, 323-4, 326
      leaks 330-4
      stones 338-9

dabigatran 44
damage control surgery 482-7, 493
deep venous thrombosis (DVT)
      bariatric surgery 465-6
      prophylaxis 206, 248-9, 454, 457, 495
defensive medicine 184, 454-5
dehiscence
      abdominal wall 145-54, 212
      after breast surgery 397-8, 406
delay, don't 51, 186, 189, 478-9
delirium, sedative-related 253-4
denial 187, 536
devascularization colitis 270-1
developing countries 203-15
diabetes mellitus 60, 452, 453
diaphragmatic injuries 480, 491
diarrhea 375

diathermy injuries 178, 210, 501
diet *see* nutrition
direct thrombin inhibitors 44
discharge procedures 33-4, 198
disclosure 190, 196-7, 214-15, 536
diverticulitis 360
documentation
      consent 189-90, 455
      medical records 16-17, 185-6, 197
      operative reports 33, 194, 303
drains 66-9
      of abscesses 67, 68, 86, 356
      anastomoses 98, 112-13, 122-3, 138, 271, 463
      appendectomy 356
      bariatric surgery 458, 463
      bile leaks 328, 331-3, 342-3, 387, 388
      blood in 48, 68
      breast surgery 397, 403, 406
      duodenal 67, 122-3, 491
      EPSBO prevention 158
      of hematomas 86
      pancreatic 67, 368, 369-70
      thyroidectomy 419
drugs
      pediatric dosages 503
      pre-existing medication 18, 40-4, 251-3
duodenal drains 67, 122-3, 491
duodenal injuries
      in cholecystectomy 340
      in pyloromyotomy 508-9
      trauma 119-21, 487, 490-1
duodenal ulcers 118-19, 121, 125
duodenal/gastroduodenal anastomoses 116-28
duration of the operation 30-1, 64, 483
DVT *see* deep venous thrombosis

early postoperative small bowel obstruction (EPSBO) 155-68, 356
elderly patients 17, 296, 317
electrolyte balance 162, 237, 475
embolism
      AAA surgery 442
      bariatric surgery 462, 465-6
      carotid surgery 440
      limb ischemia 437, 444
      vena cava filters 495
Emergency Department 476-7
emergency surgery 23, 25
      AAA rupture 435-6, 442
     - hemostasis 43-4, 50-4
      hernias 297, 299-300
      NG tube placement 159
      operating out-of-specialty 188-9
      pediatric 499

in rural practices 220-1
Third World situations 213-14
see also trauma care
endocrine surgery 413-16
adrenalectomy 426-30
parathyroidectomy 422-6
thyroidectomy 416-22
endoscopic retrograde cholangiopancreatography (ERCP)
bile leaks 332, 334, 387
obstructive jaundice 319, 339, 364
enteral nutrition 36, 70, 133, 245-6
enterostomy 131-4, 274, 275
environment of the OR 64, 193
epigastric hernias 515-16
EPSBO (early postoperative small bowel obstruction) 155-68, 356
ERCP *see* endoscopic retrograde cholangiopancreatography
esophageal surgery
anastomoses 67, 98, 103, 106-16
Nissen fundoplication 509-10
experimental treatments 189
see also new procedures

facial nerve 440
factor VIIa, recombinant 475
failure to rescue (FTR) 24-5, 445
fasciotomy, lower limb 444
FAST ultrasound 51, 476
femoral vein 301
femoropopliteal bypass 436, 443
fever, postoperative 36-7, 73-4, 213
fibrinogen concentrate 54
financial considerations 7, 199
in rural settings 226-7
in the Third World 205, 207, 215
fistulas
anal 280-1, 285-6, 289-90
aorto-enteric 449-50
cholecysto-biliary-enteric 319
colonic 142, 272-3
esophageal 115-16
gastrocolic 510-12
gastroduodenal 124, 127-8
gastrogastric 468
management in the Third World 212
pancreatic 369-70, 371
small bowel 131-4
fluid management 34-5, 49
high-output stomas 275
in the ICU 234-7
trauma patients 474-5
fresh frozen plasma (FFP) 43-4, 54, 239
frozen shoulder 405-6
functional capacity of patients 18-19

funktionslust 7, 24

gallbladder surgery 315-43
gallstones 318, 319, 322, 325
     in the bile duct 321, 324, 338-9, 341
gastrectomy
     partial 106, 121-3
     sleeve gastrectomy (LSG) 452, 456-8, 461, 464, 465, 468-9
     total 114-15, 464
gastric banding (LAGB) 456, 460, 461, 469-70
gastric bleeding, in the ICU 245
gastric bypass surgery (LRYGB) 452, 456, 458-60, 461, 463-4, 465, 466-8
gastric dilatation, acute 466
gastric emptying, delayed 106, 162, 374
gastric lavage 116-17
gastric trauma 119, 491
gastrocolic fistula 510-12
gastroduodenal anastomoses 116-28
gastroduodenal artery 117, 373
gastroduodenal fistula 124, 127-8
gastroduodenostomy 125-6
gastrogastric fistula 468
Gastrografin® contrast agent 140-1, 162, 271
gastrojejunostomy (GJ) 122, 126
     in Roux-en-Y gastric bypass 458-9, 461, 465, 468
gastroparesis 106, 162, 374
gastrostomy tubes, pediatric 510-13
glucose control 249-50, 428
goiter 416-22
'golden hour' 51, 473
grading of complications 5
granulation tissue, stomal 277
great auricular nerve 440
groin
     avoid incisions in AAA surgery 442
     hernias *see* inguinal hernias
     scrotal swelling 531
gunshot wounds 472, 480-1
gynecological surgery, complications 213-14, 527-8, 529

handovers in the ICU 254-5
head injuries 54, 237-8
healing 83, 95, 288
health status of the patient (pre-operative) 14, 16-21, 60, 147, 258
     malnourishment 18, 136
     in the Third World 205-6, 209
heart *see* entries at cardiac
hematocrit 52
hematomas 86, 308, 395, 441
     major vessel injuries 484-5
hematuria 530-1, 532
hemoglobin-based oxygen carrying fluids 475
hemorrhoids 279, 282-5, 288, 290

hemostasis *see* bleeding and hemostasis
heparin
>AAA surgery 442
>bridging therapy 42-3, 50
>prophylactic 249
hepatic arteries
>in cholecystectomy 340
>in liver surgery 385
>in pancreatic surgery (replaced RHA) 372-3
>traumatic injuries 485
hepatic conditions *see* liver
hepatic veins 382, 384-5
hernias 291-314
>incarcerated/strangulated 163, 165, 297, 298, 299-300, 304
>incisional 146, 304, 443, 505, 516
>inguinal 296-7, 300, 301-2, 303, 307-8, 310-11, 514-15
>intra-operative considerations 299-307
>parastomal 268, 275-6
>pediatric 514-16
>'planned' 151-2
>postoperative complications 307-14
>pre-operative considerations 21, 294-8
>recurrence 295, 300, 313-14
>sliding 300, 307
hetastarch 237
HIDA scans 333
history of the patient 16-19
honey, for wound care 87, 88
hospitals, variation in
>facilities/conditions 203-5, 209-11, 220
>mortality rates 24-5, 445
hubris 316, 537-8
hungry bone syndrome 422, 425
hydration levels *see* fluid management
hydrocele 311, 515
hydrogen peroxide irrigation 46
hydronephrosis 521, 533
hydroureteronephrosis 521
hyperaldosteronism 429-30
hypercalcemia 424, 425-6
hypercapnia 177
hypercortisolism 428-9
hyperglycemia 249-50
hyperkalemia 237, 504
hyperparathyroidism 422-6
hyperthyroidism 416, 422
hypervolemia 236
hypocalcemia
>hungry bone syndrome 422, 425
>hypoparathyroidism 417, 421-2, 425
hypoglossal nerve 440
hypoglycemia 250, 428
hypokalemia 162, 504

hypoparathyroidism 418-19, 421-2
hypotension
        postoperative 49-50, 107
        in traumatic brain injuries 238
hypothermia 64, 483, 500
hypovolemia 48-9, 234-5
hypoxia *see* oxygen is good

ileal pouch-anal anastomosis 138, 267
ileostomy 274, 275
ileus 155-68, 356
iliac arteries 441-2
iliac veins 265, 441
ilio-inguinal nerve 311, 312-13
iliofemoral vessels 301
imaging
        anal fistulas 280
        anastomotic leaks 104, 129-30, 140-1, 271, 462
        bile leaks 333
        ileus/EPSBO 161, 162
        parathyroid 423
        pre-operative 22-3
        in rural practices 222-3
        trauma patients 51-2, 476, 477, 478, 479
immunocompromised patients 135, 140
incisional hernias 146, 304, 443, 505, 516
incisions, choice of 22, 147-8
        AAA surgery 442
        appendectomy 83, 352-3
        liver surgery 381
        trauma laparotomy 482
incontinence, fecal 281, 284
indications for the operation 14, 15-16, 189
        see also not operating
infections 57-76
        appendectomy 354-6, 358
        arterial grafts 448-9
        bowel surgery 132, 140, 268-9
        C. difficile colitis 250-1
        central venous lines 247
        hernia surgery 294, 308-10
        in the ICU 239-43
        intra-operative period 63-9, 82-4, 268-9
        in laparoscopic surgery 211-12, 469-70
        pre-operative period 21, 60-3, 80-2
        SIRS does not equal sepsis 36, 58-9, 73-4
        Third World problems 210, 211-12
        wound *see* surgical site infections (SSIs)
inferior epigastric artery 175, 301
inflammation, not always infection 36, 58-9
inflammatory bowel disease 259, 262
infrastructure
        in rural practices 219, 220
        in the Third World 209-11

inguinal hernias 296-7, 300, 301-2, 303, 307-8, 310-11
    pediatric 514-15
instrument and sponge count 31-2
intensive care unit (ICU) 231-55
    pediatric 503
    trauma patients 486, 493
intermittent claudication 436
intra-abdominal pressure elevation 147, 151, 212, 297-8
    compartment syndrome 150, 443n, 446, 486, 494
    in laparoscopy 178, 505
intracranial pressure 238
intraoperative period, general considerations 26-32, 191-4
intravenous lines
    central 235, 246-7, 505-6
    pediatric 500-1, 505-6
    removal 35, 70
intubation 253
    VAP 241-3
intussusception 513-14
irrigation of tissues 65-6
ischemia
    bowel 270-1, 274, 299-300, 446
    in breast reconstruction surgery 395-6, 406-7
    limb 436-7, 443-4, 446-9
    liver 372-3
    mesenteric 163
    testicular 302, 307-8, 310
ischemic preconditioning in esophagectomy 107
isolation in rural practices 219

jaundice
    postoperative 337, 339
    pre-operative 319, 364
jejunojejunostomy 458-9, 463, 464, 466
judgment, errors in 6-7, 24, 187
junior staff
    OR assistants in rural practices 224-5
    supervision 192, 211, 536-7

kidney
    failure 519-21
    hydronephrosis 521, 533
    masses 522
    trauma 486, 487, 489, 526-7
Kübler-Ross model (five stages of grief) 195

lactate 235
lactated Ringer's solution 237
laparoscopy 169-82
    adrenalectomy 427
    appendectomy 346, 351, 355-6, 358
    bariatric surgery 451-70
    cholecystectomy *see* cholecystectomy

complications 164-5, 175-82, 304, 329-40, 358, 505
conversion to an open procedure 180-1, 328-9, 353
EPSBO 157, 158, 164-5
hernia repair 294, 304, 305, 311-12
pancreatic conditions 364
pediatric 500, 505, 507, 508
Third World problems 211-12
urological injuries 263-4, 304-7
laparostomy 151, 154, 443n
after trauma repair 486-7, 492
large bowel *see* colon
laryngeal nerves 417-18, 420-1, 424, 440
laxatives 282, 287
leg ischemia 436-7, 443-4, 446-9
legal issues 183-4, 185-6, 191, 199-201, 360, 410-11, 438
less-developed countries 203-15
leukocytosis 74
life expectancy 17
liver
bleeding 381-3, 384-5, 484, 488
size, in bariatric surgery 453
surgery on 377-91
trauma 478, 484, 487, 488
long thoracic nerve 405
loupes 439, 500
lower limb ischemia 436-7, 443-4, 446-9
lumpectomy 393-403, 406-7, 409
lymphadenectomy
in breast surgery 402, 403-6
in pancreatic surgery 367, 374
lymphedema 404-5

M&M conferences 537
magnifying devices 439, 500
malaria 213
malignant hyperthermia 36
malnourishment 18, 136
malpractice litigation 183-4, 185-6, 191, 199-201, 360, 410-11, 438
massive blood loss 54, 474, 477, 484-5
mastectomy 393-8, 406-7, 409
medical records 16-17, 185-6, 197
medications
pediatric dosages 503
pre-existing 18, 40-4, 251-3
mesenteric injuries 479-80
mesenteric ischemia 163
meshes used in hernia repair 293, 294, 300, 305-6, 309-10, 312
midline incisions 147-8, 149, 353, 482
minimal access surgery *see* laparoscopy
Mirizzi syndrome 318-19
mobilization of the patient 35, 162
money matters 7, 199
in rural settings 226-7
in the Third World 205, 207, 215

mortality rates, hospital-to-hospital differences 24-5, 445
MRSA (methicillin-resistant *S. aureus*) 89, 448
multidisciplinary teams in the ICU 255
multiple organ dysfunction syndrome (MODS) 59
mycobacterial infections, atypical 211-12

nasogastric (NG) tubes
        after GI surgery 35-6, 114, 158-60, 161
        insertion 167
        pediatric 503
        removal 36, 167
near misses 196
necrotizing soft tissue infections (deep SSIs) 78, 85, 89, 152, 309, 354
negligence 200-1
neonates 497, 498, 501
neostigmine 167
nephrectomy 486, 489
nerve damage
        axillary clearance 404, 405
        carotid surgery 440
        hernia repair 311-12, 312-13
        (para)thyroidectomy 417-18, 420-1, 424
new procedures 189, 207, 454
        gallbladder surgery 316, 321
        hemorrhoid surgery 282-3
NG tubes *see* nasogastric (NG) tubes
Nissen fundoplication 509-10
non-steroidal anti-inflammatory drugs (NSAIDs) 95, 99
norepinephrine 107
not operating 6
        appendix 349-50
        bariatric surgery 453, 454
        colorectal conditions 258
        gallbladder 319, 322
        hernias 21, 295, 298, 299
        liver/spleen trauma 478
        vascular surgery 433, 434, 435, 436
        see also referral
nutrition
        in the ICU 245-6
        in malnourished patients 136
        postoperative 36, 70, 133, 162
        pre-operative status 18, 94-5, 136

obesity 18
        bariatric surgery 157, 451-70
        bowel anastomosis 135, 140
        DVT prophylaxis 206, 457
        hernia repair 21, 298
        laparoscopy 171, 174
        pediatric 503
        stoma complications 274
omentopexy 118-19, 125

operative reports 33, 194, 303
opiates 162
orchiectomy 302
oximetry probes 502
oxygen is good 25-6, 34, 63
        in ARDS 244
        in TBI 238
        in trauma 473-5

P-POSSUM score 20
packing the abdomen 53, 482, 483-4, 494
pain
        anal 279, 287
        breast cancer 403-4, 408
        hernias 296-7, 311-13
pain control 35, 162, 253-4
pancreas
        drains 67, 368, 369-70
        iatrogenic injury 118
        pancreatitis 320, 365
        surgery 361-76, 489-90
        trauma 480, 486, 488, 489-90, 495
pancreatic duct injuries 488, 489
pancreatojejunostomy 367
papillary stenosis 341
paralytic ileus 155-68, 356
parathyroid glands
        parathyroidectomy 413-16, 422-6
        after thyroidectomy 418-19, 421-2
parenteral nutrition 36, 70, 136, 162, 245
patient attitudes in rural areas 221-2
patients' pre-operative status 14, 16-21, 60, 147, 258
        malnourishment 18, 136
        in the Third World 205-6, 209
pediatric surgery 497-517
pelvic bleeding
        pelvic fractures 52-3, 486
        rectal surgery 264-5
penetrating trauma 119, 472, 476-7, 480, 481, 491
peptic ulcers 118-19, 121, 125
percutaneous endoscopic gastrostomy (PEG) 126, 510-13
pericarditis 409
peritoneal irrigation 65-6
peritonitis 72, 134, 140, 206
pest infestations 204-5, 210
phaeochromocytoma 417, 426, 427-8
phlegmon of the appendix stump 358
piles (hemorrhoids) 279, 282-5, 288, 290
plastic surgery, breast reconstruction 398-400, 406-7
platelet transfusions 43, 54
pneumonia (VAP) 241-3
pneumoperitoneum 177-8, 513
pneumothorax 247, 473-4, 477

portal hypertension 175, 365, 379
portal vein
          injured during liver surgery 385
          resection 368, 375
          stenosis/occlusion 366
          thrombosis 374-5
positive end-expiratory pressure (PEEP) 244
post-cholecystectomy syndrome 340-1
postoperative period, general considerations 33-7, 194-201
post-renal failure 520-1
potassium 162, 237, 504
pre-incisional check list 27
pre-renal failure 520
pre-sacral veins 265
preventability of complications 9-12
primary survey 476-7
Pringle maneuver 382, 390, 485
prostate, BPH 297, 530
pseudomembranous colitis 250-1
pulmonary artery catheters 235
pulmonary embolism (PE) 462, 465-6, 495
pyloric exclusion 126-7, 490
pyloric mobilization 108-9
pyloromyotomy 507-9
pyrexia, postoperative 36-7, 73-4, 213

radiation enteritis 166
radiotherapy in breast cancer 408-9
rectum
          bleeding per 270
          colorectal anastomoses 98, 134-43, 261-2, 265-7, 271-2
          pelvic bleeding 264-5
          trauma 491
          see also colon
recurrent laryngeal nerve 417-18, 420-1, 424, 440
re-feeding syndrome 508
referral 188-9, 198, 207
          bile duct injuries 336
          from rural practices 220-1, 223-4, 226
          liver surgery 379-80
          neonates 497
renal arteries 485
renal conditions see kidney
renal vein, left 441
reportable complications 7-8
respiratory complications
          ARDS 236, 243-4, 495-6
          VAP 241-3
responsibility 8-9, 34, 198
resuscitation
          in the ICU 234-8
          trauma patients 54, 474-5
retention sutures 150

risk assessment 16-21
Roux-en-Y gastric bypass (LRYGB) 452, 456, 458-60, 461, 463-4, 465, 466-8
rural practices 188, 217-27

saline
      hypertonic 475
      isotonic 237
saphenofemoral junction 444
SBO (small bowel obstruction)
      early postoperative (EPSBO) 155-68, 356
      gastric bypass surgery 157, 459-60, 466-8
Scopinaro procedure 460
scrotal swelling 531
      hernia repair 303, 307-8, 310-11
second opinions 198, 536
secondary survey 477
sedatives, in the ICU 253-4
sepsis 36, 58-9, 75-6
      leaking bowel anastomosis 132, 140
seromas, breast surgery 396-7, 406
shaving of the operative site 61
s**t happens 1-538
shock, hypovolemic 48-9, 234-5
shoulder disability after breast surgery 405-6
SIRS (systemic inflammatory response syndrome) 36, 58-9, 73-4
skin
      iatrogenic injuries 210, 408, 501
      suturing 83, 151-2
skin flaps in breast surgery 395-6
sleeve gastrectomy (LSG) 452, 456-8, 461, 464, 465, 468-9
sliding hernias 300, 307
small bowel
      anastomoses 128-34
      enterostomy 131-4, 274, 275
      EPSBO 155-68, 356
      obstruction after gastric bypass surgery 157, 459-60, 466-8
      trauma 479, 487-8, 490-1
      see also entries at duodenal
smoking cessation 60, 95, 107, 297-8
soft tissue, deep incisional SSIs 72, 78, 85, 89, 152, 354
specialty, not operating out of 14, 188-9
      advantages of specialized centers 380, 433, 473
      implications for rural practices 219
      Third World problems 206, 207-9
sphincterotomy 284, 288-9
spleen
      effect of splenectomy on gastric perfusion 117
      iatrogenic injuries 263
      trauma 478, 489
splenic vein 368
sponge count 31-2
SSIs see surgical site infections
stab wounds 119, 476-7, 480, 481, 491

staplers 97, 137
statins 252, 432
stents
>   colonic 258
>   esophageal 113
>   transanal 138
>   ureteric 264
>   vascular 372
steroids
>   adrenal gland disorders 428-9
>   anti-inflammatory 135
stomach *see entries at* gastrectomy; gastric; gastro-
stomas
>   closure 277-8
>   colostomy 83, 137-8, 141, 258, 262-3, 267-8, 273-8
>   enterostomy 131-4, 274, 275
stool softeners 282, 287
Streptococcus pyogenes 85
subcostal retractors 381
sump syndrome 341-2
superior laryngeal nerve 418
superior mesenteric artery (SMA) 373
superior mesenteric vein thrombosis 374
supervision of junior staff 192, 211, 536-7
suprapubic catheterization 523
surgeons
>   *funktionslust* 7, 24
>   keeping within specialty 14, 188-9, 208-9, 219
>   reactions to complications 194-8
surgical site infections (SSIs) 77-89
>   appendectomy 354
>   breast surgery 394
>   causing abdominal wall dehiscence 152
>   colorectal surgery 268-9
>   deep (necrotizing) 78, 85, 89, 152, 309, 354
>   hernia repair 308-10
>   *see also* infections
sutures/suture material
>   abdominal wall closure 149-51, 212, 516
>   bowel anastomoses 97
>   in pediatrics 516
>   skin 83, 151-2
system failures 8-9, 37, 201, 209-10, 220
systemic inflammatory response syndrome (SIRS) 36, 58-9, 73-4

tamponade 476-7
teamwork
>   in the ICU 255
>   in rural practices 219, 224-5
>   in the Third World 207-8
tension pneumothorax 473-4, 476
tertiary survey 479, 493

testicular damage during/after hernia repair 302, 307-8, 310-11
thermal injuries 178, 210, 501
Third World 203-15
thoracic leaks of esophageal anastomoses 106, 111-13
thoracodorsal nerve 405
thoracotomy, emergency 477
thromboembolism
       arterial (limb ischemia) 436-7, 444, 447
       bariatric surgery 465-6
       prophylaxis 206, 248-9, 454, 457, 495
thrombolysis 437, 447
thyroidectomy 413-22
thyrotoxic crisis 416
timing of the operation 23, 25
       appendectomy 349, 499
       avoid delay 51, 186, 189, 478-9
       duration 30-1, 64, 483
       gallbladder 319-20
       IBD 259
       pediatrics 499
       trauma surgery 478-9, 483, 493-4
total parenteral nutrition 36, 70, 136, 162, 245
tourniquets 474
tracheomalacia 420
trainee supervision 192, 211, 536-7
training, a continuous process 283, 316, 321
transfusions
       avoid if possible 30, 35, 53-4
       in the ICU 238, 239
       in massive blood loss 54
       Third World shortages 210
       in trauma patients 483
trauma care 471
       abdominal surgery 479-96
       before reaching hospital 472-5
       bleeding/hemostasis 50-4, 474-5, 477, 483-7, 493, 526-7
       in the ED 476-7
       gastroduodenal injuries 119-21, 487, 490-1
       missed injuries 472, 479, 493
       post-traumatic hematomas 86
traumatic brain injury (TBI) 54, 237-8
'trephine' sigmoid colostomy 278
trocar insertion 171, 175-6, 505

ulcerative colitis 259
ultrasound, FAST 51, 476
umbilical hernias 515
unnecessary surgery 6-7, 15-16, 21
upper limb 405-6, 437
ureteric injuries 527-8, 532
       in AAA surgery 443
       in bladder surgery 531

in colonic surgery 263-4
delayed 531
trauma 486, 491
ureteric misidentification 525
ureteric obstruction and resection 525-6
urethral catheterization 522-4, 530
urinary bladder *see* bladder, urinary
urinary leaks 527, 529, 531, 533
urinary retention 529-30, 533
urinary tract obstruction 297, 521, 525-6
urological surgery 214, 519-34
uterine perforation 213

vacuum wound therapy 87
vagus nerve 440
VAP (ventilator-associated pneumonia) 241-3
varicose veins 437-9, 444
vas deferens transection 303
vascular surgery 431-50
veins
in AAA surgery 441
in carotid surgery 441
thromboembolism *see* deep venous thrombosis
varicose 437-9, 444
vena cava, bleeding 384-5, 485
ventilator-associated pneumonia (VAP) 241-3
ventral hernias 308
violence towards surgeons 211, 215
vitamin D 422, 423
vitamin K 44
voice changes, after thyroidectomy 416-17, 420-1
vomiting, in children 503, 507, 509

walk/climb test 19
warfarin 42-3, 43-4, 50
Whipple procedure 489-90
see also pancreas, surgery
white blood cell count, high 74
wound dehiscence
abdominal wall 145-54, 212
after breast surgery 397-8, 406
wound healing 83, 95, 288
wound infections *see* surgical site infections (SSIs)
wrong-site surgery 26, 498

X-rays, ileus/EPSBO 161